W. Blauth · F. Schneider-Sickert

Congenital Deformities of the Hand

An Atlas of Their Surgical Treatment

Translated by U.H. Weil

With 426 Figures, Most in Color

Springer-Verlag
Berlin Heidelberg GmbH 1981

Professor Dr. WALTER BLAUTH, Direktor der Orthopädischen Universitätsklinik und Poliklinik, Klaus-Groth-Platz 4, 2300 Kiel

Dr. FRANK R. SCHNEIDER-SICKERT, Jasperallee 6, 3300 Braunschweig

Translator:

Professor Dr. U.H. WEIL, New Haven Orthopaedic Group, Orthopaedic Surgery, The Temple Medical Building, 60, Temple Street, New Haven, Connecticut 06510, USA

Translation of the German edition:
Handfehlbildungen

ISBN 978-3-642-67656-7 ISBN 978-3-642-67654-3 (eBook)
DOI 10.1007/978-3-642-67654-3

Library of Congress Cataloging in Publication Data. Blauth, Walter. Congenital deformities of the hand. Translation of Handfehlbildungen. Bibliography: p. Includes index. 1. Hand–Abnormalities. 2. Hand–Surgery. I. Schneider-Sickert, F., 1944– joint author. II. Title. [DNLM: 1. Hand–abnormalities–Atlases. 2. Hand–Surgery–Atlases. WE17 B645h] RD778.B5713 617'.575 80-15119

Softcover reprint of the hardcover 1st edition 1980

Reproduction of figures: Gustav Dreher GmbH, Stuttgart

2121/3130-543210

Author's Preface to the German Edition

In the past 10–15 years marked progress has been made in the surgical treatment of congenital anomalies of the hand. More and more, the reluctance to operate on these deformities has been abandoned. One reason for this – at least in the German-speaking countries – was the thalidomide catastrophe (1959–1962), which involved the birth of many children with deformed upper limbs. These previously rare severe abnormalities resulted in many problems and required new ways of thinking in terms of their treatment by all persons concerned with their care. At the same time hand surgery was beginning to come of age and the combination of these two events increased the interest in the field of hand anomalies, particularly by orthopaedic surgeons who had always been involved in it.

The idea and preparation for this book go back to 1964. Since that time nearly all operations on anomalous hands were systematically charted by us. They were photographically recorded from skin incision to wound closure. Regular follow-up examinations were performed. This atlas represents our experience gained in over a thousand operations.

The book has been written by practitioners. We hope that a hand surgeon looking for additional advice will find answers in regard to therapy and surgical suggestions. This intent influenced the book's compilation and structure:

- Only those operations that have given us good long-term results will be discussed.
- We felt it insufficient to describe only some standard procedures for more common anomalies, but also thought that it would be impossible to report on a specific operation for every possible anomaly. We wanted to present proven methods and realized that this would limit the scope of this publication. We wanted further to report exemplary procedures for most of the more common types of hand anomalies.
- Each chapter opens with an introduction. We have tried to keep the information contained therein to a minimum. It should enable the reader to classify deformities, mainly in regard to operative technique, to critically analyze surgical feasibilities, and to develop a plan of treatment. We felt that functionally important concomitant deformities had to be included and that facts obtained from personal experience and our perusal of the literature should be reported. In the introductions we also give general directives on treatment and the optimum times for surgical intervention.
- Due to the fundamental morphological and operative problems they pose, we decided to include a few very rare anomalies on which we have not yet formed a final opinion. These cases have not been illustrated by drawings. We shall discuss them only, as we do not yet have enough personal experience to evaluate surgical feasibilities.

- We have tried to present operations in such a manner that other surgeons will be able to replicate them. Serial drawings will explain their important phases and the text will give further details. Errors and their consequences will be pointed out.
- The drawings constitute an attempt to represent the entire operative field and to illustrate all important structures that the surgeon will encounter. These drawings were made possible because every means of recording, i.e., operative reports, hospital charts, x-rays, and photographs, was available for their production.
- We stress the importance of postoperative care. It alone guarantees any long-term surgical success.
- In indicating errors and their consequences we hope to impart knowledge gained from our own and other surgeons' operative results.
- We have deliberately tried to keep references to literature sources to a minimum. This book has been written for the practitioner and presents our own surgical experiences. A small number of publications will be quoted for each chapter. These publications have either been mentioned in the text or we felt that they would be useful to elucidate some problems.

The authors hope to provide a book of reference for the surgeon who occasionally sees a patient with a hand anomaly and a compendium with many details for the experienced hand surgeon. In addition we intend to give an overview of proven operative methods. Hopefully it can be used as a text for surgery of the hand.

The voluminous preparations were supported by our colleagues P. HIPPE and H. MEVES. We express our thanks for their important contributions, without which the book would not have been written so quickly.

We are particularly grateful to Mr. J.S. PUPP, the artist who created all of the drawings. We admire his sensitivity and understanding of the difficult field of hand anomalies. We also thank Mrs. H. KRAMMETBAUER, who was responsible for the manuscripts and proof corrections.

Last but not least we thank Springer-Verlag, which was always open to our ideas and which is responsible for the generous layout of this book.

Kiel, July 1976

W. BLAUTH
F. SCHNEIDER-SICKERT

Translator's Preface

Three years ago Professor W. BLAUTH asked me to translate this book on congenital anomalies of the hand and their treatment. After seeing the atlas I was very happy to comply with his request. I feel that the book is an extremely valuable addition to the library of every surgeon who deals with hand deformities.

We live in an age of rapidly progressing science. Thus in future editions of this book, the authors will undoubtedly expand their discussion of the new microvascular techniques (groin flaps, random flaps, axial pattern flaps) which they introduce briefly here. In coming years, microvascular techniques in combination with toe transplants will also be used increasingly in the construction of posts in monodactylous or symbrachydactylous hands.

I want to thank my secretary, Ms. P. COSGROVE, for her invaluable help in preparing the manuscript for this translation.

New Haven, Connecticut ULRICH H. WEIL

Contents

1 Introduction

Surgery to correct congenital deformities of the hand is particularly rewarding and attractive, but the difficulty of these operations and the great responsibility of the surgeon should not be underestimated. Orthopaedists and other surgeons interested in this field will gain only limited personal experience, because these deformities are rare and vary greatly in appearance. The rapid progress in hand surgery has made it impossible to give up-to-date information in textbooks and surgical manuals. Frequently they still describe operations that have been proven to be of doubtful value or have been replaced by better procedures.

The prerequisites of a physician contemplating surgical correction of hand deformities are an extensive knowledge of the basics of orthopaedic and plastic surgery and a critical evaluation of his own capabilities. In addition, the physician should have the ability to think in a manner that HACKENBROCH has termed the "sensus orthopaedicus."

Critical reflections on the expected functional improvement as a result of surgery, the amount of residual disability of the nonoperated hand deformity due to the patient's probable adaptation to it, as well as some knowledge of the future development of the deformity due to growth are part of this process, as are the psychological and aesthetic reactions of the patient and his environment to the malformation. All decisions will be further influenced by the patient's age, his ability to cooperate, his intelligence, and the presence of concomitant deformities.

From these considerations one can derive the following axioms:

Not every hand deformity requires surgical intervention.

Hand deformities should never be treated by someone with little experience in this field.

It is more important to avoid the risk of further loss of function than to hope for an uncertain improvement of function.

1.1 General Directives

Indications for corrective surgery of congenital deformities of the hand should be distinguished from those for reconstructive hand surgery necessitated by trauma or neurologic disorders for three reasons:

- In most instances operations are not urgent and immediate intervention is not required: it is possible to await optimal surgical conditions.

– Surgery to improve function has to be weighed against its risks, as in cases of congenital hand deformities adaptive amelioration is better than in situations caused by trauma or by sequelae of nerve paralysis.

– Aesthetic considerations and the still persisting discriminative social stigma of a malformation play an important role.

Indication for surgery depends in each instance on many factors, some of which have already been mentioned. To achieve optimal results and to avoid future disappointments one should consider the additional following *general prerequisites:*

– The deformity has to be recognized in all its components and should be precisely classified according to its genetic and morphological characteristics. Erroneous interpretation of these factors could result in pathologicoanatomic misconceptions of the original state of the malformation and of its developmental tendencies.

– In contrast to acquired deformities of the hand, one has to consider that congenital deformities often involve more structures than those readily visible. Aplasias of vessels, nerves, and muscles, insertion anomalies of tendons, and dys- and aplasias of joints must be taken into account, otherwise unexpected findings during the operation will lead to its failure.

– Improvement of *function is more important* than improvement of *appearance.* If surgery is performed for aesthetic reasons only, one has to be sure that no loss of function will result.

– *Function* should *be tested* thoroughly by an experienced physiotherapist and/or occupational therapist prior to any operation. This examination should produce adequate information concerning (a) the functional status of muscle groups, (b) adaptive mechanisms, and (c) the usefulness of the affected limb. It should also inform us of the patient's ability to cooperate and to carry out a rehabilitation program after operation.

– The result of the aforementioned initial examination is extremely important for the *timing of the operation.* Few congenital deformities of the hand require early surgical intervention; examples of those that do are malformations that increase rapidly due to growth and those in which circulatory disturbances can be expected. The *preschool age is the best time for most operations,* i.e., the 4th–6th year of life. Anatomic structures are more readily identifiable, growth tendencies can be more adequately predicted (serial x-ray and photographic measurements), and the patient's cooperation is quite well-developed. Also, psychic aberrations caused by pronounced malformations can be more easily prevented if the operation is carried out during this period. Moreover, important time in school is not lost, nor are vacations sacrificed for operations that require long-term hospitalization. The timing of surgery also depends on the number of necessary surgical interventions. On the other hand, postoperative functional adaptability declines with increasing age. Procedures that can damage the epiphyseal plate (e.g., resection arthrodesis) have to be postponed until the second decennium.

– *Exact radiographic pictures* are part of the preoperative requisites; pre-, intra-, and postoperative *photographs* are an important part of proper documentation.

It must again be emphasized that the distinction between *congenital* and *acquired* hand deformities is of utmost importance. In treating congenital hand deformities it is not the aim to restore lost functions that had been imprinted and stored in the cortical and subcortical areas of the brain; instead, the creation of new functions is required. Therefore, the intelligence of the patient and his willingness to cooperate are of the utmost significance. All persons involved in his recovery, the surgeon, the physiotherapist, the occupational therapist, and the patient's family, have to exercise a high degree of patience. The learning and reeducation process may require a long period, particularly if the patient is older at the time of surgery, i.e., when he may have become accustomed to his deformity.

The possibility of prosthetic treatment – immediately or later – has to be carefully considered if the deformities are of a more severe nature. The employment of prostheses in infancy should be severely limited as their disadvantages are well-known (problems of proper use, continuous adjustment due to growth, lack of sensation, etc.).

1.2 General Surgical Suggestions

The following *minimum requirements* have to be fulfilled if one considers surgery of congenital malformations of the hand:

- Utmost *asepsis* in the operating room.

- The surgeon must have adequate *experience* in general orthopaedic surgery and in plastic surgery.

- *Special surgical kits* must be available for each operation. One has to have proper instruments for every possible intraoperative complication.

- *Well-supervised postoperative physiotherapy* must be available to safeguard the results of the operation.

Our standard method of surgery is as follows:

1.2.1 Skin Preparation

On the evening prior to surgery the fingernails must be thoroughly cleansed and trimmed. Shaving of a sufficiently large area of skin has to include the site for the removal of skin transplants. This is followed by surgical disinfection of a generous area of the skin (use a soft brush to avoid superficial skin abrasions).

The hand and arm are then wrapped in sterile sheets soaked with alcohol or similar agents. This dressing should only be removed on the following morning in the operating room.

1.2.2 Positioning

A hand board, which should be wide enough to allow resting space for the hands and forearms of the surgeon and his assistants, is fixed to the operating table.

1.2.3 Anesthesia

The type of anesthesia (general or conduction) depends on the particular factors of each individual case (and on the experience of the anesthesiologist). Plastic surgery requiring tubed or cross flaps and procedures requiring skin transplants are usually done under general anesthesia, which is our method of choice for all operations during childhood. Further details can be found in standard textbooks of anesthesiology (FREY et al. 1972; KILLIAN 1973; MOORE 1971; see also A. WILHELM 1972).

1.2.4 Exsanguination

Exsanguination of the involved limb with an Esmarch bandage and a pressure-recording pneumatic tourniquet is a prerequisite for nearly all operations described in the following chapters. It alone guarantees anatomic dissection of the involved structures and a meticulous surgical technique. The duration of exsanguination should be restricted to 2 h. If necessary, one can continue with the operation after the tourniquet has been released for 10–15 min. Tourniquet pressure should be between 220 and 250 mmHg, i.e., about 100 mmHg above the systolic pressure. After the tourniquet has been released, the operative site is compressed with moist tapes and elastic bandages until reactive hyperemia has subsided (approx. 5 min).

1.2.5 Instrumentarium

Special instruments for hand surgery are required for each operation. This alone permits "atraumatic" surgery. Additional instruments will have to be added to the basic kit in certain situations. We recommend the use of a sterile *marking pen* to outline the incisions and of *surgical telescopes* as important aids for careful dissection.

1.2.6 Operative Technique

The fragility of the structures of the hand and fingers requires an *atraumatic operative technique*. This begins with a properly placed *incision:* General rules have to be observed (avoidance of scars in areas subject to tensile forces; such scars would result from incisions within the flexor creases or at an oblique angle between them or from incisions in the middle of the lateral aspects of the fingers). The section on recurrent syndactylies will point out the problems caused by improperly placed incisions. The many examples in the following chapters will give our recommendations for their correct placement.

It is better to retract skin with fine sutures or hooks to expose an operative area than to use forceps, which have crushing tendencies. Atraumatic surgical technique also requires the parsimonious use of moist sponges and regular moistening of the operative site to avoid drying out of the tissues. To obtain exact hemostasis one should use *bipolar electrocoagulation* (to limit electronecrosis to the tissue between the two electrodes).

Continuous optimal exposure of the involved structures is important, but unnecessarily large incisions are to be avoided. Complex congenital deformities of the hand show great variety in the development and course of vessels and nerves. For this reason, and also because of their close anatomic proximity, one should not hesitate to expose them adequately. This gives additional security in regard to the topography of the operative site. To dissect these structures adequately we have found very narrow, long dissecting scissors with blunt points to be useful.

Following osteotomies we try to obtain rigid osteosynthesis to shorten the time of joint immobilization.

For skin transplants we use *three-quarter thickness grafts* (PADGETT 1939), i.e., thick-split thickness grafts of 0.5–0.6 mm with a thick portion of cutis. Thin-split thickness grafts heal well, but have, for example, a tendency to shrink. We prefer the thick-split thickness graft to the full-thickness graft (Wolfe-Krause graft) because of the latter's tendency to heal more poorly and to contract more due to small necrotic areas (ANDINA 1970, a.o.).

Whenever possible we prefer the use of *flaps raised near the operative site,* primarily swivel pedicle flaps and Z-plasties. It is important *not* to remove the subcutis of the pedicle flap as this can impair its circulation and mobility. Tubed pedicle *flaps raised far away* from the site of their insertion require staging and are problematic in respect of their future sensibility. Nevertheless, we still use them for several operations (see Sects. 4.2.2, 3.10 etc.).

Atraumatic surgery requires use of the finest atraumatic needles and of suture materials which ensure minimal granulation tissue reaction. Great care is required in closing the skin. Wound edges should be loosely adapted and never tightly pulled together in order to avoid necrosis of the edges caused by unavoidable postoperative edema.

1.2.7 Postoperative (Wound) Care

Postoperative wound care can be decisive for the success of the operation. Compression dressings to avoid postoperative hematoma formation are absolutely necessary; frequently one has to use a thin suction drainage system. The operative site should be covered with vaseline gauze. Skin transplants require a graduated pressure dressing to avoid collection of wound secretions under the transplant. The fingernails must be exposed to allow control of circulation of the fingers.

In children the *immobilization of the limb* requires a long-arm plaster-of-Paris cast with the elbow at right angles and the forearm in midpronation, as short-arm casts can be removed by small patients.

It is obvious that wrist and finger joints should be kept in a position of function in the cast. Compression dressings should be split down to the skin no later than 2 h after they have been applied, as even cast padding can create circulatory strictures. In the first few postoperative days it is advisable to *elevate* the hand to avoid edema formation.

In general the *first dressing change* will be carried out between the 5th and 7th day; however, if a free transplant has been used then it should not be done until between the 8th and 10th day. The first dressing change is the responsibility of the surgeon and should not be delegated to other members of the team.

1.2.8 Postoperative Exercises

A satisfactory postoperative result is obtained and safeguarded by a proper exercise program. It is therefore important to have an experienced physiotherapist available who can work closely with the patient and supervise progress. Physiotherapy and occupational therapy are directed toward improvement of grasp, power, and manual dexterity. Exercise instruction sheets (for an example, see Sect. 4.2.4), exercise splints, dynamic traction and night splints are necessary and useful. The operative result must be *regularly inspected* over a long period to allow the prompt introduction of countermeasures if any unsatisfactory development should be noted.

1.3 Review of Frequent Errors of Therapy and Their Consequences

Each single error, whether made prior to, during, or after an operation, can lead to an unsatisfactory result, as already mentioned in Sect. 1.1. In the descriptions of the different operations we shall point out the most frequent errors made in each individual case. However, the following mistakes occur in a wide range of operations (**E**, error; **C**, consequence):

E. The severity of a defect has been underestimated as a result of its external appearance and/or the radiogram. Not all components of the malformation have been recognized, leading to its wrong classification.
C. Errors of this type may result in wrong operative indications or in intraoperative technical difficulties.

E. The preoperative management has been insufficient.
C. Preoperative physiotherapy or occupational therapy is required, particularly in operations involving muscles and tendons in which creation or improvement of grasp is intended. Without these measures one has to expect a suboptimal result.

E. Proper staging of operations has been neglected in the correction of complex deformities.
C. Circulation and proper wound closure may be problematic; postoperative complications, i.e., infections, involve an unnecessarily large area around the incision.

E. The special surgical kit and suture material is incomplete or insufficient.
C. Atraumatic surgery may be impossible.

E. The operation is performed without exsanguination of the limb.
C. Meticulous dissection of the involved structures is impossible.

E. Skin flaps are formed in an improper manner:

a) Placement of the incision does not take postoperative tension or shrinking of the scar tissue sufficiently into consideration.

b) Skin flaps have angles that are too pointed, too long, or too narrow; this results in trophic disturbances. It is impossible to recommend proper angles or lengths for each individual case. The expected amount of tension, the course of the blood vessels, the age of the patient, and other pertinent points have to be considered. Generally one can state that the angle at the apex of a triangular flap should be no less than 40–45°. The ratio of length to width for commissure and most pedicle flaps should be between 1:2 and 1:2.5 (see operative example, Sect. 2.1.6a.o.). Only the so-called groin flap (McGregor and Jackson 1972; Buck-Gramcko and Epping 1974) and the so-called flag flap of Villain do not require these proportions as their blood supply is much better.

c) The raising of the skin flap is carried out in a wrong stratum (subcutaneous fatty tissue has been removed).

d) Improper surgical technique has damaged the vessels providing the necessary blood supply of the flaps. The bases of the flaps have not been sufficiently mobilized and are sutured under tension during wound closure.

E. The entire flap has been handled too roughly during surgery.

C. Vessels and nerves, particularly on the volar aspect, are damaged, crushed, or strangulated.

E. While deepening the web space, structures limiting the operative field have not been properly dissected. A branch of a blood vessel has not been severed and ligated. A bifurcating nerve has not been separated interfascicularly.

C. The depth of the web space will be insufficient.

E. Mistakes have been made during or after wound closure.

a) Compression of the wound is not maintained long enough (5 min) after release of the tourniquet and complete hemostasis has not been accomplished (microcautery).

b) In spite of a relatively large wound cavity, suction drainage has not been employed.

c) Free skin transplants have not been used, resulting in (too much) tension of the skin flaps.

d) In the presence of circulatory embarrassment of the tips of the skin flaps, skin sutures that hold the flaps under tension have not been released.

e) Thin-split thickness grafts have been used instead of thick-split thickness grafts; this results in graft shrinkage due to contracture.

E. The postoperative compression dressing is too loose or too tight; it has been loosened too late, circulation has not been watched carefully; the suction drainage tube is kinked in the (plaster) dressing.

E. The corners of the flaps, particularly in the depth of the web space, have not been protected by a proper compression dressing at the time of its original application or during subsequent dressing changes.

C. Maceration by wound secretions.

E. Postoperative elevation of the limb has not been carried out or was insufficient; inadequate attention has been given to the postoperative edema.

E. The hand has been insufficiently immobilized, or the immobilizing dressing or Kirschner wire fixation has been removed too soon.

E. Kirschner wires below skin level have been inadequately padded.

C. So-called internal decubiti may develop.

E. Kirschner wires penetrating the skin have been incorporated into the cast.

C. Immobilization is insufficient, as minimal movements of the hand are transmitted fully through the cast.

E. Night splints have not been employed or they have been removed too soon.

E. Wound healing, postoperative therapy, or long-term results have not been supervised for a sufficient amount of time. Postoperative physiotherapy or occupational therapy was insufficient. The physiotherapist was improperly informed about the deformity, the operation, and the postoperative goal. Physiotherapy was not supervised on a regular basis by the physician. Motivation of the patient and his family has been overestimated prior to surgery.

2 Syndactylies

Syndactyly has been one of the most common hand deformity in our patients (see also BUNNELL 1959; KELIKIAN 1974; a.o.). Its incidence in blacks is reported to be ten times less frequent (DAVIS and GERMAN 1930).

For morphological and operative reasons one can distinguish two main types of syndactyly: soft tissue syndactylies, which we shall call *"cutaneous syndactylies,"* and fusion of fingers with involvement of bony components, which we shall designate as *"osseous syndactylies."*

Syndactyly can be observed both as an isolated deformity and in complex deformities of the hand; in the latter case, the syndactyly may be either an essential part of the condition or merely an accompaniment. Examples of such complex deformities are acrocephalosyndactyly, symbrachydactyly, numerical variation, cleft hand, and peripheral hypoplasia. Such conditions can also be designated as *combined syndactylies;* most osseous forms belong to this group. Syndactyly is also present in other deformity syndromes (e.g., Down syndrome, Laurence-Moon-Bardet-Biedl syndrome, and Klippel-Feil syndrome).

Acro- and bridge syndactylies constitute a *special group* of peripheral hypoplasias. Due to certain concepts of developmental mechanisms they have been classified as exogenous (W. MÜLLER 1937) or *secondary syndactylies* (LÖSCH 1970).

In this chapter we shall discuss only the noncombined cutaneous syndactylies, the deformities noted in Apert syndrome, and the so-called recurrent syndactylies. Recommendations for the care of combined forms will be found in other chapters (3, 4, 8, 9), but we shall discuss these syndactylies in detail only if particular problems exist or if approaches other than the standard skin incisions described in this chapter may be required.

2.1 Cutaneous Syndactylies

2.1.1 Introduction

2.1.1.1 General Remarks

An uninterrupted skin and soft tissue bridge between two or more fingers is *characteristic.* The fusion extends for longer or shorter distances distally into the interdigital space, and on the basis of this criterion *partial, subtotal, and total syndactylies* are distinguished. In some cases the interdigital space is tight and narrow, in others it is loose and wide.

Cleeland's ligaments are of great importance for reasons of operative technique. They originate from the ligamenta vaginalia and the lateral borders of the phalanges.

In cases of syndactyly, Cleeland's ligaments interlace in the common interdigital space and form a septumlike separating layer which "ascends" to the palmar aspect, where they insert into the skin (see Sect. 2.1.2, Fig. 4). Only in the dorsal proximal interdigital space are the palmar vessels and nerves not protected by the Cleeland's ligaments (Lösch 1970); therefore, special attention has to be paid to these structures during surgery. The bifurcations of the aa. and nn. dig. palm. prop. may be displaced distally. Differences in their size and occasional aplasia of a vessel may be present (Azzolini 1975; own observation). Peripheral fusion of two digital nerves into one unit has also been described (see Bonola and Morelli 1972, Fig. 135).

More pronounced pathologic abnormalities of the tendons of the fingers are an exception. Occasionally, the tendon of m. flex. dig. prof. fans out at the distal phalanx and interdigitates with its neighbor.

Syndactylies occur *most often between the middle and ring finger* (McKusick: type I; in the older literature, zygodactyly) and between the *index and middle finger*. They are frequently *symmetrical* (for references see Bunnell 1959; Kelikian 1974). Males are more commonly affected. Numerous hereditary forms have been recognized (see McKusick 1975; Grebe 1964; Kelikian 1974) and almost without exception they are autosomal dominant (with variable penetrance and expressivity).

If fingers of *different lengths* are involved (ring and little fingers) one has to expect flexion contractures and ulnar deviation during growth because the adjacent joints are located at different levels and the shorter finger will pull the longer toward it.

2.1.1.2 Timing of Surgery

In cases of syndactyly of fingers of equal length we usually operate during preschool age (i.e., the 4th–5th year of life). If more than two fingers are involved we recommend surgery at a somewhat earlier age, during the 3rd–4th year. Treatment should be completed prior to the child reaching school age. A fusion of fingers of unequal length with impairment of function or with a tendency toward abnormal growth and contractures should be separated during the 1st–2nd year.

2.1.1.3 General Surgical Directives

The new *commissure* has to be of sufficient width and depth and should incline obliquely in a proximal-dorsal to distal-palmar direction. Its site depends on the position of the adjacent normal web folds. One can form one, two, or three swivel flaps with local pedicles. *We prefer a palmar* (so-called leaf flap) *or a dorsal flap* since scar formation in the area of tension of the web space is avoided and the natural inclination of the commissure can be followed (Blauth 1972). In employing a dorsal (two-tailed) flap (see Sect. 2.1.4), one does not create such an extensive wound surface on the palmar aspect of the finger as in employing a palmar swivel flap (see Sect. 2.1.3). These skin flaps should be neither too short nor too narrow. Our goal is to bring the tip of a palmar flap as close as possible to the skin folds of the proximal interphalangeal (PIP) joint.

In the presence of a narrow web *between the thumb and the index finger* we recommend the following three procedures:

- In cases of little involvement, a *Z-plasty* (see Sect. 2.2.5 a.o.).
- In most cases with more pronounced narrowing, an *extended Z-plasty* (with additional dorsoradial or dorsoulnar swivel flaps; BLAUTH 1975) (see Sects. 5.4; 2.2.3 a.o.).
- In the occasional severe case, a *tubed pedicle flap* (see Sects. 4.2; 2.2.2).

For the *separation of the long fingers* we employ a zig-zag incision (BLAUTH 1972; BUCK-GRAMCKO 1975; CRONIN 1956; EBSKOV and ZACHARIAE 1966; KINMOTH 1975; MEISSL et al. 1975; MILLESI 1970, 1971) which has to extend at least to the midline of the flexor and extensor surface of the adjacent fingers (BLAUTH 1972). Longitudinal or undulatory incisions are to be avoided (see later).

Skin defects on the sides of the fingers are covered with *thick-split thickness transplants*. The amount of locally available skin is always insufficient, even in syndactylies with wide interdigital bridges. Every attempt to close the wound without the use of skin transplants will lead to recurrence. We prefer using several small transplants as they compensate better for their tendency to contract (see Sect. 1.2).

Syndactylies of more than two fingers should never be separated during one operation. Surgery should be performed in stages and with different techniques in forming the commissure. In this way, it is possible to construct each web space with scar-free skin.

Even today the difficulties of separating syndactylies are frequently underestimated! Supple web spaces without contracted scars (as long-term results) can be created only by proper incisions. It is well known that *longitudinal incisions over the flexor (or extensor) finger surfaces must be avoided,* since they will definitely result in scar tissue contractures.

Incisional scars in children grow at a rate different from the rest of their skin; thus, undulatory skin incisions may change into longitudinal scars or may become contracted (see Sect. 2.3) (MILLESI 1961; MEISSL et al. 1975). In regard to possible errors we refer the reader to our introduction (Sect. 1.3), to the section on recurrent syndactylies (Sect. 2.3), and in particular to our remarks concerning the surgical example in Sect. 2.1.2.

2.1.1.4 Postoperative Care

We recommend the following steps after the wound has been closed:

The wound is covered with *vaseline gauze* and the interspace between the extended and abducted fingers is filled with *fluffs or steel wool.* A *light pressure dressing* is applied with a small elastic bandage, followed by a padded *long-arm cast* with inclusion of all fingers; only the fingertips are exposed to permit observation of circulation (Meves 1975). The dressing and elastic bandage is to be split on the extensor surface no later than 2 h after surgery. The limb is elevated for 5–7 days.

The first *dressing change* is carried out after 8–10 days if no complications have occurred. Encrusted fluffs are carefully soaked off with physiologic saline or similar solutions.

Active exercises are allowed only after complete healing of the incision and incorporation of the transplants. Night splints or specific physiotherapy measures are usually unnecessary.

2.1.2 Total Syndactyly of Fingers of Equal Length (III/IV)

Goal of Surgery

Removal of the interdigital skin and soft tissue bridge and creation of a web space in anatomic position by using swivel flaps with local pedicles.

Fig. 1 Preoperative appearance and incision, dorsal aspect.
The zig-zag incision extends approximately to the midline of the extensor surfaces of the fingers.

Fig. 2 Palmar aspect.
The tip of the "commissure flap" *(1)* should extend close to the flexor creases of the PIP joints. The triangles lateral to flap *(1)* outline areas that will be excised prior to the insertion of thick-split thickness skin transplants at a later stage of the operation (Fig. 8). This improves the course of the scars on the palmar aspect: longitudinal scars are avoided.

Fig. 3 One has to protect all main vessels, including veins, in raising the skin flaps. Subcutaneous fatty tissue is left undisturbed. One enters the digital space via a dorsal approach, the vertically positioned Cleeland's ligaments acting as a guide. They form a dividing wall and fuse with the connective tissue of the palmar skin. These structures are located between the two main veins (Fig. 4). Transverse venous anastomoses near the main veins should be ligated, not coagulated.

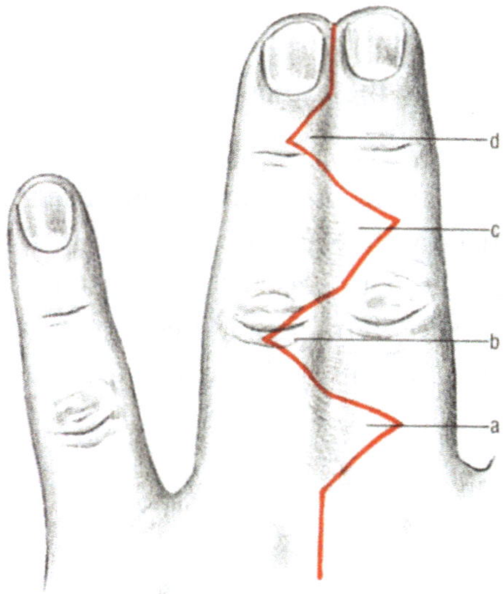
d
c
b
a

1

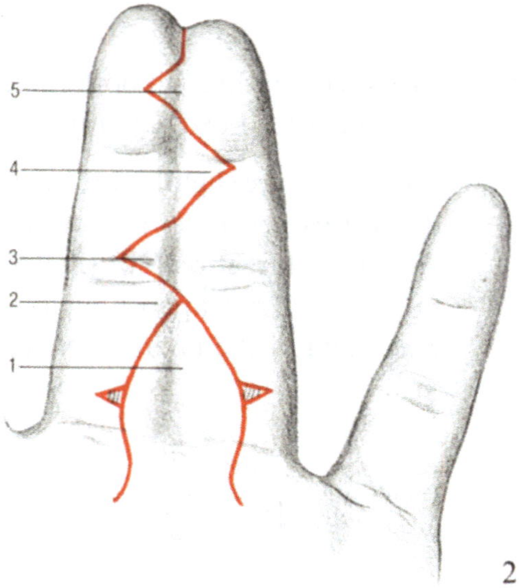
5
4
3
2
1

2

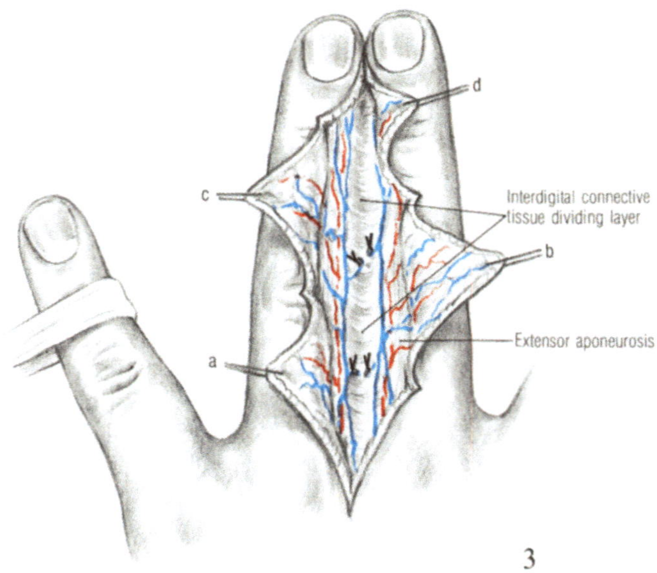
d
c
Interdigital connective tissue dividing layer
b
Extensor aponeurosis
a

3

Fig. 4 Cross section through both fingers at the level of the proximal phalanges (schematic drawing after Lösch, 1970).

Fig. 5 The fingers are slightly spread apart after the palmar flaps have been raised, bringing the soft tissues under tension. Beginning distally they are separated until the neurovascular bifurcation (not shown) is visible. The neurovascular bundles are carefully protected. Trial apposition of the commissure flap *(1)*; if necessary, additional deepening of the interdigital space by transection of the lig. capit. transversum.

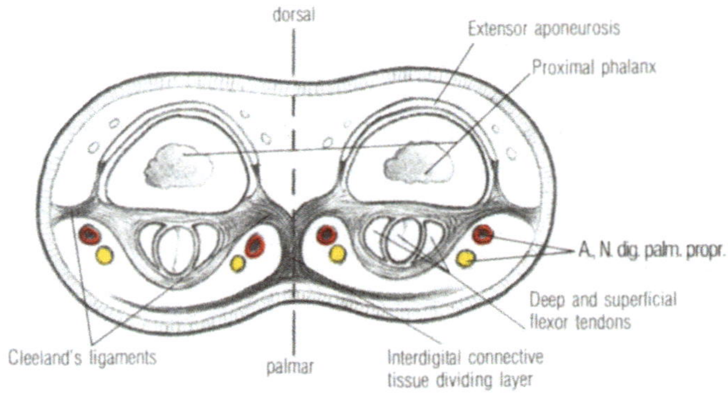
dorsal
Extensor aponeurosis
Proximal phalanx
A. N. dig. palm. propr.
Deep and superficial
flexor tendons
Cleeland's ligaments
palmar
Interdigital connective
tissue dividing layer

4

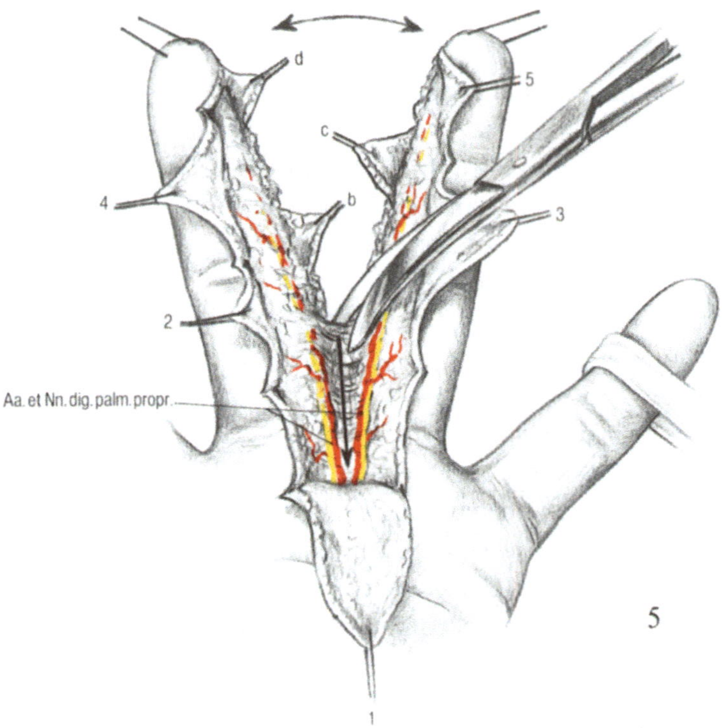
d
5
c
4
b
3
2
Aa. et Nn. dig. palm. propr.
1

5

Figs. 6–8 Postoperative appearance; dorsal, palmar, and lateral aspects of the fingers. Because of its shape, flap *(1)* extends slightly to the lateral aspects of the fingers. This prevents scar formation in the area of the commissure. Defects are covered with thick-split thickness skin transplants *(Tr)*.

Postoperative Care. See Sect. 2.1.1.4.

Errors and Their Consequences

E. The incision has not been properly delineated at the beginning of the operation (no sterile marking pen has been used).
E. The swivel flaps on the lateral aspects of the fingers are too short: the zig-zag incision does not extend to the midline between the extensor and flexor surfaces.
E. The commissure flap is not long enough or the depth of the web space is insufficient (see later).
C. The tips of the flaps or suture lines are placed in the area of tensile stress of the commissure.
E. The dissection of the skin flaps has been carried out in the wrong layer: Subcutaneous fatty tissue *has* to remain on the pedicle flaps.
E. Palmar vessels and nerves have been damaged during dissection; dorsal veins have been inadequately protected.
E. An arterial branch has not been ligated and the nerve has not been split interfascicularly in the presence of an unusual distal position of the neurovascular bifurcation (see Sect. 2.1.3).
E. Hemostasis is insufficient.
C. Postoperative tension under the skin flaps will increase.
E. The swivel flaps have been sutured under tension; circulation of the skin flaps has not been sufficiently checked after removal of the tourniquet.
E. Skin sutures holding the flaps under excessive tension have not been removed after the tips of these flaps have become ischemic. Ischemic areas have to be resected and replaced by thick-split thickness transplants if circulation remains insufficient.
E. The transplants used were not *thick*-split thickness grafts.
C. Thin-split thickness grafts shrink! (see Sect. 1.2.6).
E. The thick-split thickness skin transplants and pedicle skin flaps have been dressed under too much or too little compression.
E. The area of the wound has been inadequately immobilized (e.g., no plaster cast). The duration of immobilization was too short (the first dressing must not be changed prior to the 8th postoperative day).
E. The commissure has not been spread sufficiently by the dressing (but avoid tension!)
E. The interdigital space has not been filled with fluffs to its deepest point.
C. Agglutination and skin maceration may result.

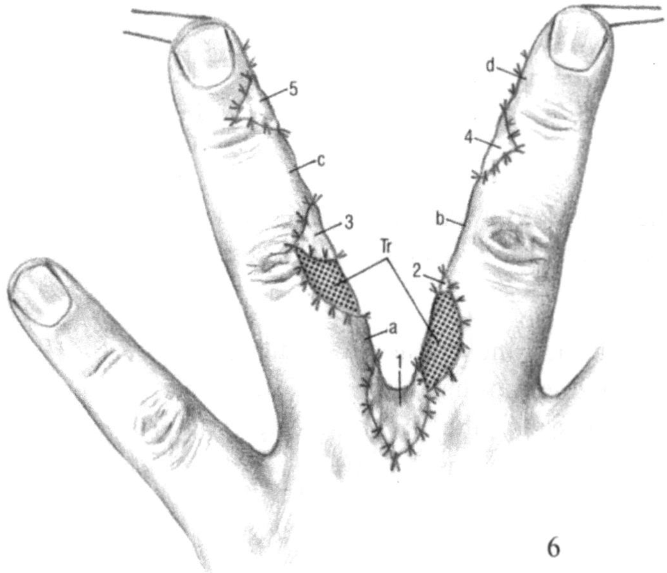

6

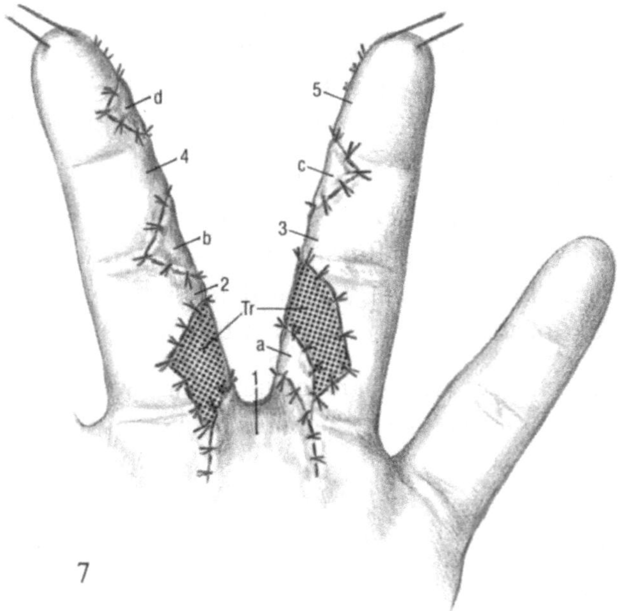

7

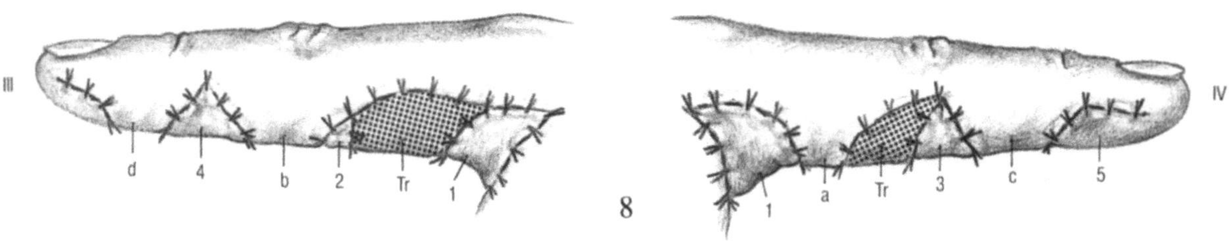

8

2.1.3 Subtotal Syndactyly of Fingers of Unequal Length (IV/V)

Goal of Surgery

Removal of the interdigital skin and soft tissue bridge and creation of a web space in anatomic position by using swivel flaps with local pedicles.

Fig. 1 Preoperative appearance and incision, dorsal aspect.
The zig-zag incision does not have to extend across the midline of the distal phalanx of the ring finger because the involved fingers are of different length and the interdigital soft tissue bridge is relatively wide. Occasionally one has to employ an additional horizontal incision *(broken line)* to reapproximate the skin flaps (Fig. 4).

Fig. 2 Preoperative appearance and skin incision, palmar aspect.
Flap *(3)* appears to be somewhat short, but the interdigital skin bridge is wide enough to permit its displacement to the extensor surface of the ring finger without tension. The triangles lateral to flap *(1)* outline areas which will be excised prior to the insertion of the thick-split thickness skin transplants at a later stage of the operation (Figs. 4 and 5). This improves the position of the scar.

Fig. 3 Palmar aspect after dissection of the dorsal and palmar skin.
With the fingers spread apart, the interdigital soft tissue bridge is carefully separated from distal to proximal. In addition, interfascicular splitting of the trunk of the main nerve is carried out (using surgical telescopes). No tension should persist in the soft tissues of the commissure when the fingers are maximally spread apart!

Figs. 4, 5 Postoperative appearance after shaping and suturing of the flaps *(c, 3)* and coverage of the open areas with thick-split thickness skin transplants *(Tr)*.

Postoperative Care

See Sect. 2.1.1.4.

Errors and Their Consequences

See Sect. 2.1.2.

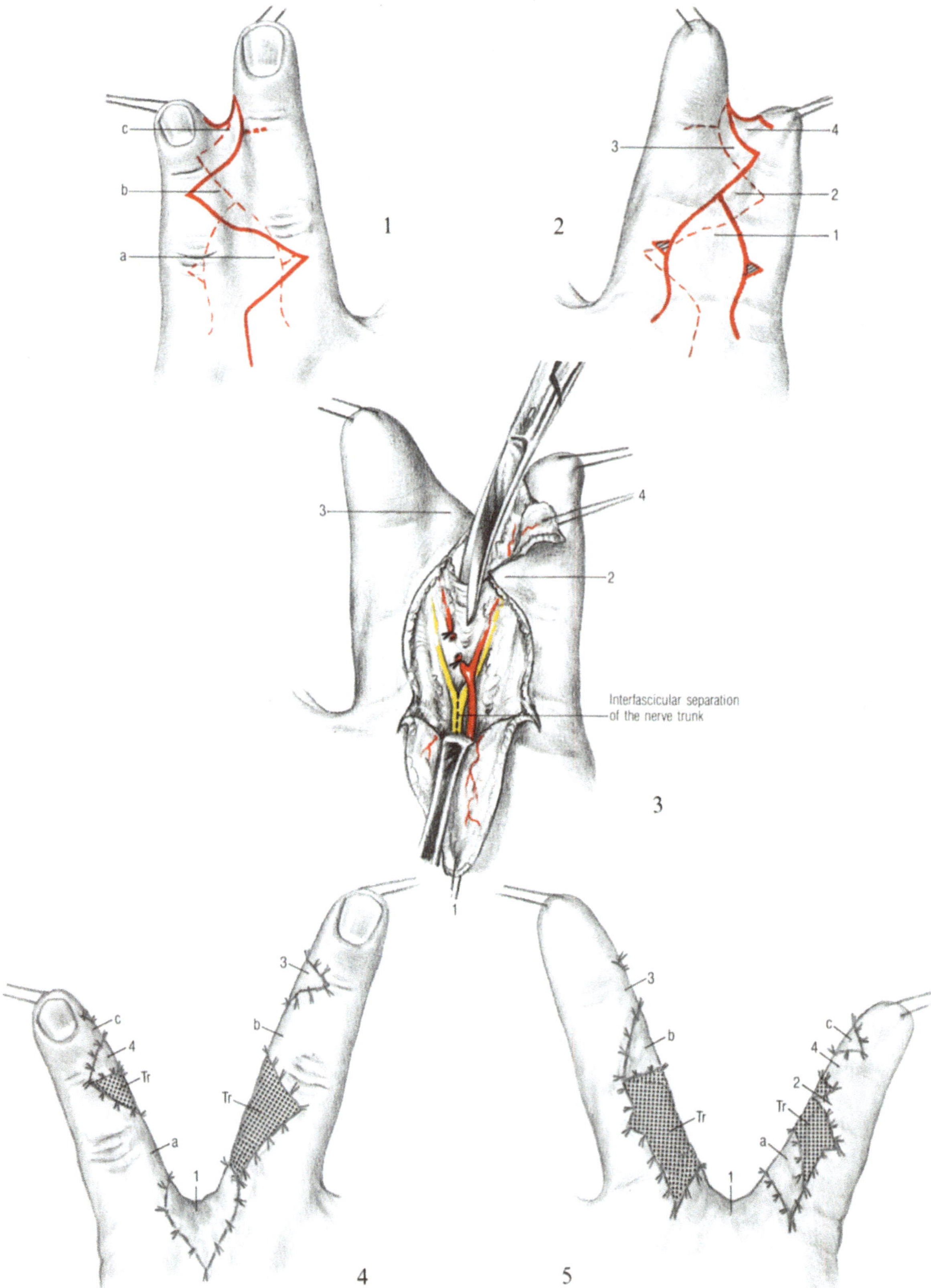
c
b
a
1
3
4
2
1
2
3
4
2
Interfascicular separation of the nerve trunk
1
3
3
c
b
4
Tr
Tr
a
1
3
b
Tr
c
4
2
Tr
a
1
4
5

2.1.4 Total Syndactyly of Several Long Fingers

Goal of Surgery

Removal of the interdigital skin and soft tissue bridges and construction of web spaces in anatomic positions by using swivel flaps with local pedicles.

The separation of the fingers is done in stages with a period of at least 3 months between operations.

Fig. 1 Preoperative appearance and incision, dorsal aspect.
Separation of middle and ring fingers by employing a dorsal pedicle flap to cover the commissure (see also Sect. 4.3.1). The web space between the ring and little finger is reconstructed with a dorsal and a palmar triangular flap *(broken line)*. This is done during a second operation at a later date.

Fig. 2 Preoperative appearance and skin incision, palmar aspect.
Separation of interdigital spaces using zig-zag incisions.

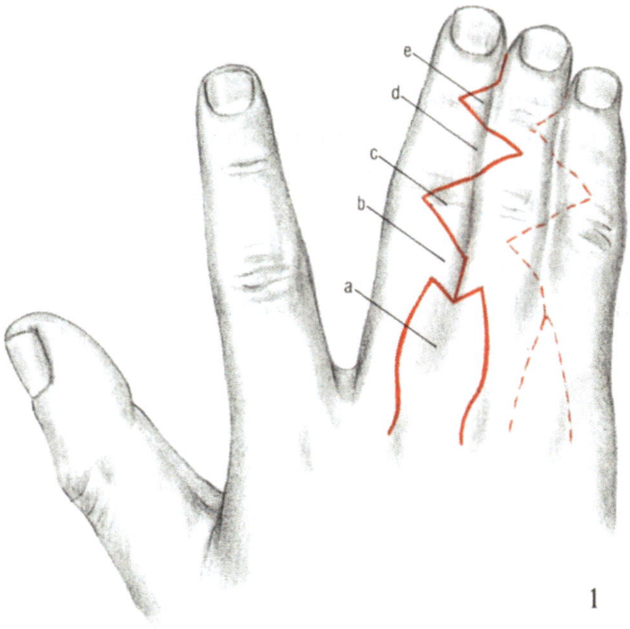

1

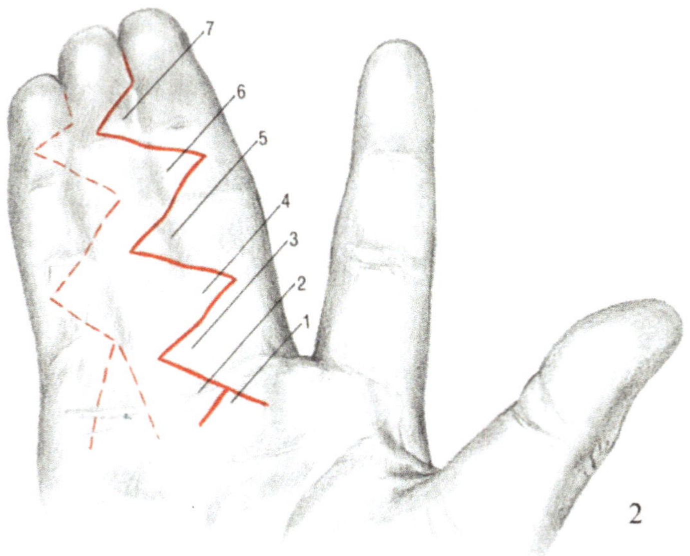

2

Fig. 3 Postoperative appearance, dorsal aspect.
The local pedicle flaps have been sutured into their proper position. Skin defects on the lateral aspects of the fingers have been covered with thick-split thickness skin transplants *(Tr)*.

Fig. 4 Postoperative appearance, palmar aspect.
The skin of the dorsal commissure flap *(a)* extends slightly onto the lateral aspect of the fingers.

Postoperative Care

See Sect. 2.1.1.4.

Errors and Their Consequences

See Sect. 2.1.2.

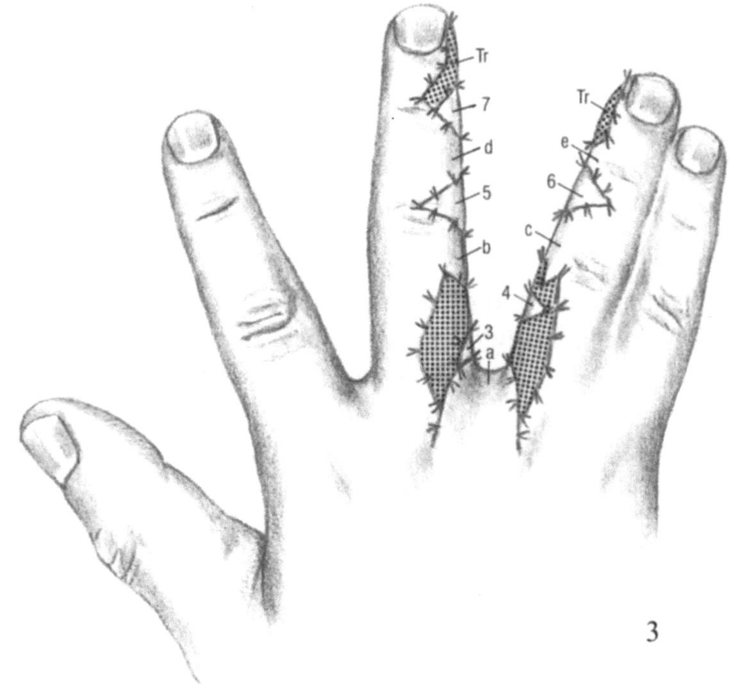

3

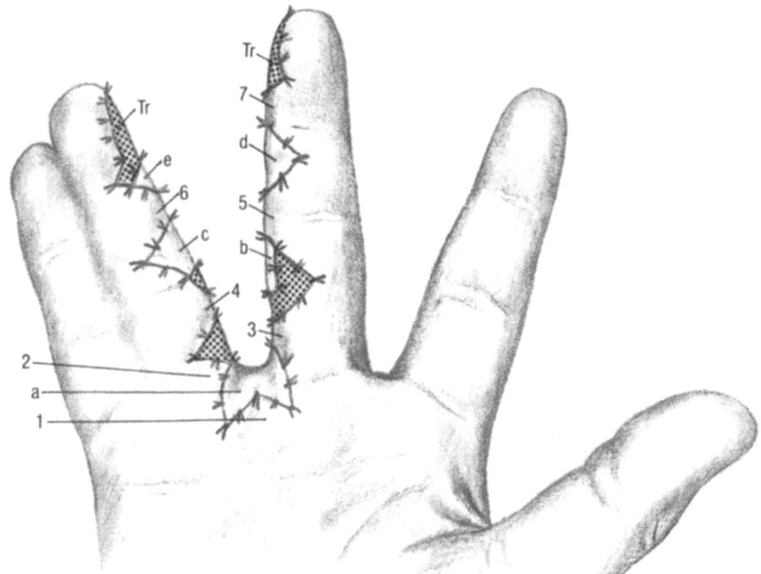

4

2.1.5 Partial Syndactyly ("Short Type")

Goal of Surgery

Construction of a web space in anatomic position.

Fig. 1 Preoperative appearance and incision, dorsal aspect.
Separation of the interdigital skin bridge using zig-zag incision. The commissure is constructed by employing a proximally based palmar, pedicle flap *(1)*. Its tip extends past the apex of the web to the dorsal side. Main vessels and nerves must be preserved during the dissection of the dorsal and palmar flaps. Incision of the opposite side is demarcated by *broken lines*.

Fig. 2 Preoperative appearance and skin incision, palmar aspect. The basis of the commissure flap *(1)* may have to be extended at a later stage to permit tension-free closure (*thick broken lines*). Dorsal incision demarcated by *thin broken lines*.

Fig. 3 Postoperative appearance, dorsal aspect.
Skin sutured without tension. The remaining defects at the lateral aspects of the fingers have been covered with thick-split thickness skin transplants.

Fig. 4 Postoperative appearance, palmar aspect.
In this case it would have been impossible to suture flap *(b)* without tension in the corner of the commissure. Therefore the exposed area was covered with a larger thick-split thickness skin transplant. *Broken lines:* suture lines of the dorsal side.

Postoperative Care

See Sect. 2.1.1.4.

Errors and Their Consequences

See Sect. 2.1.2.

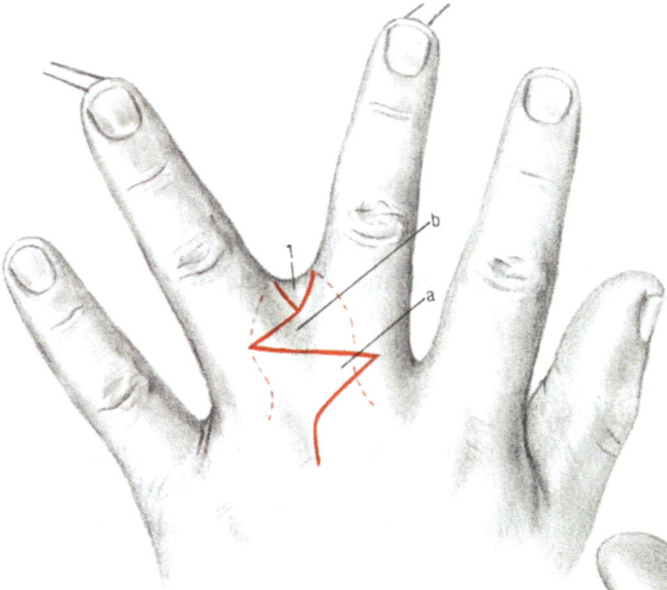

1

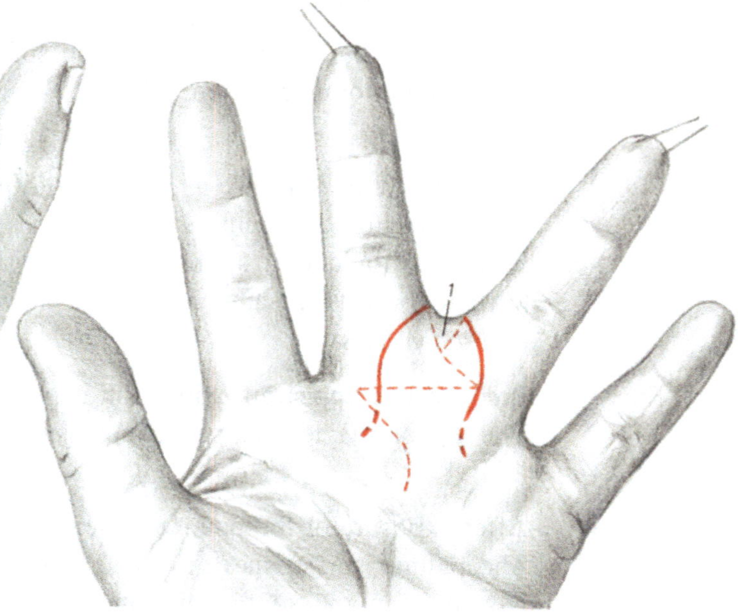

2

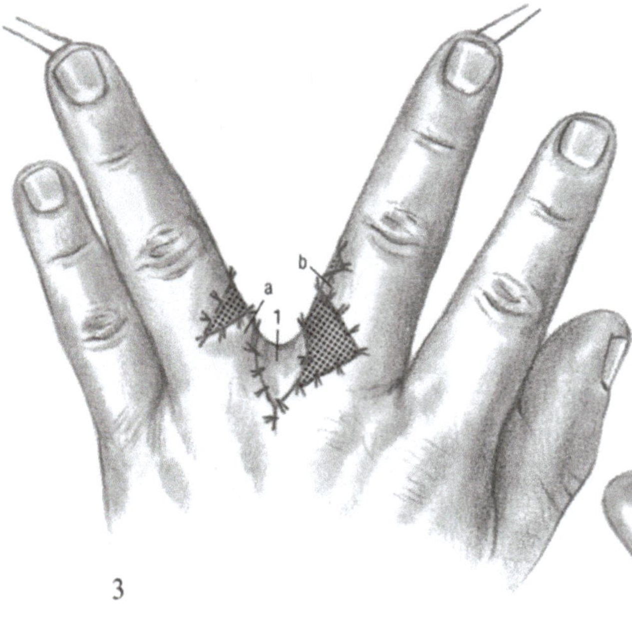

3

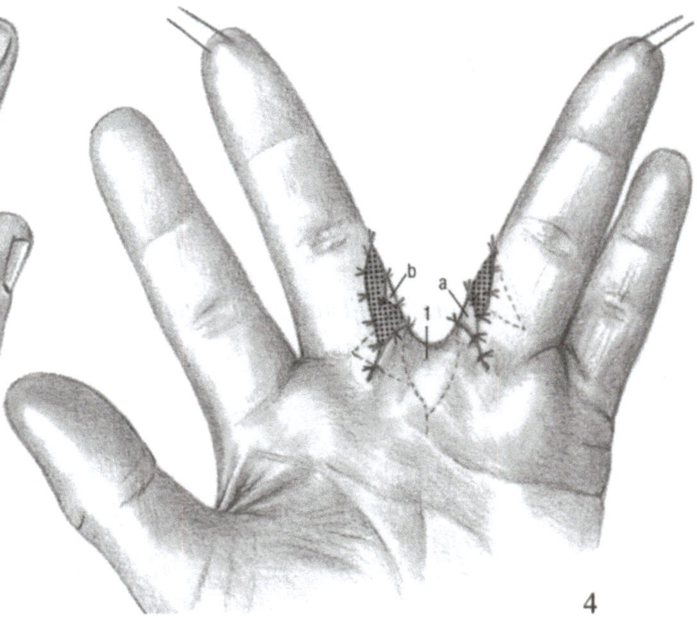

4

2.1.6 Partial Syndactyly ("Long Type")

Goal of Surgery

Removal of the interdigital skin and soft tissue bridge and construction of a web space in anatomic position.

Fig. 1 Preoperative appearance and incision, dorsal aspect.
The separation of the interdigital space is accomplished by using a zig-zag incision. Flap *(d)* should correspond to flap *(3)* (Fig. 2); therefore, the tips of both flaps have to be at the same level. The incision of the opposite side is demarcated by *broken lines*.

Fig. 2 Preoperative appearance and skin incision, palmar aspect.
The tip of the leaf-shaped commissure flap *(1)* extends to the level of the PIP joint.

Fig. 3 After exposure of the palmar vessels and nerves.
The palmar soft tissues are being transected. Dissection of the interdigital space has to be made so far proximal that maximum spreading of the fingers does not result in any soft tissue resistance. During this stage dissection is carried out alternately on the palmar and dorsal sides. The figure shows the situation from the dorsal aspect.

Figs. 4, 5 Postoperative appearance.
Flaps have been sutured without tension. Skin defects at the lateral aspects of the fingers have been covered with thick-split thickness skin transplants.

Postoperative Care

See Sect. 2.1.1.4.

Errors and Their Consequences

See Sect. 2.1.2.

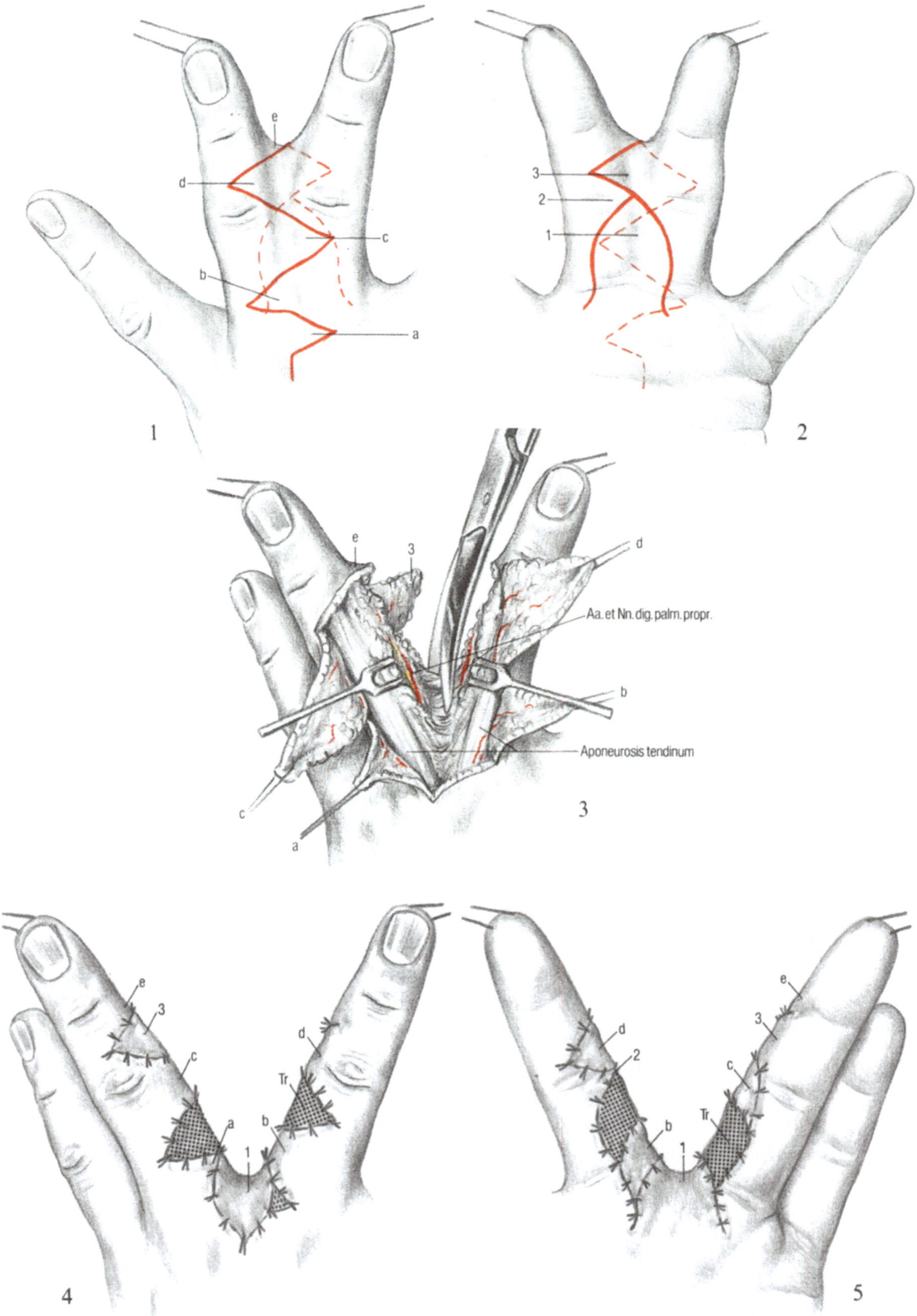
1
2
3
4
5
a
b
c
d
e
Tr
Aa. et Nn. dig. palm. propr.
Aponeurosis tendinum

2.2 Osseous Syndactylies

The highest incidence of osseous syndactylies is found in patients afflicted with *Apert syndrome*. Only cases pertaining to it shall be discussed in this chapter.

In the past some combinations of skull deformities and syndactylies on a familial basis have been classified as variants of Apert syndrome (see PFEIFFER 1969); however, today they are recognized as a separate entity (see MCKUSICK 1975: acrocephalosyndactyly type II–VI etc., acrocephalopolysyndactyly type I–III). All these types, and particularly the two most important ones, Pfeiffer syndrome (PFEIFFER 1964) with dominant heredity (partial syndactylies with pollex varus) and Carpenter syndrome (TEMTAMY 1966) with recessive heredity (preaxial polysyndactyly), generally consist of pure soft tissue syndactylies as described in Chap. 2.1.

Therapy for osseous syndactylies associated with other complex deformities requiring markedly different surgical techniques or modifications is described elsewhere (for oligodactyly, see Sect. 4.3; for polydactyly, see Sect. 4.5.5).

2.2.1 Introduction: "Apert Hand"

2.2.1.1 General Remarks

Characteristic and frequently specific hand deformities are part of Apert syndrome [acrocephalosyndactyly (ACS) type I according to MCKUSICK, "typical" ACS according to BLANK]. The syndrome (APERT 1906) consists of rather *uniform deformities* despite the large number of abnormalities present. Therefore, it can be easily distinguished from other dyscraniodysphalangies. *Cranial changes* (acrocephaly of the brachysphenocephalic type: turricephaly, exophthalmus, hypertelorism, anomalous positions of the teeth with a high palate, and occasional cleft palate) are striking and are combined with *pronounced syndactylies* of all four limbs. Other segments of the skeletal system are always affected, but to a lesser degree. Changes of the upper limbs involve the shoulder (usually slight loss of abduction) and the elbow joint (limitation of extension and cubitus valgus), but apparently never the wrist joint. *Impaired mental development* is nearly always noted, and extreme mental debility has been observed in some cases.

The hand deformities involve *all* fingers. With few exceptions mirrorlike alterations of both hands are present. Numerical variations are not typical.

Morphologically, functionally, and therapeutically one can distinguish *three grades of severity*. Common to all grades is a tight total syndactyly involving fingers II–IV with fusion of the fingertips and a common nail band. Peripheral synostoses (acrosynostoses II–IV) are frequently present, and there is at least a partial syndactyly of the Vth finger. Brachydactyly of the long fingers caused by an assimilation hypophalangy or a symphalangy (for remarks on terminology, see Sect. 6.1.1) with an abnormally long proximal element is regularly observed. Prior to the 4th year of life one has to be aware of an *apparent* three-jointedness of single fingers in the presence of a radiologically observable additional ossification center (joint hypoplasia). True three-jointedness has sporadically been reported (mild joint hypoplasia), but osseous symphalangies with marked loss of motion of the distal interphalangeal (DIP) joints of all long fingers will develop during the first few years of life.

The most frequently observed form, *type I,* shows a well-defined delineation of the thumb from the remaining hand plate. However, the range of motion of the thumb is usually impaired by the insufficient depth and width of the web space. The little finger also appears to be well-segmented on inspection. Only a partial interdigital soft tissue bridge tethers it to the adjacent fingers.

In *type II* (obstetrician's hand) the little finger is conjoined to the other long fingers by a tight, total, nonosseous syndactyly.

Type III (spoon hand) consists of a total syndactyly of all fingers. Their tips are located at the same level. The fingers form a palmar concavity, giving the hand the appearance of a spoon. The common nail band is markedly raised, and some parts of it may show a rooflike deformity.

The following *skeletal* and *soft tissue deformities* will have to be considered:

In types I and II the *thumb* is markedly shortened and broadened. More or less pronounced radial deviation is noted at the first metacarpophalangeal (MP) joint. In approximately one-half of all cases two short dysplastic phalanges are present. A synchondrotic–synostotic fusion of the interphalangeal joint does not appear to occur at a later age. If only one phalanx is present it is usually longer and thicker (assimilation hypophalangy).

In comparison, the thumb of type III is longer. The thenar musculature is usually normal. A side-to-side synostosis of the proximal segments of the fourth and fifth metacarpal bones has been observed in nearly all cases.

As previously described in cases of *simple* cutaneous syndactyly, in Apert hands one also has to reckon with an abnormal distal bifurcation of the nerves and vessels in the interdigital spaces. Occasionally one notices hypoplasias of palmar digital arteries, or finds only one vessel or nerve in the interdigital space. Such anomalies appear to be more common between the IIIrd and IVth finger. In correspondence with the diminished distance of the skeletal and soft tissue parts, the vessels supplying the thumb may be markedly *shortened,* particularly in type III (Lösch 1970).

In a majority of cases, *muscles and tendons* are normally developed. Occasionally one observes irregular insertions of the flexor tendons; this is probably caused by the abnormal differentiation of the distal hand blastema. The chiasm of the superficial flexor tendons at the level of the MP joint is absent in such cases. Therefore, the deep flexor tendons cannot pass through this area in a normal manner; to continue distally they have to wrap themselves around each other. At the level of the DIP joints they fan out and interdigitate with the tendons of neighboring segments in an arcadelike fashion to form a wide, common tendinous arch. In type III the tendon of m. flex. poll. long. joins this arch. In one case of type I we found it fused with a tendon of the index finger up to the level of the commissure (see operative example, Sect. 2.2.5).

Aplasias, hypoplasias, and insertion anomalies of the mm. lumbricales and mm. interossei have been observed.

The *palmar aponeurosis* extends farther distal than normal and ends in archlike, transversely running tight bands. This can result in a tight tethering of the thumb to the rest of the hand. The extensor tendons of syndactylous fingers join distally into a common dorsal aponeurosis, which may be fused to underlying bony parts. Strong, transversely running connective tissue bands are found at the extensor surface of the interdigital spaces.

In type III, tight tendinous bands (connexus intertendinei, juncturae tendinum) can be observed between the extensor tendons of the Ist and IInd rays.

2.2.1.2 Timing of Surgery

Release of the syndactylies should be carried out early if pronounced tethering of the thumb to the index finger is present. In Apert hands of type III, surgery should therefore be initiated during the 2nd and 3rd years of life to assure differentiated functions of grasp at an early age. In patients with types I and II we do not like to postpone surgical interventions beyond the 6th year, as improvement of the thumb commissure and correction of the radial thumb deviation require no formidable expenditure of time or operative technique.

2.2.1.3 General Surgical Directives

The *"loosening" of the Ist ray* by separation (Sect. 2.2.2) or by deepening and widening of a poorly developed commissure (Sect. 2.3.3) has absolute *precedence* over separation of the long finger syndactylies (Sect. 2.2.4) (Blauth 1972). The next goal is to improve the *squeeze-type grasp* between thumb and the rest of the hand to a *pinch-type grasp* by corrective osteotomies of the Ist and IInd rays. During this stage it is important to eradicate the radial clinodactyly of the thumb (Sect. 2.2.5). Concurrent surgical rotation of the distal phalanx of the thumb should be considered to achieve optimal positioning.

We feel that formation of a supple functional web space in cases of type III deformities is only possible by employing a *tubed pedicle jump flap,* as a large skin and soft tissue defect will be present after separation of the thumb and incision of its adductor muscles (Blauth 1969, 1972).

In operating on syndactylous *long fingers* one should in general separate only the index and little fingers. In selected cases, particularly in forms of type I, separation of all fingers may be indicated. The plan for a series of such surgical procedures has to be established at the time of the first operation. This plan has to be kept in mind while deciding which vessel branch to ligate when a distally displaced bifurcation is encountered. One has to expect severe circulatory impairment if, at the time of the final separating procedure, another distally displaced bifurcation requiring additional ligation of a vessel is found. In considering indications for *separating the Vth finger* one has to be aware of the fact that increased abduction at the fifth MP joint may result if one finds the synostotic fourth and fifth metacarpals to be closely approximated (m. interosseus anomaly?)

In selected cases one may consider *"flexion osteotomies"* of the long fingers after the 4th year of life, as motion essentially takes place only at the MP joints (see Chap. 6). For further information we refer the reader to the directives given in Sect. 2.1.

2.2.1.4 Postoperative Care

Excessive sweat collection has to be expected due to the typical hyperhidrosis noted in Apert hands. Porous pressure dressings (i.e., steel wool) should be employed.

Otherwise, we refer the reader to the individual operations and to the general remarks in Sect. 2.1.

2.2.2 Total Syndactyly Between Thumb and Long Fingers

Goal of Surgery

Staged separation of the thumb ray and construction of a web space by using a tubed pedicle flap.

Fig. 1 Preoperative appearance and incision, dorsal aspect.
Total syndactyly of all fingers with a common nail band (type III). The deepest point of the future commissure should be level with the MP joint of the thumb. This point is marked by a needle.

Fig. 2 Preoperative appearance and incision, palmar aspect.
The skin is folded and puckered on the palmar side, especially in the area of the fingertips. This provides a certain amount of excess skin.

Fig. 3 The dorsal and palmar skin bridge and soft tissues have to be separated with care; vessels and nerves must be protected! Parts of the palmar aponeurosis, contracted fasciae, and muscle strands of the m. add. poll. are severed or indented while increasing the abduction of the Ist ray. The neurovascular bundle is protected by an elevator.

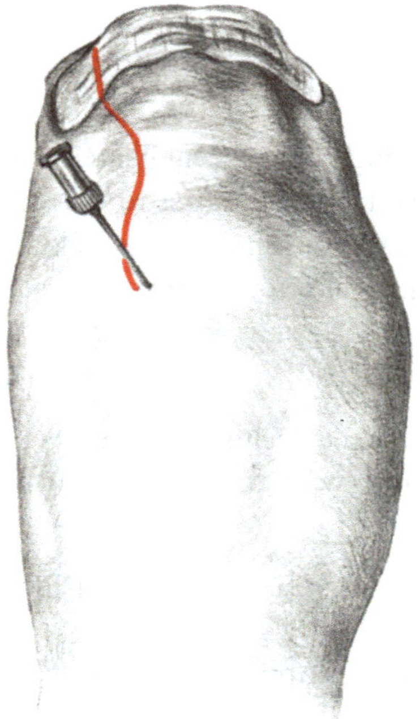

1

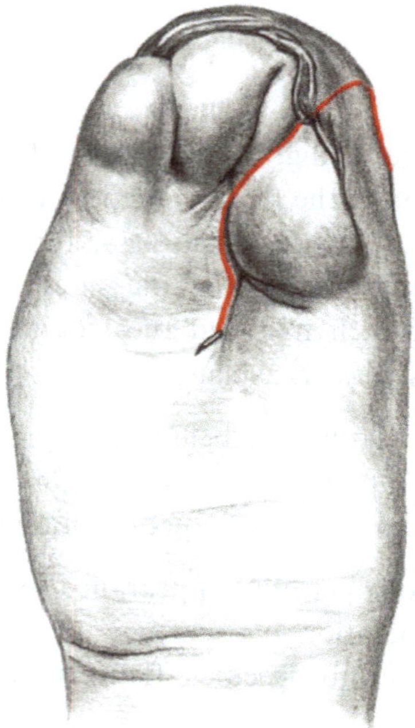

2

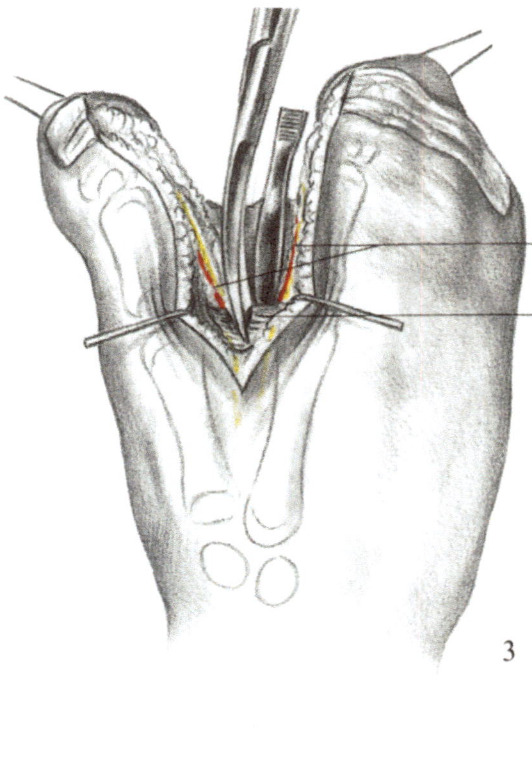

3

Fig. 4 The a. dig. palm. propr. of the index finger has been ligated and transected to obtain the required depth. Temporary fixation of the first to the second metacarpal bone in the position of function with two Kirschner wires. Excess subcutaneous fatty tissue from the sides of the fingers has to be removed. After preparation of each nail bed the wound is covered with skin from the palmar side as well as with transplants of thick-split skin *(Tr)*.

Fig. 5 The tubed pedicle flap is prepared (BUNNELL technique: see Sect. 4.2.2) to cover the palmar side of the commissure defect with one triangle and the dorsal side with the other. Suction drainage.

Fig. 6 Postoperative appearance, dorsal aspect after first stage, and incision for second operation.
The tubed pedicle flap can be separated after approximately 4 weeks.

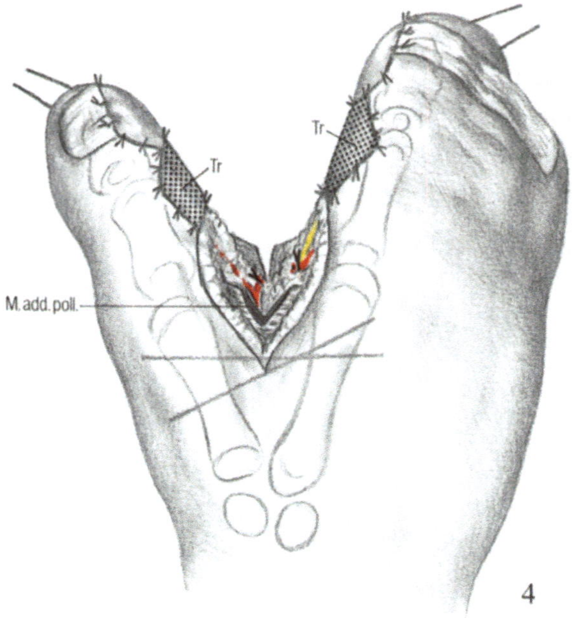

4

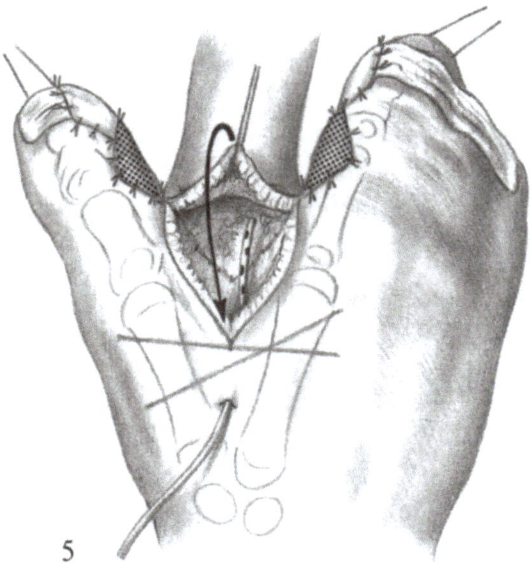

5

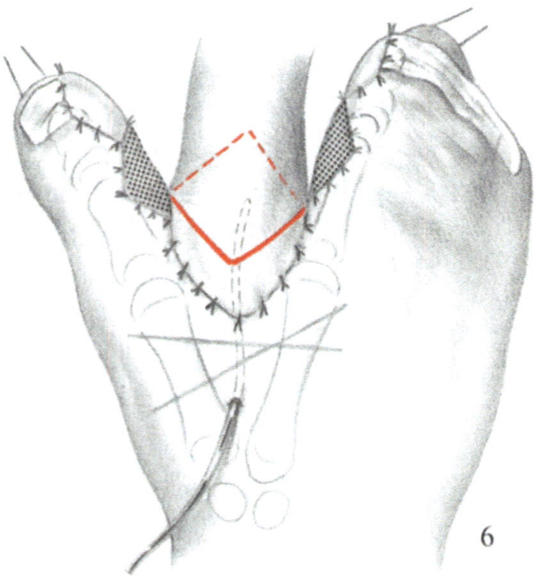

6

Fig. 7 *Second stage*. Separation of the tubed pedicle flap.
The palmar part of the tubed pedicle flap has to be longer to avoid transverse web space scars (see Fig. 6). Suction drainage.

Figs. 8, 9 Postoperative appearance.
For subsequent separation of the long fingers, see Sect. 2.2.4.

Postoperative Care

See Sect. 2.1.1.4.

Errors and Their Consequences

See also operative example (Sect. 2.1.2).
E. Routine approach: additional anomalies have to be expected during each phase of the dissection.

E. Omitting suction drainage of the wound.
C. Hematoma may cause circulatory impairment in the area of the transplanted flap.

E. Failure to fix the separated Ist ray temporarily in a position of function with crossed Kirschner wires.
C. Adduction malalignment with subsequent contracture; the flap may telescope and its circulation is apt to suffer.

E. Faulty bandaging technique causes the tubed pedicle flap to be under excessive tension, strangulated, or kinked (see Sect. 4.2.2 for additional information regarding errors and their consequences when using a tubed pedicle flap plasty).

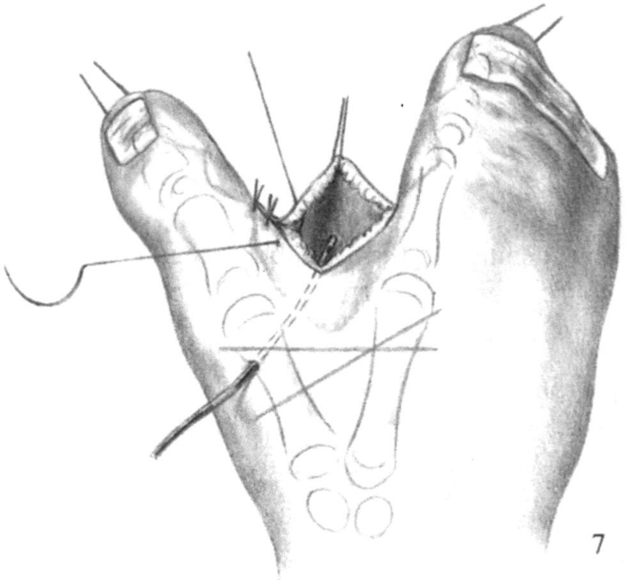

7

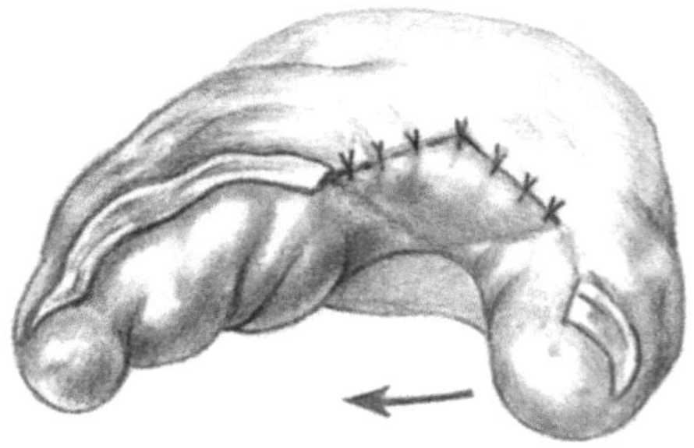

8

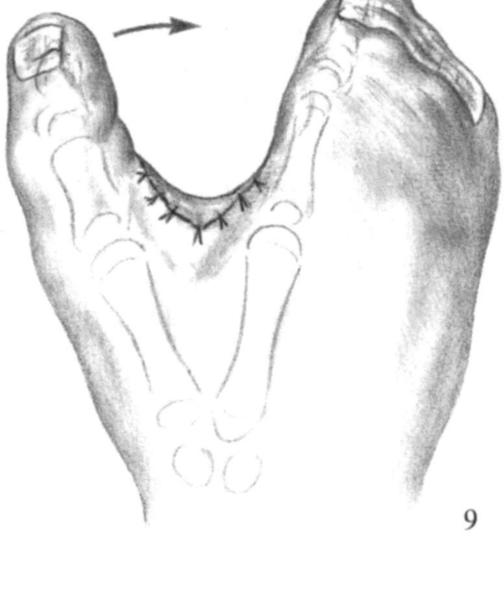

9

2.2.3 Partial Syndactyly Between Thumb and Index Finger

Goal of Surgery

Deepening and broadening of the thumb commissure by using a local pedicle swivel flap.

Figs. 1, 2 Preoperative appearance and incision.
The needle marks the depth of the future commissure. Its apex should be approximately level with the MP joint of the thumb.

Figs. 3, 4 Postoperative appearance.
Dorsal and palmar fasciae as well as m. add. poll. have been incised (use elevator to protect the palmar neurovascular bundles). Fixation in desired functional position with two crossed Kirschner wires from the first to the second metacarpal. Skin defects on the IInd ray are covered with a thick-split thickness skin transplant.

Postoperative Care

See Sect. 2.1.1.4.

Errors and Their Consequences

E. The local pedicle swivel flap is too short to form a web space of sufficient width and depth. The existing width of the syndactyly has to be evaluated very critically prior to surgery. Radial clinodactyly of the thumb can simulate relatively good abduction of the Ist ray. In case of doubt it is preferable to use a tubed pedicle flap (see Sect. 2.2.2).

E. The swivel flap originating from the index finger is too long or too narrow (the ratio of flap width to flap length should be between 1:2.5 and 1:3).
C. Skin sutures are under tension.

We also refer the reader to the corresponding comments in Sects. 2.1.2 and 2.2.2.

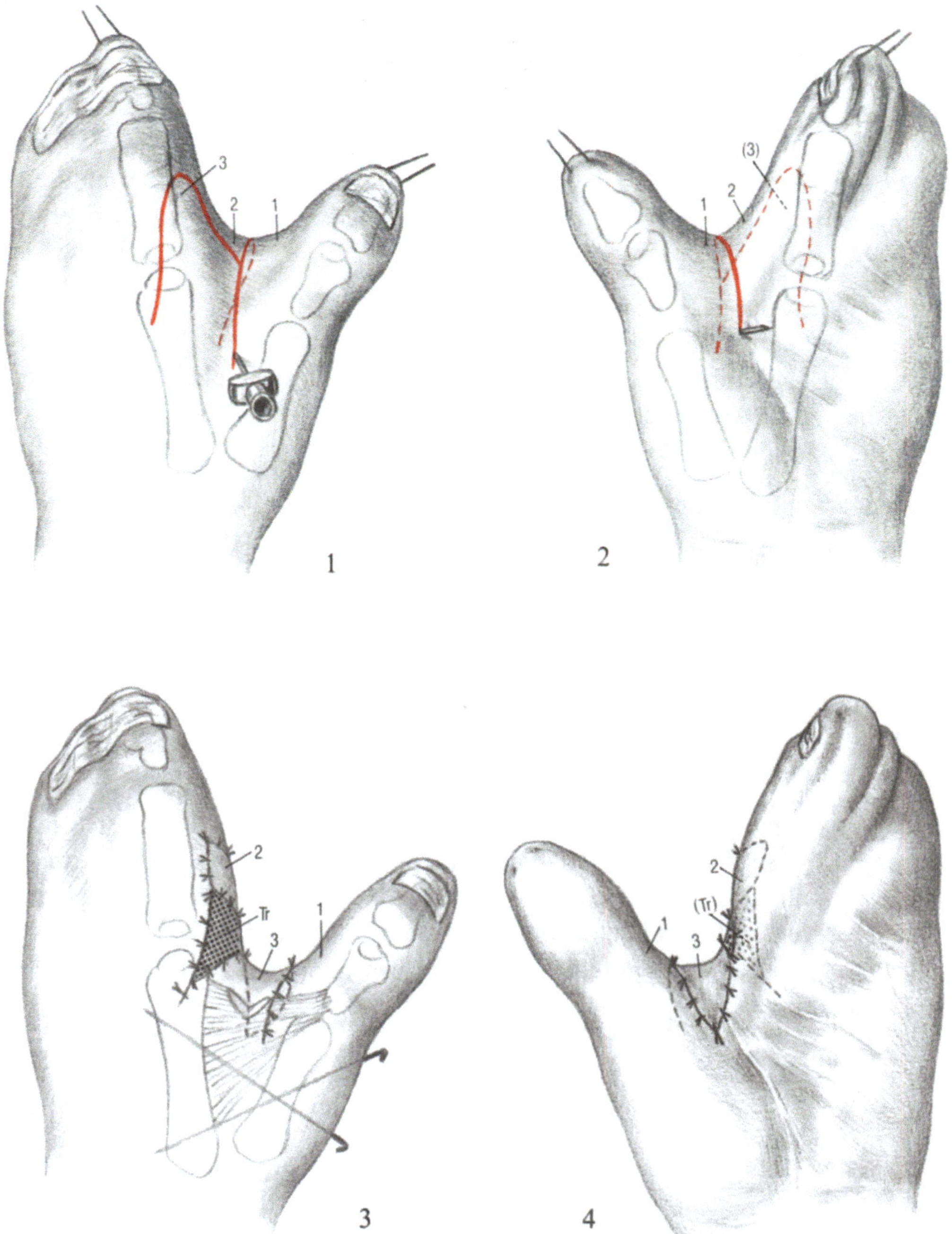
3
2
1
(3)
2
1
1
2
2
Tr
1
3
2
(Tr)
1
3
3
4

2.2.4 Total Syndactyly of the Long Fingers with Acrosynostosis

Goal of Surgery

Correction of the cutaneous and osseous syndactyly between the middle and ring finger (preceded by separation of the index finger during an earlier operation).

Fig. 1 Preoperative appearance, dorsal aspect.
A needle marks the basis of flap *(1)* (Fig. 2) and the site of the future web space. Parts of the common nail band and, later on, the hatched areas of bone and cartilage will be resected (see Fig. 3). Occasionally a slight proximal extension of the skin incision becomes necessary (*broken line*).

Fig. 2 Preoperative appearance, palmar aspect.
The commissure will be covered with a local palmar flap *(1)*. The triangles (*) define the radial and ulnar skin areas to be excised prior to implanting the thick-split thickness grafts to prevent scar formation along the axis of the finger (see Fig. 6). Incisions on opposite side are marked by *broken* line.

Fig. 3 The proximal edge of the interdigital skeletal bridge is visible after dissection of the dorsal skin flaps. The space proximal to it is filled with loose fatty tissue. The common nail band is transected in its center, and the hatched area is removed.

Fig. 4 The opposing sides are reduced to normal phalangeal width by osteotomizing the bones (*broken lines*). The DIP joints are opened during this step. A partial resection of the nail matrix is performed (see *hatched area*). The main vessels and nerves can be seen in the subcutaneous fatty tissue on the palmar side. The lig. capit. transversum has to be notched or severed if it interferes with finger abduction.

Fig. 5 The interdigital joint and the resected area of the distal phalanx are covered with subcutaneous fatty tissue.

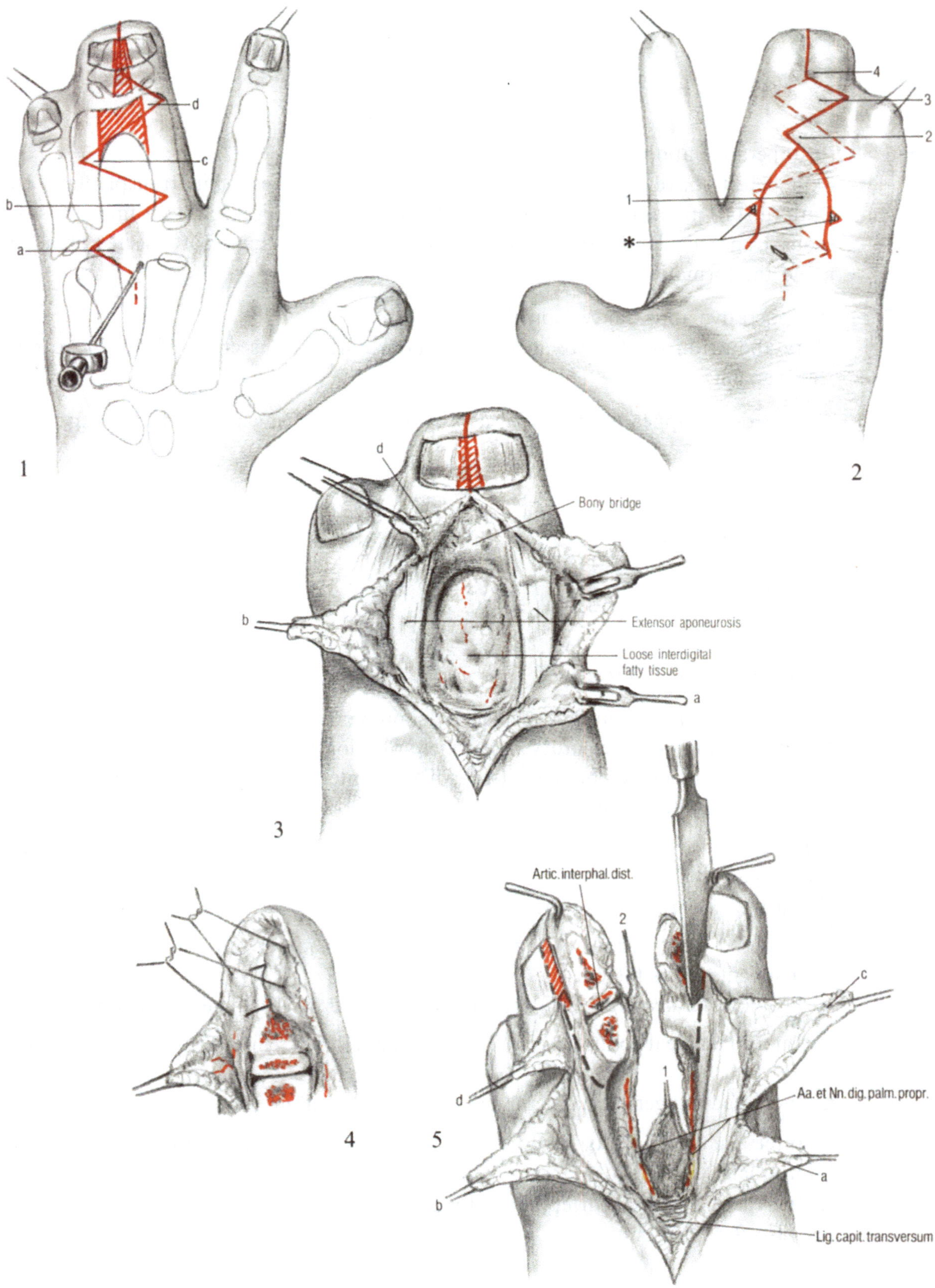

a
b
c
d
1
4
3
2
1
*
2
d
Bony bridge
b
Extensor aponeurosis
Loose interdigital fatty tissue
a
3
4
5
Artic. interphal. dist.
2
c
1
d
Aa. et Nn. dig. palm. propr.
a
b
Lig. capit. transversum

Fig. 6 Postoperative appearance, palmar aspect.
Skin defects have been covered with thick-split thickness skin transplants *(Tr)*. Both (distal) interphalangeal joints are temporarily immobilized with thin transosseous–transarticular Kirschner wires. Two additional triangles of resected skin (*) avoid the formation of longitudinal scars.

Fig. 7 Postoperative appearance, dorsal aspect.
Note abduction of the two metacarpal bones after transection of the lig. capit. transversum.

Fig. 8 Postoperative appearance, lateral aspect of the IVth finger and dorsal aspect of the IIIrd.

Postoperative Care

See Sect. 2.1.1.4.

Errors and Their Consequences

E. Separating more than one syndactyly simultaneously.
C. Great danger of circulatory impairment, tension in swivel flaps etc. As a matter of policy, syndactylies between two adjacent interdigital spaces should never be separated simultaneously!

E. The nailbeds of the individual fingers have not been properly shaped after their separation.
C. Further deformation of the nails.

E. Exposed bone (areas of synostoses) and DIP joints have not been covered with subcutaneous fatty tissue.
C. Problems in healing of the skin transplants; increased danger of infection.

E. Interphalangeal joints have not been immobilized temporarily with Kirschner wires.
C. Increased danger of malalignment and wound healing problems.

E. Interphalangeal joints have been fixed with Kirschner wires that are too thick (more than 0.6 mm).
C. Increased potential for epiphyseal plate damage.
See also Sect. 2.2.2.

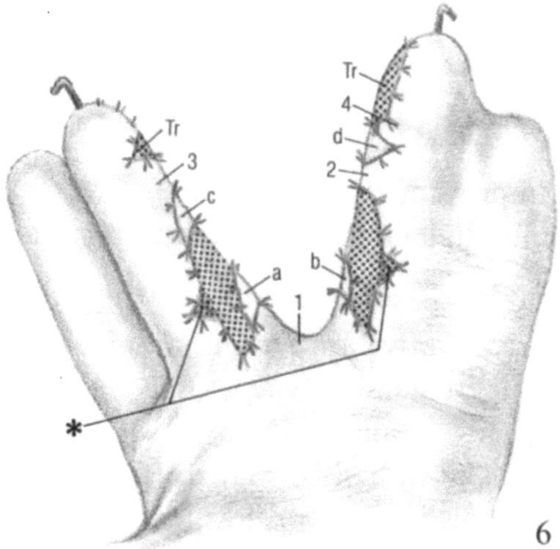
Tr
4
d
2
Tr
3
c
a
b
1
*

6

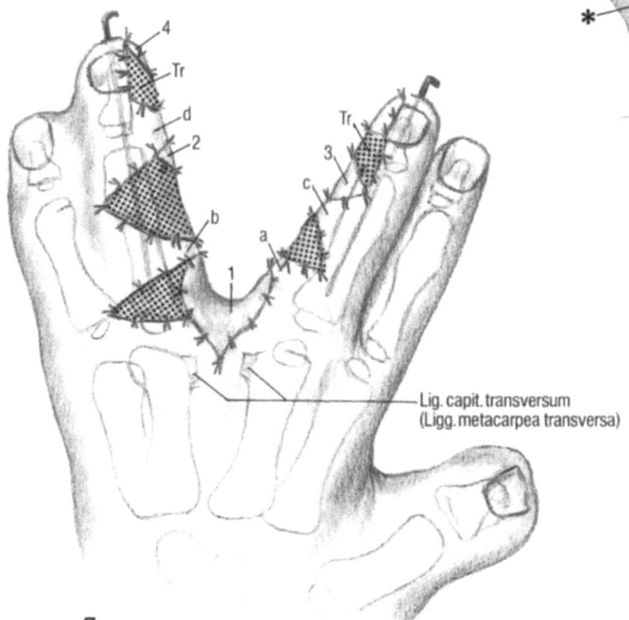
4
Tr
d
2
b
1
a
c
3
Tr
Lig. capit. transversum
(Ligg. metacarpea transversa)

7

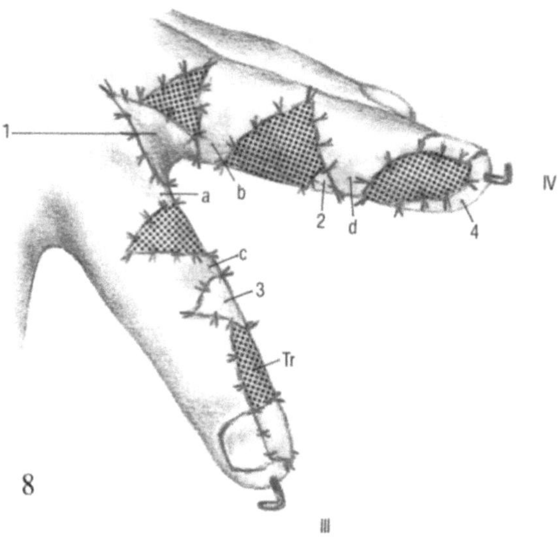
1
a
b
2
d
4
IV
c
3
Tr
III

8

2.2.5 Radial Clinodactyly of the Thumb

Goal of Surgery

Improvement of grasp by correcting the thumb deviation and by deepening the interdigital space between thumb and index finger.

Fig. 1 Preoperative appearance and incision, dorsal aspect.
"Apert hand," type I: the plump thumb is well defined; however, the first web space is shallow. The dysplastic proximal phalanx of the thumb is roughly trapezoidal and radially deviated. Its epiphysis is abnormal (Fig. 2). The tip of the thumb cannot be used for grasp because of the radial clinodactyly.
Two swivel flaps created by a Z-plasty suffice to deepen the commissure. Correction of the longitudinal thumb axis results in surplus skin on its extensor surface which is resected at the end of the operation *(hatched area)*.

Fig. 2 Palmar aspect, partial view.
Both swivel flaps *(a, 1)* as well as palmar vessels and nerves are prepared. Bifurcation of the vessels occurs far distal within the web space. The main radial palmar artery of the index finger has to be ligated in order to deepen the interdigital space sufficiently. If necessary, fascia and parts of the m. add. poll. have to be incised (not shown, see Sect. 2.2.2).
The proximal phalanx of the thumb is exposed subperiosteally (see Fig. 3) and an ulnar-based wedge of bone will be removed (*hatched area*).

Fig. 3 Dorsoulnar aspect, partial view.
The proximal phalanx of the thumb is visible. A narrow osteotome is used to remove the bone wedge. The shape of the bone wedge should permit slight overcorrection to prevent future radial deviation during growth.

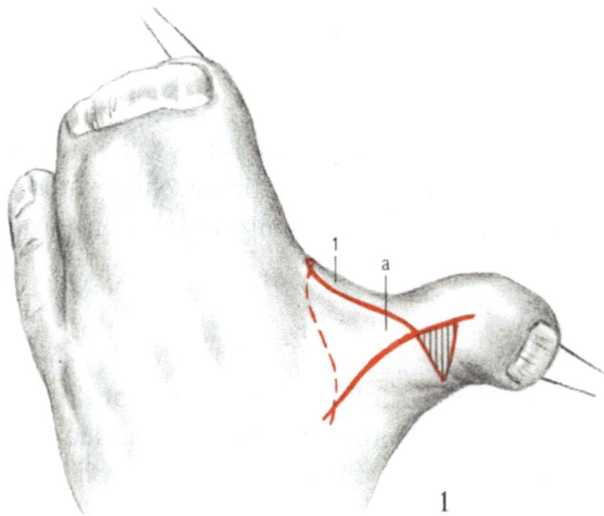

1

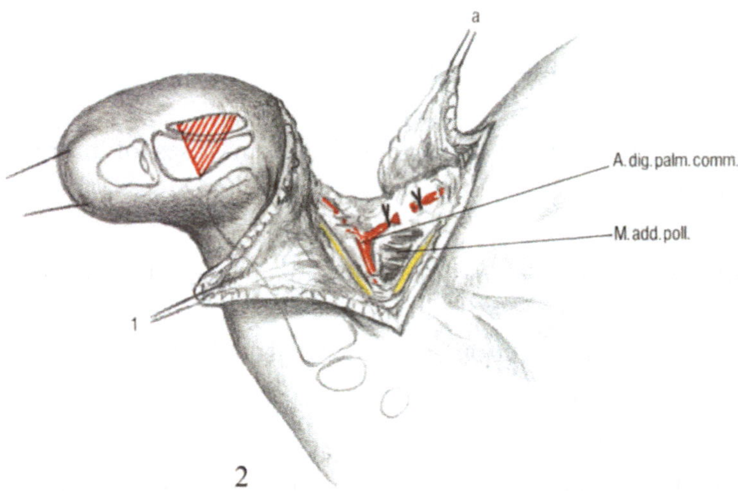

2

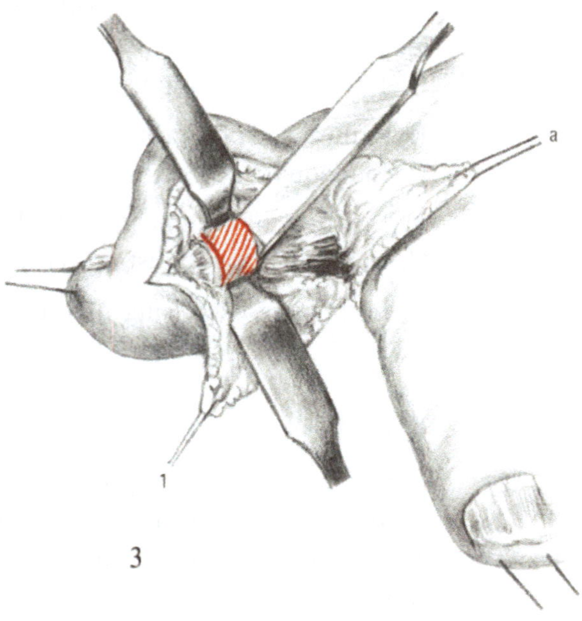

3

Figs. 4, 5 Postoperative appearance, dorsal (4) and dorsoulnar (5) aspects. Transarticular-transosseous fixation with Kirschner wires with the MP joint in slight flexion and approximately 20° of thumb tip rotation toward the index finger.

Postoperative Care

Long-arm cast for 3–4 weeks followed by removal of Kirschner wires and application of a dorsal splint holding the thumb in maximal abduction and medium opposition. When 6 weeks have elapsed since surgery, the splint is used only at night (for a further 6 months).

Errors and Their Consequences

E. Injury of palmar vessels and nerves during dissection of soft tissue between thumb and index finger.

E. Ligation of the main artery at the side of the index finger in cases of more distal bifurcation has been omitted.
C. Insufficient depth of the web space.

E. The size of the bone wedge was incorrect or it was removed from the wrong location.
C. Fusion of the joint, under- or overcorrection, secondary growth impairment.

E. Failure to rotate thumb during osteotomy.
C. Inadequate correction of functional impairment.

E. Fixation of fragments with Kirschner wires that are too thick (over 0.6 mm).
C. Epiphyseal plate disturbances are probable.

E. Permitting exercising of the thumb too soon, neglecting to use a night splint.

Remarks

A certain decrease in growth of the proximal phalanx and the possibility of a recurrence of the deviation has to be expected. Therefore, one should not operate in early childhood but during school age, when the degree of malfunction can be more reliably assessed.

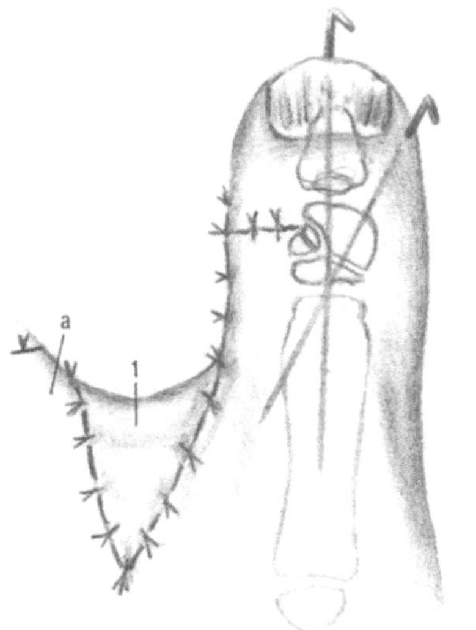

4

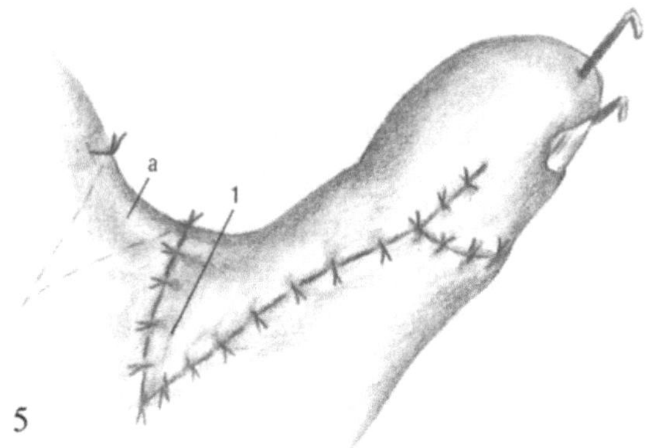

5

2.3 Recurrent Syndactylies

2.3.1 Introduction

2.3.1.1 General Remarks

Recurrent syndactylies are not genuine recurrences but *interdigital bridges caused by postoperative scar tissue formation* ("cicatricial syndactyly"). However, the expression is so commonly used that we would rather not change it.

As a rule, recurrent syndactylies are the result of *improperly placed incisions, erroneous assessment of morphological variations of the bifurcation of vessels and nerves,* or *secondary healing processes* (BLAUTH 1970; BUCK-GRAMCKO 1975; MILLESI 1961).

Timing of the original operation is but a minor factor in recurrent syndactyly. However, operations performed at a very early age and with poor technique result in the worst recurrences.

Basically, one can distinguish two types (BLAUTH and HIPPE 1973):

a) The *"short" type* with interdigital scar tissue formation limited to the proximal phalanges (Sects. 2.3.2 and 2.3.3). For purposes of operating technique we distinguish between a "narrow" and a "wide" short type depending on the width of the soft tissue bridge. Occasionally, strands of scar tissue course from the web to the distal phalanges, raising the skin like a sail on the lateral aspects of the fingers (Sect. 2.3.4). Slight cases not affecting normal function, rotation and flexion deformities with inadequate abduction and extension, and severe deformities with corresponding markedly limited function have been observed.

b) The *"long" type* is characterized by scars filling the interdigital space from the proximal to the distal phalanx (Sect. 2.3.5). As in the short type, strands of scar tissue sometimes radiate from the apex of the web to the distal phalanges (Sect. 2.3.6) or even to the nails; they can cause deformation of the nails and yokelike bending of the fingers. On occasion we have seen secondary growth disturbances of the phalanges.

The rigid web is particularly *susceptible to trauma;* it tears easily, *develops scabs and fissures*, and is apt to become more rigid as a result of such chronic mechanical irritations.

2.3.1.2 Timing of Surgery

Recurrent syndactylies should be corrected *as soon as possible* (BLAUTH 1970). Nonintervention increases the danger of aggravating the deformity because the areas of scarred skin are unable to keep pace with normal skeletal growth.

2.3.1.3 General Surgical Directives

Each type of recurrence requires a particular operation.

However, certain *basic rules of treatment* apply to all cases. They are similar to or identical with those of syndactyly operations (see Sect. 2.1.1.3). The most important rules are repeated here:

- *Skin incisions should be outlined with a sterile marking pen.* Even experienced surgeons depend on this aid in making complicated incisions.
- *As a rule, do not excise scars!* The scarred skin areas should become part of the swivel flaps. They should only be excised if, at the end of the operation and after the tourniquet has been released, their blood supply is unsatisfactory or surplus skin is present.
- *Web spaces* should be wide and deep. They should be formed from *local* swivel flaps!
- *Dissect palmar neurovascular bundles with extreme care!* Surgical telescopes facilitate recognizing these important structures. One of the two volar finger arteries has to be ligated if an a. dig. palm. comm. is bifurcating more distally. One chooses the artery of the finger with the better blood supply. The *common nerve trunk* has to be separated *interfascicularly* in a proximal direction.
- *Release tourniquet before closing wound!* Cover wound with moist sponges and apply an elastic pressure bandage for approximately 5 min. Subsequently use bipolar microcoagulation to assure *complete hemostasis!*
- *Suture skin edges without tension!* Avoid suture lines along the long axis of the finger. Cover skin defects at the lateral aspects of the fingers with thick-split thickness skin transplants.

2.3.1.4 Postoperative Care

See Sect. 2.1.1.4.

2.3.2 Recurrent Syndactyly of the Long Fingers (Narrow "Short" Type)

Goal of Surgery

Removal of the interdigital scar tissue bridge and formation of a web space in anatomic position.

Figs. 1, 2 Preoperative appearance and incision.
Recurrence of a partial cutaneous syndactyly in a patient with oligodactyly (and a relatively narrow commissure caused by scar tissue). Dorsal and palmar triangular flaps *(a, 1)* are used to construct the commissure. Zig-zag incisions are made at the lateral aspects of the adjacent fingers.

Fig. 3 Palmar aspect, detailed view.
Protecting main nerves and vessels, the skin flaps of the web space covered with scar tissue have been raised. The bifurcation of the vessels is located more distal than normal (not corrected during previous operation!). One of the palmar arteries of the finger must be severed and ligated to obtain a commissure of sufficient depth. The size of the incision to be made for flaps *(2)* and *(3)*, as well as *(4)* and *(5)* (*broken lines*), is determined after approximation of the skin flaps.

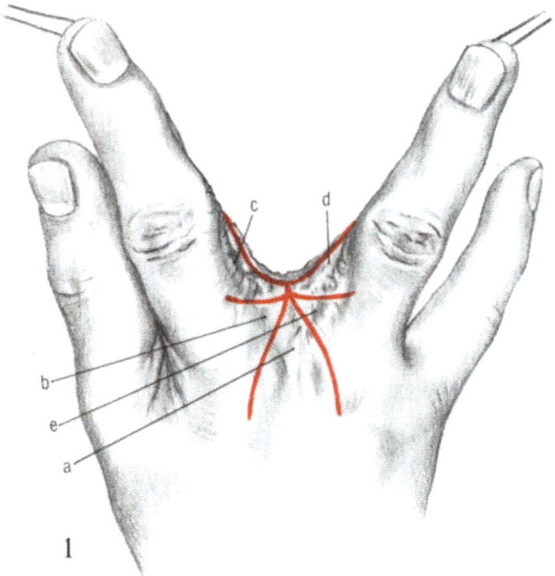

1

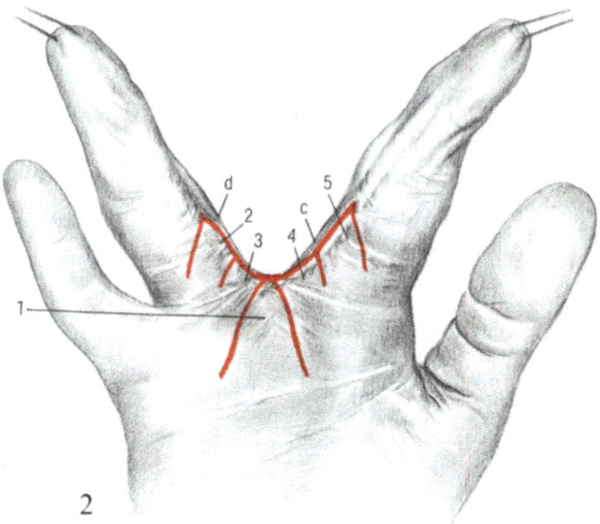

2

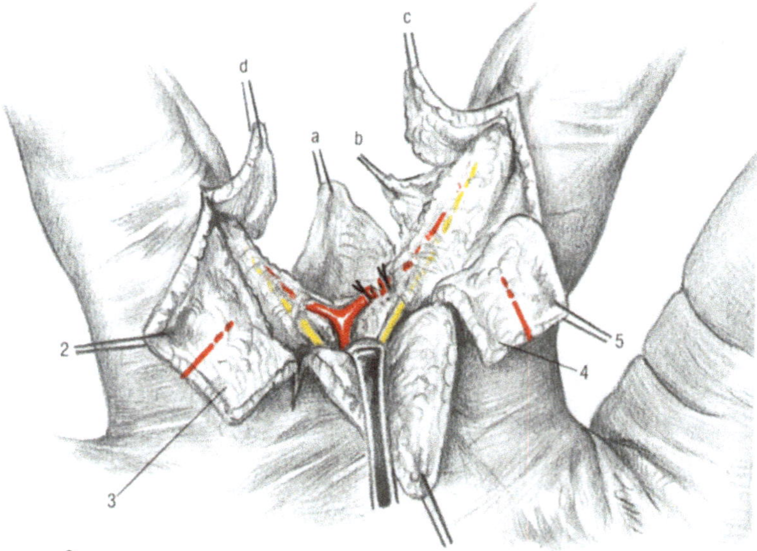

3

Figs. 4, 5 Postoperative appearance after the swivel flaps have been sutured.
Thick-split thickness skin transplants are required if tension cannot be avoided on one or the other flap. Occasionally one should consider using a palmar flap for the formation of the commissure, as shown in Sect. 2.3.3.

Postoperative Care

See Sect. 2.1.1.4.

Errors and Their Consequences

See Sect. 2.1.2.

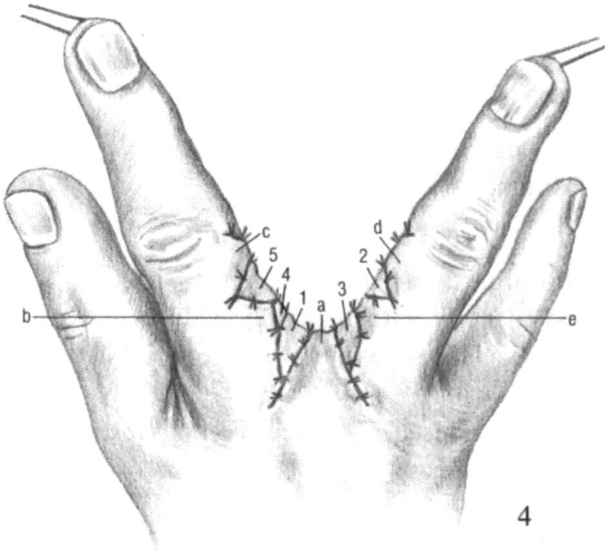

4

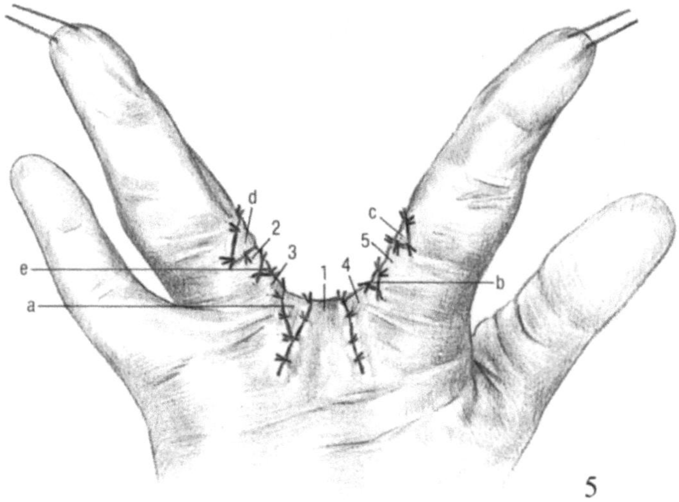

5

2.3.3 Recurrent Syndactyly of the Long Fingers (Wide "Short" Type)

Goal of Surgery

Removal of the syndactyly caused by scar tissue and formation of a web space in anatomic position.

Fig. 1 Preoperative appearance and incision, dorsal aspect.
Recurrence of syndactyly with relatively wide commissure in a patient with first-degree symbrachydactyly (caused by improper skin incision during previous surgery).
Scars should not be excised. The new commissure is to be formed by a palmar flap. Due to the narrowness of the bridge scar tissue, the flap will have to extend across its apex to the dorsal side.
Dissect on the dorsal side when opening the interdigital space! Do not damage palmar nerves and vessels!

Figs. 2, 3 Postoperative appearance, dorsal (2) and palmar (3) aspects.
Skin defects on the lateral aspects of the fingers have been covered with thick-split thickness transplants. The fingers now appear to be longer than before.
The procedure described in Sect. 2.3.2 can be considered as an alternative.

Postoperative Care

See Sect. 2.1.1.4.

Errors and Their Consequences

See Sect. 2.1.2.

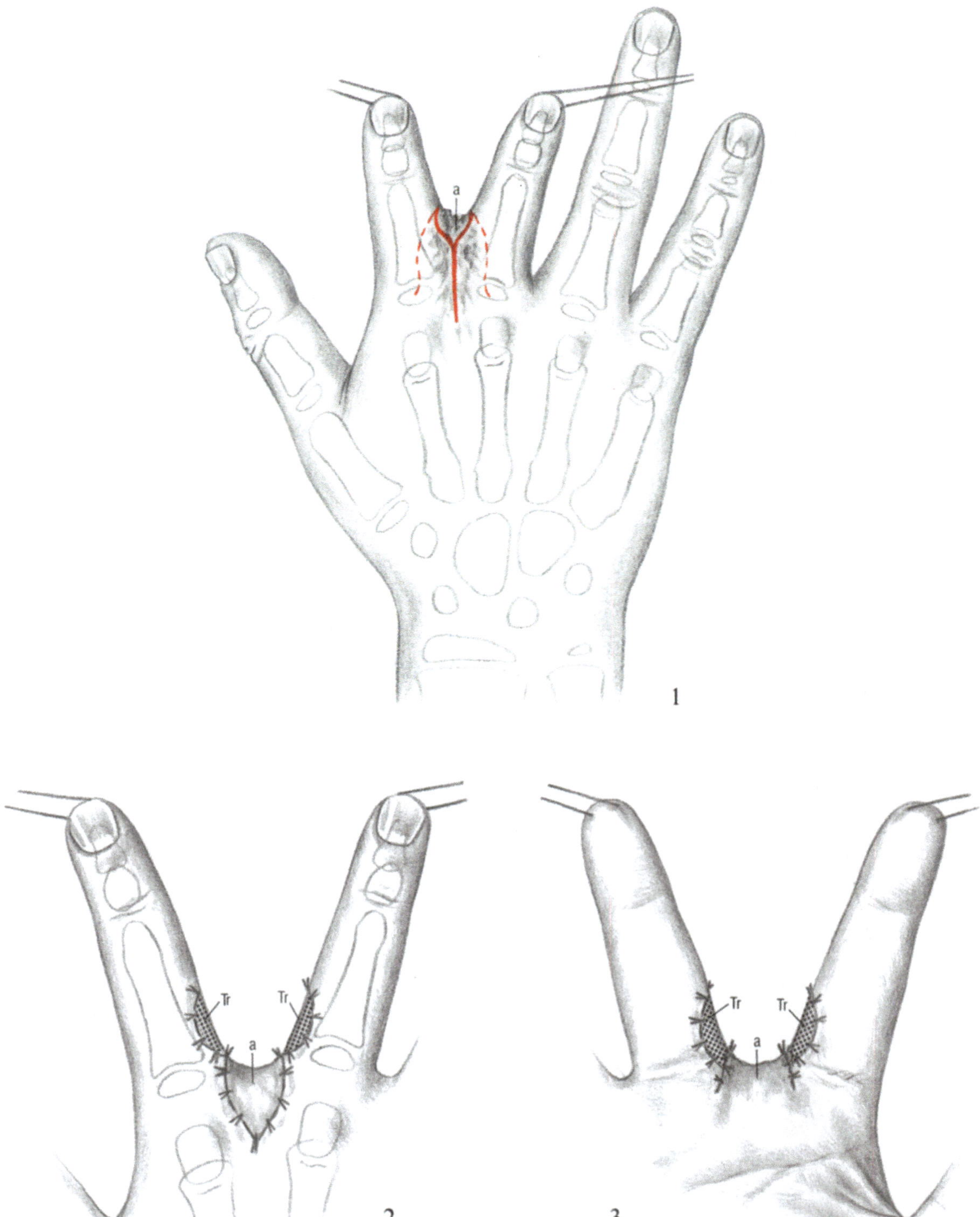
a
1
Tr
Tr
a
2
Tr
Tr
a
3

2.3.4 Recurrent Syndactyly of the Long Fingers ("Short" Type) with Scars Extending to the Distal Phalanges

Goal of Surgery

Removal of the interdigital bridge of scar tissue and the strands of scar tissue on the lateral aspects of the fingers. Formation of a web space in anatomic position.

Figs. 1, 2 Preoperative appearance and incision (adapted from ISELIN, 1959).
In contrast to the previous example, additional scarring is present on the lateral aspects of the fingers. The scar is not to be excised (*see above*). The commissure is created with two triangular flaps (*a, 1*). The skin on the lateral aspect of the fingers is raised like a sail and excessive skin makes the commissure too wide. The skin has to be rearranged with multiple Z-plasties; thus more skin becomes available along the longitudinal axis of the finger.

Figs. 3, 4 Postoperative appearance.
Following dissection of the palmar vessels and nerves of the fingers and severing of the scar tissue between the bases of the proximal phalanges III and IV, the skin flaps can be sutured tension-free. Some flaps may require additional adjustment. Remaining exposed areas on the lateral aspects of the fingers will have to be covered with thick-split thickness skin transplants (*hatched areas*).

Postoperative Care

See Sect. 2.1.1.4.

Errors and Their Consequences

See Sect. 2.1.2.

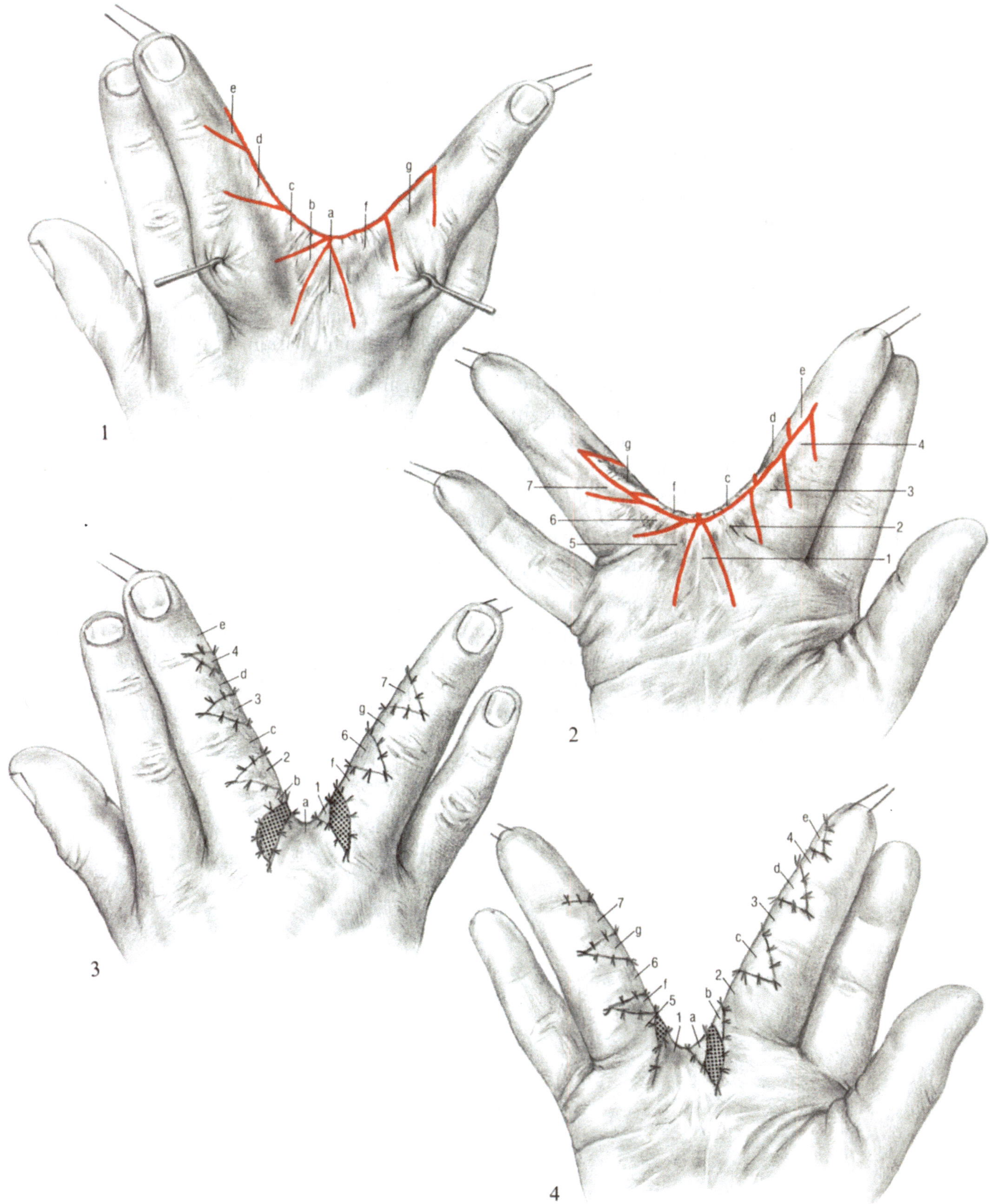

e
d
c
b
a
f
g
1
e
d
g
4
7
f
c
3
6
2
5
1
2
e
4
d
3
c
2
b
a
1
7
g
6
f
3
e
4
d
3
7
g
c
6
2
f
5
b
1
a
4

2.3.5 Recurrent Syndactyly of the Long Fingers ("Long" Type)

Goal of Surgery

Removal of the interdigital bridge of scar tissue and formation of a web space in anatomic position.

Fig. 1 Preoperative appearance and incision, dorsal aspect.
Keeping the main arteries in mind, the two dorsal flaps are raised and dissected from the extensor aponeurosis. *Broken line:* palmar incision.

Fig. 2 Preoperative appearance and incision, palmar aspect.
The incision runs from the tip of the triangular flap (*3*) across the apex of the scar tissue bridge toward the dorsal aspect. The base of the triangular flap (*thick broken lines*) has to be moved proximally if the commissure proves to be too "shallow" after a trial fitting of the dorsal flaps. *Thin broken lines:* dorsal incision.

Fig. 3 Dorsal flaps (*a*) and (*b*) have been raised. The horizontal (scarred) strands of connective tissue of the interdigital space have to be severed (*black broken line*).

Fig. 4 Start dissecting from normal tissue using surgical telescopes to expose palmar vessels and nerves! The a. dig. palm. comm. bifurcates more distally than normal (not corrected during previous surgery). Severing and ligation of an a. dig. propr. is required to create a sufficiently proximal located web. Individual digital nerves are present in this example. Interfascicular division may be necessary if this is not the case.

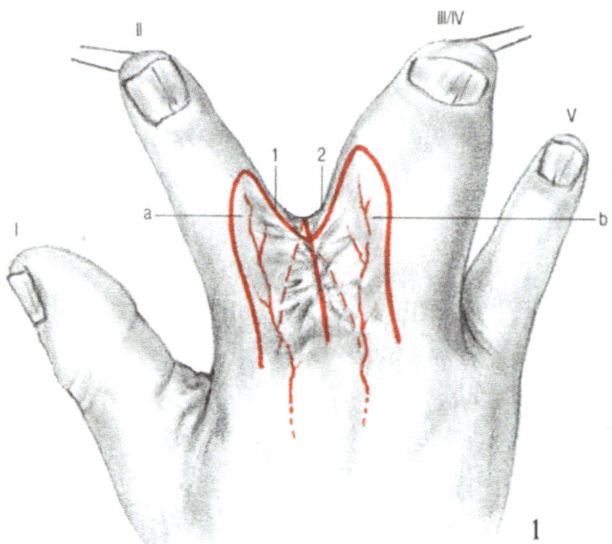
II
III/IV
V
I
1
2
a
b

1

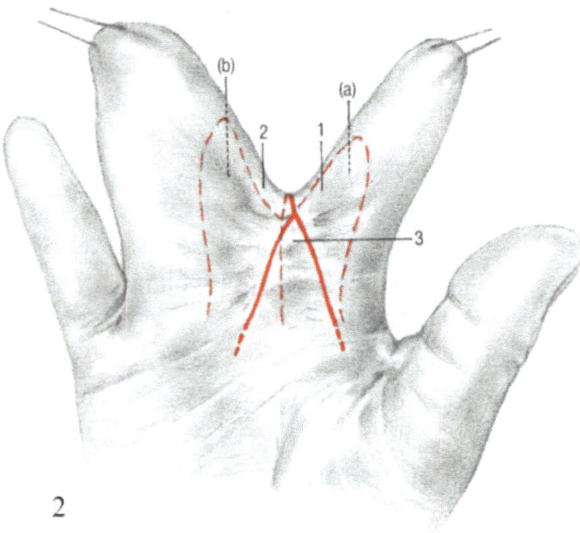
(b)
(a)
2
1
3

2

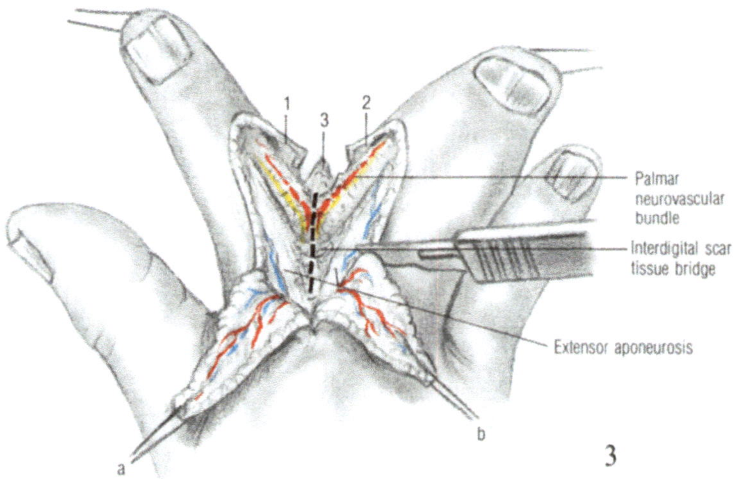
1
3
2
Palmar neurovascular bundle
Interdigital scar tissue bridge
Extensor aponeurosis
a
b

3

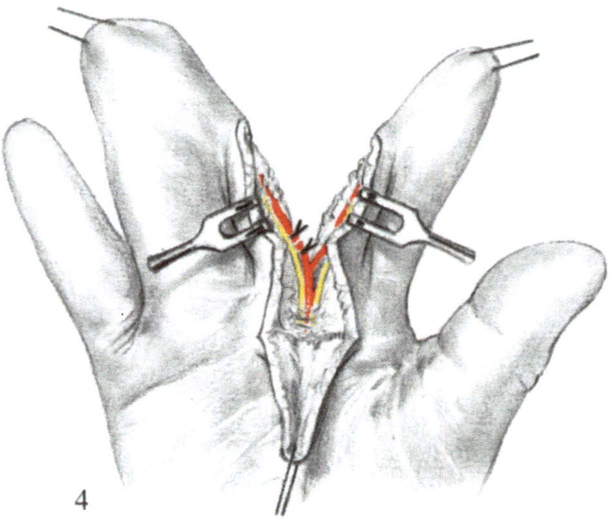

4

Fig. 5 Postoperative appearance, dorsal aspect.
Skin defects on the dorsal sides of the fingers have been covered with thick-split thickness skin transplants (*Tr*). Sutures of the opposite side are demarcated by *broken lines.*

Fig. 6 Radial lateral aspect of the middle finger.

Fig. 7 Postoperative appearance, palmar aspect.

Postoperative Care

See Sect. 2.1.1.4.

Errors and Their Consequences

See Sect. 2.1.2.

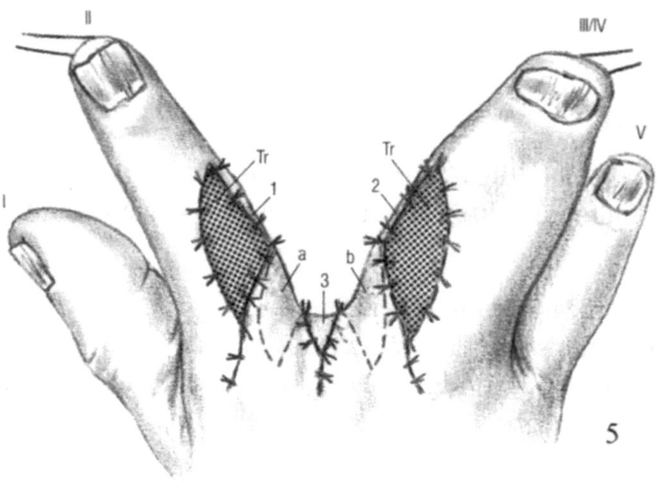

5

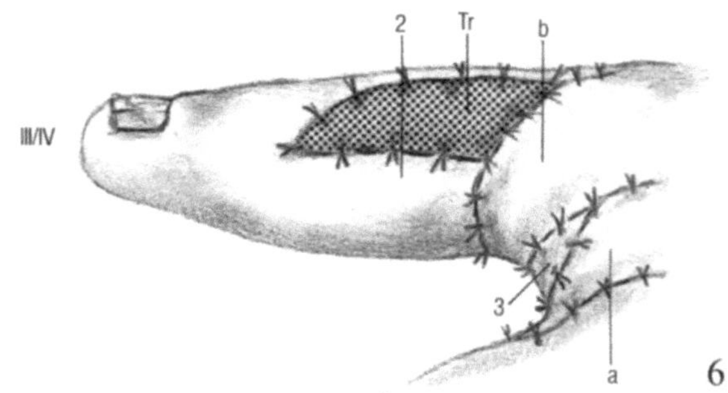

6

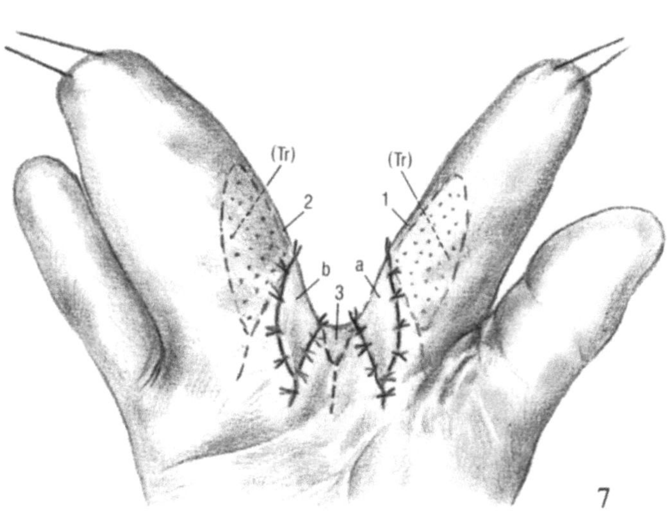

7

2.3.6 Recurrent Syndactyly of the Long Fingers ("Long" Type) with Scars Extending to the Distal Phalanges

Goal of Surgery

Removal of the interdigital bridge of scar tissue and the longitudinal scars on the fingers' lateral aspects; formation of a web space in anatomic position.

Figs. 1, 2 Preoperative appearance and incisions.
The palmar commissure flap (*1*) extends slightly onto the extensor surface of the interdigital scar tissue bridge. The length of the incision between flaps (*c*) and (*d*) (*dotted line*) will be determined after the flaps, especially flap (*5*), have been rearranged.

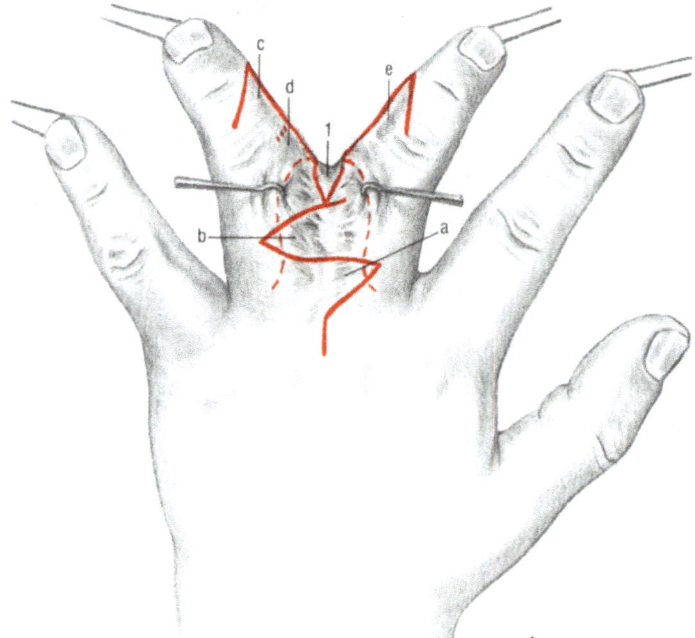

1

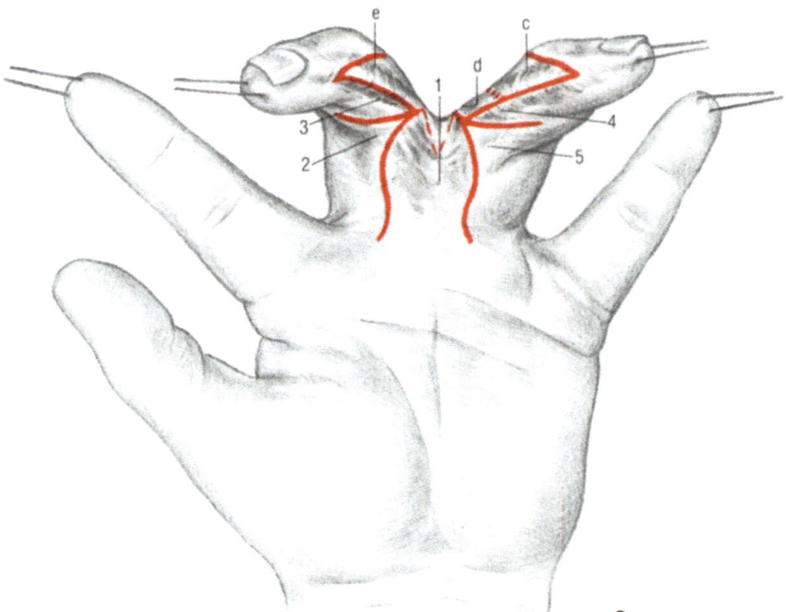

2

2.3.6 Recurrent Syndactyly of the Long Fingers ("Long" Type) with Scars Extending to the Distal Phalanges

Fig. 3 View of the interdigital soft tissue structures after the skin flaps have been raised. The point of bifurcation of the neurovascular bundle is located very distally; it had not been corrected during a previous operation.
Ligation and transection of a palmar finger artery; interfascicular division of the nerve trunk in a proximal direction, using surgical telescopes (*black broken line*).

Figs. 4, 5 Postoperative appearance.
Skin defects on the lateral aspects of the fingers have been covered with thick-split thickness skin transplants (*Tr*).

Postoperative Care

See Sect. 2.1.1.4.

Errors and Their Consequences

See Sect. 2.1.2.

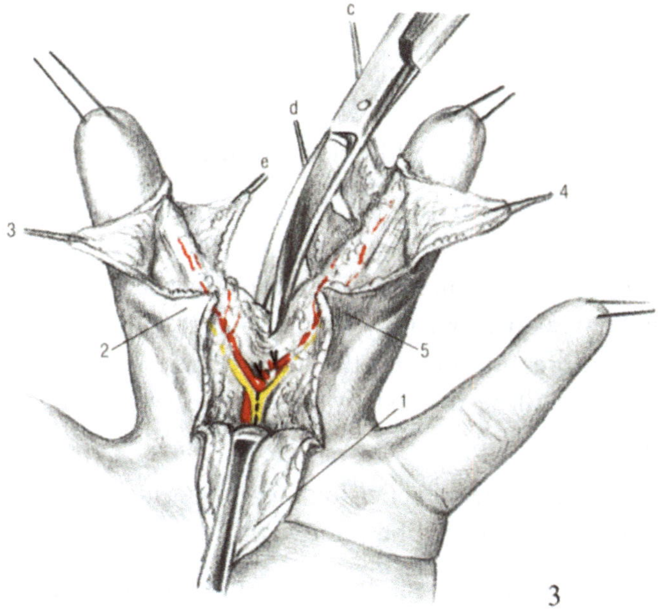

3

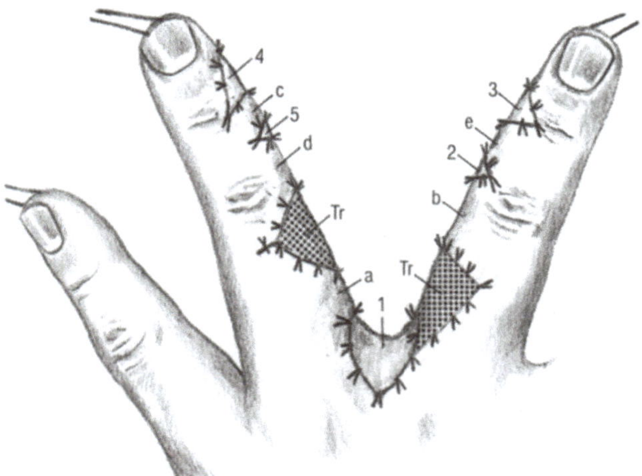

4

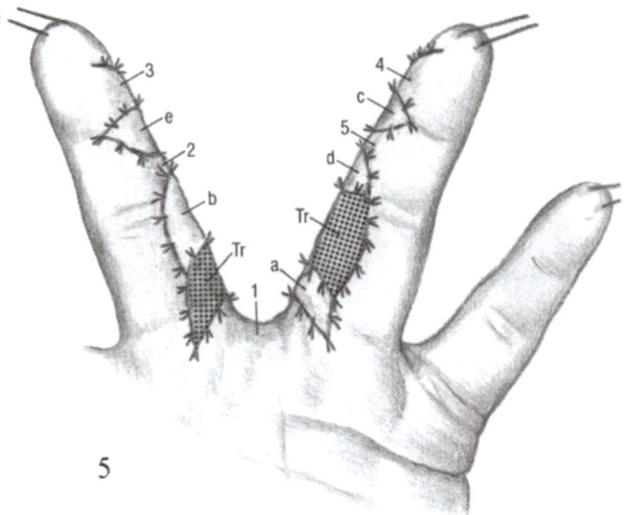

5

2.3.7 Recurrent Syndactyly Between Thumb and Index Finger

Goal of Surgery

Removal of the cicatricial adduction contracture of the thumb, and deepening of the thumb commissure.

Fig. 1 Preoperative appearance and incision, dorsal aspect
This is a patient with a partially treated Apert hand, type I; additional recurrent syndactylies are present between the long fingers.
The commissure will be formed by two dorsal swivel flaps (*a, b*). Scar tissue will not be excised.

Fig. 2 Preoperative appearance and incisions, palmar aspect.
The dotted areas of skin will be removed at the time of wound closure.

Fig. 3 The fascia (note dissecting scissors) is split longitudinally (*broken line*) after the dorsal flaps have been raised.

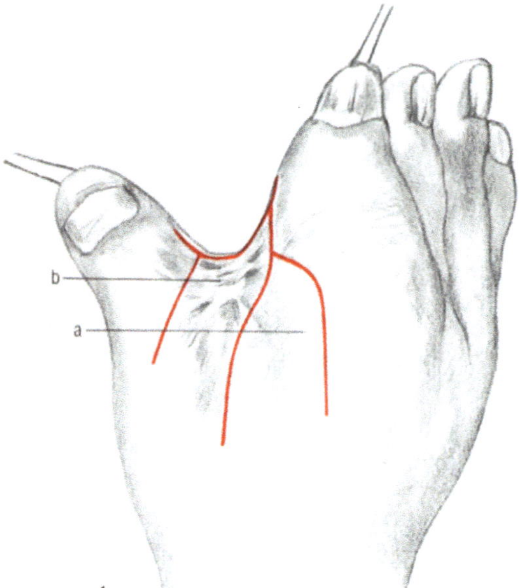

1

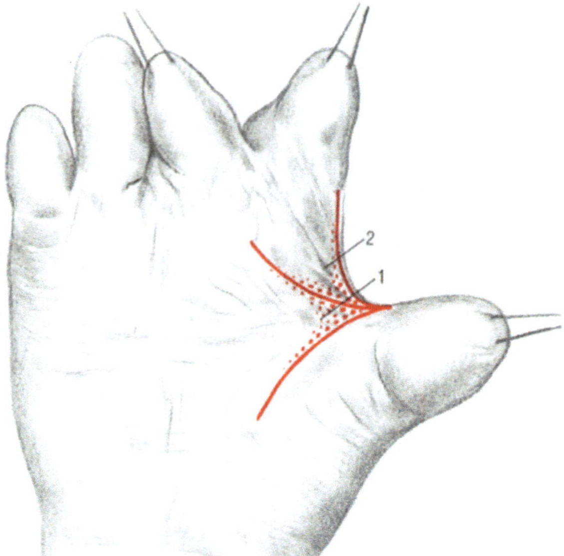

2

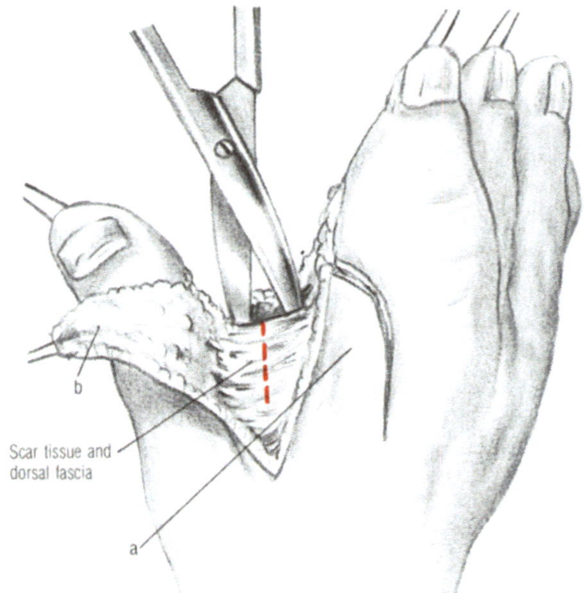

3

Fig. 4 The palmar soft tissues are separated and the m. add. poll. is indented until adequate thumb abduction is obtained. Vessels and nerves are carefully protected during this step.

Figs. 5, 6 Postoperative appearance after suturing of skin flaps and covering of open skin areas with thick-split thickness skin transplants (*dotted areas*).

Postoperative Care

See Sect. 2.1.1.4.

Errors and Their Consequences

See Sect. 2.1.2.

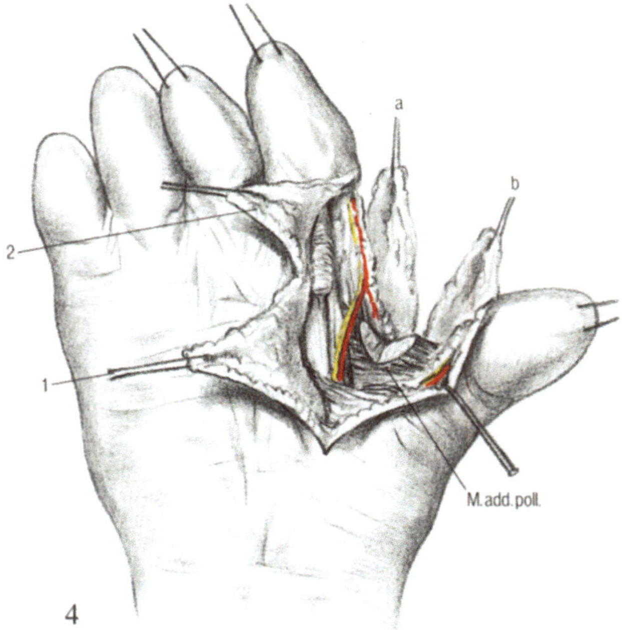

4

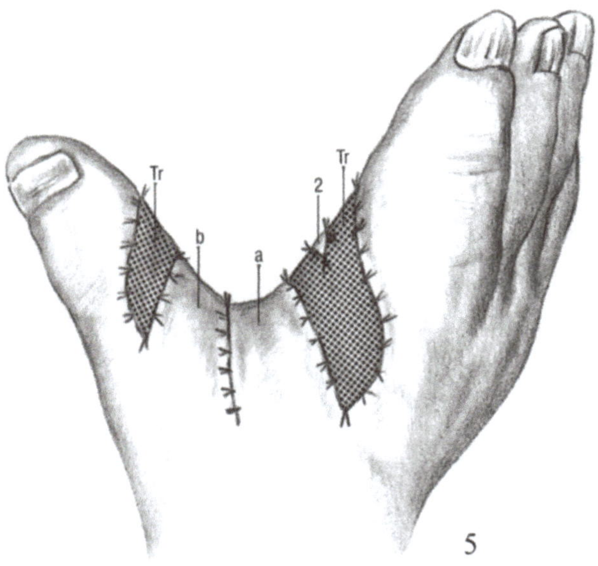

5

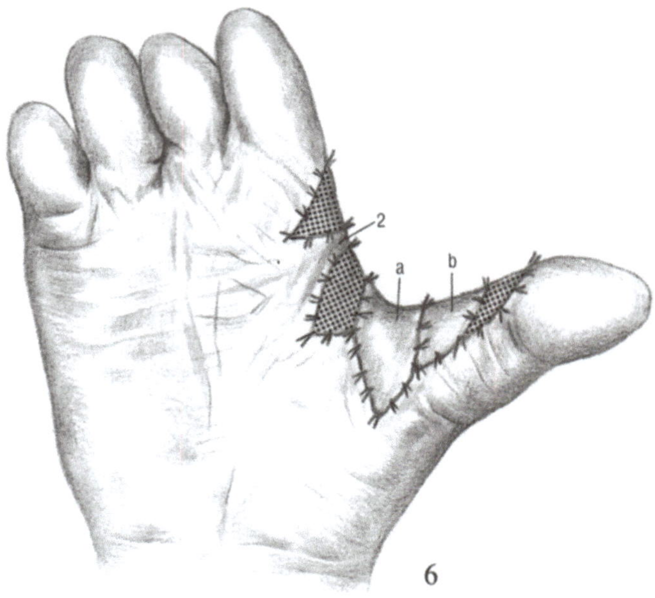

6

3 Peripheral Hypoplasias

3.1 Introduction

3.1.1 General Remarks

The concept of "peripheral hypoplasias" (GRUBER 1937) includes malformations of the hand such as the congenital *constriction band syndrome, anular grooves, amputationlike finger defects, diffuse nonpitting soft tissue swelling*, or excessive soft tissue pads ["anular grooves and allied acral absences" (KELIKIAN 1974)] and various types of *syndactylies*. To date these deformities, diversiform in their etiologic pathogenesis and morphology, have still not been categorized in any useful manner. For purposes of morphology and operating technique, unilateral amputation-like finger defects, also called *perodactylies*, might best be classified as a separate entity. However, this is unnecessary for our discussion of methods of treatment; operative problems can be outlined quite accurately according to the main characteristics of the anomalies.

Partly on the basis of heredofamilial incidence, it is now assumed that horizontal finger stumps without anular grooves (perodactylies) are caused by *endogenous* mechanisms (SCHADE 1937, 1940; MACARTHUR and MCCULLOUGH, 1932; KELIKIAN 1974, in which additional literature is cited).

The possibility of amniogenic and other *exogenomechanical* causes is undeniable for certain malformations, such as anular grooves and peripheral syndactylies (GRUBER 1937; WERTHEMANN 1952; GREBE 1964; KINO 1975; a.o.).

The malformations can be uni- or bilateral. Perodactyly usually occurs unilaterally, but defects consisting of "amputated" digits, anular grooves, soft tissue pads, and syndactylies occur more frequently bilaterally. Type, size, and site of involvement seem to affect various fingers indiscriminately. At times, only some fingers of a hand are deformed. Toes are frequently involved in a similar manner. We have seen combinations with additional proximal anular grooves (i.e., forearm: see Sect. 3.12), as well as with foot deformities (i.e., club foot).

Amputation-like finger defects. Such defects are the most frequent morphological changes seen in peripheral hypoplasias.

It seems to have no preferred site of involvement, but from personal observation it is our impression that the thumb is affected somewhat less frequently. Each finger can be involved at any level, and the location of the deformity can vary from finger to finger. Bony stump tips may be shaped like pointed cones, covered by very thin, insufficiently padded skin (see Sect. 3.8). Fingers lacking more than a nail's length show no trace of a nail. The *absence of fingernails* is characteristic of peripheral hypoplasias (differential diagnosis: symbrachydactyly a.o.), but is not obligatory; in so-called finger end defects only a part of the distal phalanx is missing and a corresponding diminution of the length of the fingernail is noted.

In general one can expect normal soft tissue and skeletal conditions to be present proximal to the particular finger defect. Occasionally, one can observe hypo- or dysplasias of the interphalangeal joints; this is more frequent in cases of perodactyly. We also have seen a patient with a dysplasia of the first carpometacarpal joint. The impaired function caused by this dysplasia was so severe that the possibility of satisfactory improvement by surgery appeared remote.

The distal phalanx is frequently reduced to a minimal piece of cartilage and bone (even in the presence of a well-developed distal phalangeal joint).

Syndactylies. Peripheral hypoplasias are frequently associated with syndactylies. Four different forms can be observed:

a) *Proximal syndactylies,* which show the typical appearance of partial cutaneous syndactylies (see Sect. 2.1). This type of webbing can be observed in both abnormal and normal fingers. It may cause marked functional limitation of the thumb (see Sect. 3.4).

b) So-called *acrosyndactylies,* which are particularly characteristic. They consist of cutaneous fusions of the ends of two or more fingers or of amputation stumps. The cutaneous bridges can be extremely small and may remind one of a garland-like structures. More common is extensive cutaneous bridging. As a rule only a cutaneous channel is present proximally (see Sect. 3.2), which allows the insertion of a probe. These channels are sometimes barely recognizable as funnel-like skin indentations. Their course is not always horizontal to the long axis of the finger, it can be oblique or tortuous. The channels are located somewhat more distal than a normal web space.

c) A third form are the rare *"bridge syndactylies."* These soft tissue connections are seen in the middle part of the fingers. The fingertips are not involved. Cutaneous channels can be found proximally between the hypoplastic fingers (see Sect. 3.3).

d) The fourth syndactyly type is characterized by peculiar *triangular or cone-shaped finger stumps* with a wide basis. In these cases one finds two or three rudimentary fingers enclosed in a common skin cover. They arise from the metacarpal area. These phalangeal remnants become smaller distally and are frequently in close approximation (similar to the example in Sect. 3.5).

Anular Grooves and Excessive Soft Tissue Pads. As a rule, anular grooves encompass the fingers in a circular manner. Their depth can extend all the way down to bone or it may be more superficial. In such cases they usually involve only the dorsal aspect of the finger. Anular grooves of the distal end of the finger frequently appear as budlike finger rudiments with a soft tissue stem in which skeletal elements can be found ("defect pseudarthrosis").

More proximal grooves may be present in the same limb and can cause additional circulatory disturbances. An anular groove of the forearm (see Sect. 3.12) can be associated even with a circumscribed radioulnar synostosis (see Sect. 14.3).

Certain types of peripheral hypoplasias are associated with circumscribed excessive soft tissue pads that are usually found distal to the anular groove (see Sect. 3.2).

The *function* of hands affected by peripheral hypoplasias can be more or less severely impaired. This depends on the morphological changes. Most pronounced loss of function is noted in perodactylies and in hands in which the finger rudiments have coalesced or in which they cross over each other and interdigitate. Less pronounced deformities may be more a cosmetic than a functional problem.

3.1.2 Indications for Surgery

Few deformities are as noticeable as most of the peripheral hypoplasias. Due to this cosmetic factor, one should be generous in one's indication for surgery. Excellent surgical technique is required in such situations. The surgeon should be experienced in treating these deformities.

One has to evaluate critically the expected improvement through surgery, as these operations are frequently very extensive. The staging of procedures, the extent of the operation, surgical risks, the time required for postoperative therapy, and the psychological aspects of hospitalization all require careful consideration.

The limits of reasonable improvement resulting from surgery can best be recognized in proposing bone lengthening operations for perodactyly or bridge plasties in the presence of distal peripheral grooves. The functional gain of these procedures will justify an operation only in a very few cases (see Sect. 3.10).

While there are many conditions that warrant an operation, there are *differences in the degree of its urgency.*

Surgical intervention is imperative in hands presenting with coalesced rudimentary fingers and with digiti superducti, which result in grotesque deformities. They are separated solely by cutaneous channels that allow the insertion of a probe. Without treatment the function of these hands is extremely limited (see Sect. 3.2). The same degree of urgency is present in patients in whom deep anular grooves cause peripheral circulatory impairment (Sects. 3.8, 3.12), in cases of congenital defect pseudarthroses of functionally important finger phalanges (Sect. 3.10), and in the amputationlike shortening of the thumb with soft tissue excess (Sect. 3.9). In the latter case it is important to have good motion in the carpometacarpal joint of the Ist ray. Only then can one expect improvement of function with a bone-lengthening operation. Surgical intervention is also generally indicated in the presence of acrosyndactyly of several fingers or in hands with a very tight thumb commissure (see Sect. 3.4).

Less urgent are operations to improve the appearance of the hand. Indication for surgery is present in shallow anular grooves (see Sect. 3.7), partial cutaneous syndactylies (see Sect. 3.3), in most cases of dorsal excessive soft tissue pads (see Sect. 3.7), in the presence of annoying skin appendages, and in total syndactylies of two finger stumps (see Sects. 3.6, 3.5).

3.1.3 Timing of Surgery

Operations requiring long recovery periods should be performed prior to the patient entering school. Less time-consuming soft tissue corrections can be carried out during school age or even later. Anular grooves with impending circulatory disturbances should be operated on very early, if necessary even during the 1st year of life. The same age level is indicated in patients with acrosyndactyly with marked functional impairment and malposition of the fingers, to retard further functional loss due to abnormal growth.

3.1.4 General Surgical Directives

In view of the multiplicity and differences of the abnormalities, the type and staging of surgical intervention depend on the localization and severity of the deformity. In general, we recommend *"operating in small steps."*

For example, separation of an *acrosyndactyly* distal to the cutaneous channels usually does not create a commissure of sufficient depth and width. The cutaneous bridge proximal to the channel must be removed in a second operation. Only then has one formed a functional web space.

Another example of operating in stages can be given in treating a *deep anular groove*. The dangers of postoperative circulatory impairment forbids its complete excision in one step (see Sect. 3.7).

In general one has to consider the following:

Treatment of *proximal cutaneous syndactylies* of the long fingers has been discussed in Sect. 2.1 and the recommendations given there should be followed. As a rule, widening and deepening of the functionally important thumb commissure will have to be carried out by employing additional swivel flaps (see Sect. 3.4). Commissurotomy by employing a Z-plasty alone will result in a deeper but not in a wider web space.

Acrosyndactylies with crossed-over finger rudiments will have to be analyzed carefully by x-rays, probing of the cutaneous channels, and inspection of the cutaneous indentations prior to separation of the fingers. On occasion it is advisable to sacrifice less important skeletal parts and to employ thick-split thickness skin grafts to obtain tension-free closure of the incision.

Some acrosyndactylies are characterized by a very small garlandlike cutaneous bridge only, which can be easily transected. The remaining skin defects are small and can be closed with one or two sutures.

Dorsal excessive soft tissue finger pads are best treated in combination with a semicircular excision of the proximally located anular groove, as this avoids additional circulatory disturbances (see Sects. 3.7, 3.8).

Anular grooves have to be removed in two stages and surgical telescopes have to be employed. Very careful dissection is of utmost importance to prevent damage of vessels and nerves that are located in the confined space between skin and bone.

Soft tissue pits, budlike finger tips, or constricted finger parts containing *defect pseudarthroses* should not be removed routinely. Bony augmentation procedures or bridge plasties may give more length or better stability to the finger and therefore improve its function. Bony augmentation operations in patients with *perodactyly* should only be considered if the gain in finger length is useful to the patient.

Incorrect soft tissue resection or length of the bone graft make the results of such procedures uncertain. If circulatory disturbances become evident after the release of the tourniquet, the bone graft has to be shortened to avoid irreversible damage.

A metacarpolysis combined with removal of a metacarpal bone may be indicated *if all long fingers are absent.* It is of no value if mobility of the border rays is insufficient.

3.1.5 Postoperative Care

It depends on the type of surgery and will be discussed under the respective operations.

Goal of Surgery

Separation of the crossed fingers (with partial resection of the rudimentary phalanges of the IVth ray) and deepening and widening of the interdigital space (two stages).

First stage:

Fig. 1 Preoperative appearance and incision, dorsal aspect.
The plump and shortened IIIrd finger is surrounded by a mass of soft tissue. X-rays and the probing of two cutaneous channels (α, β), which end at the palmar aspect of the lateral borders of the middle finger basis, clarify the deformity. A complete fusion of the IInd and IVth finger dorsal to the extensor surface of the middle finger (with peripheral hypoplasia) is noted. A rudimentary Vth finger (with a rudimentary proximal phalanx and a suggestive cutaneous channel) is part of the mass.
Rudimentary nails are present on the thumb and middle finger. Additional deformity is caused by excessive subcutaneous fatty deposits.
The skin incision extends to the cutaneous channel (β) on the ulnar side, which has been marked with a probe; later it will be extended to the cutaneous channel on the radial side (α). *Hatched areas* of bone will be removed (see Fig. 4).

Figs. 2, 3 Palmar and apical aspects.
The rudiments of the long fingers have been pulled apart in dorsal and palmar directions. The palmar exits of the cutaneous channels hidden radially (α') and ulnarly (β') by a soft tissue groove are found next to the middle finger. The area of "coalescence" between the IIIrd and IInd/IVth finger (*hatched area*) will be separated by sharp dissection to the level of the marking probe.

Fig. 4 Palmar-ulnar aspect.
The rudimentary proximal phalanx of the IVth finger has been exposed in the dorsal soft tissue mass and will be resected (see Fig. 1). A hypoplastic palmar vessel that seems to be part of the IVth finger will be ligated (not demonstrated in the figures). The "coalescence" will be separated further by approaching the cutaneous channel on the ulnar side (*β, β' in Fig. 2*). The separated IInd finger will finally rest without tension between thumb and index finger (*arrows*). The transected area of coalescence between the IIIrd and IInd/IVth finger is marked by *red dots*.

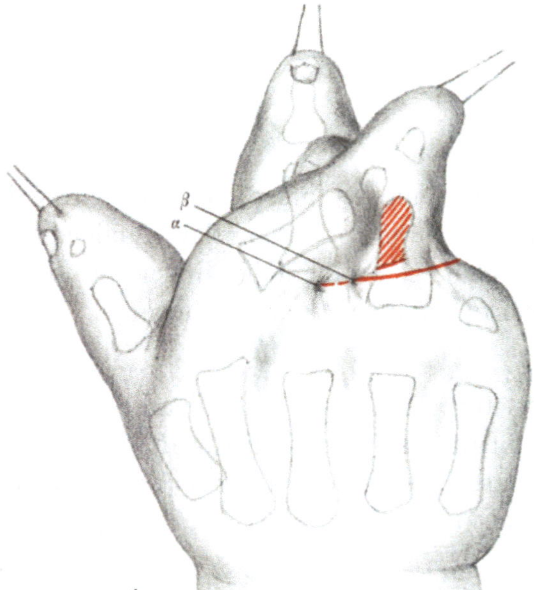

1

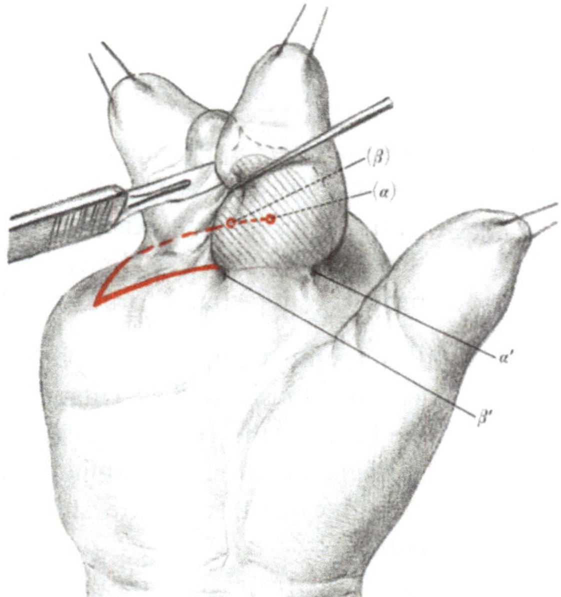

2

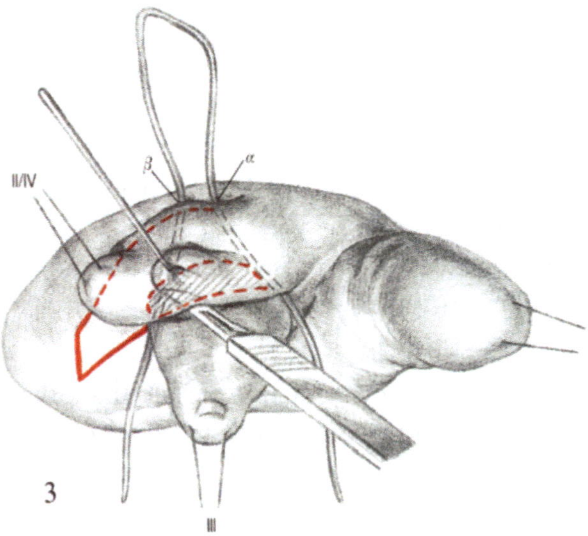

3

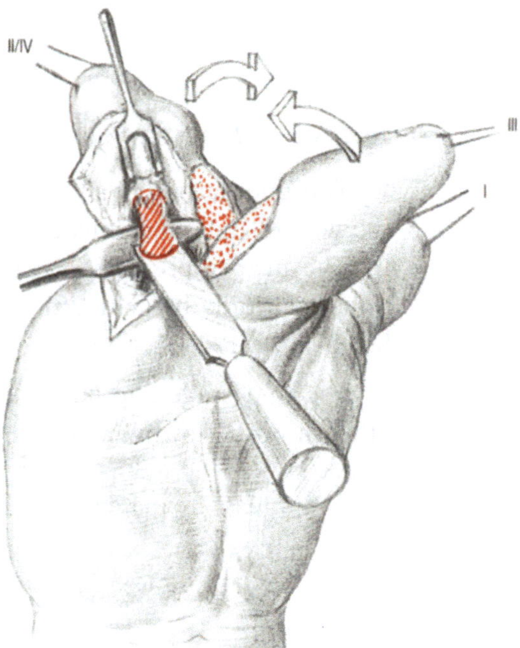

4

Fig. 5 Postoperative appearance, dorsal aspect.
The area of the separated coalescences of the middle finger has been covered with a thick-split thickness skin transplant (*Tr*). The soft tissue flap obtained by the excision of the rudimentary proximal phalanx of the IVth finger has been properly shaped and forms the ulnar border of the index finger rudiment.

Fig. 6 Postoperative appearance, palmar aspect.
The previously probed cutaneous channels form the radial and ulnar border of the basis of the IIIrd finger (or the depth of the second commissure). The fingers are held in proper position by using transarticular Kirschner wires (not shown). Dorsal wound edges are shown as a *broken line*. The area of the transplant is *dotted*.
The IInd finger can be diminished in size at the time of surgery by resection of some of the excessive fat pads (see retractor in Fig. 3).

Postoperative Care

See Sect. 2.1.2 a.o.

Errors and Their Consequences

E. The middle finger and the separated index finger have not been separated all the way to the cutaneous channels marked by the probes.
C. The proper position of the middle finger while being passed across the index finger can only be achieved by placing tension on vessels and nerves.
See also Sect. 2.1.2.

The second stage should be carried out relatively soon (but not earlier than the 6th–8th postoperative week), otherwise scar contractures may result in finger deviation.

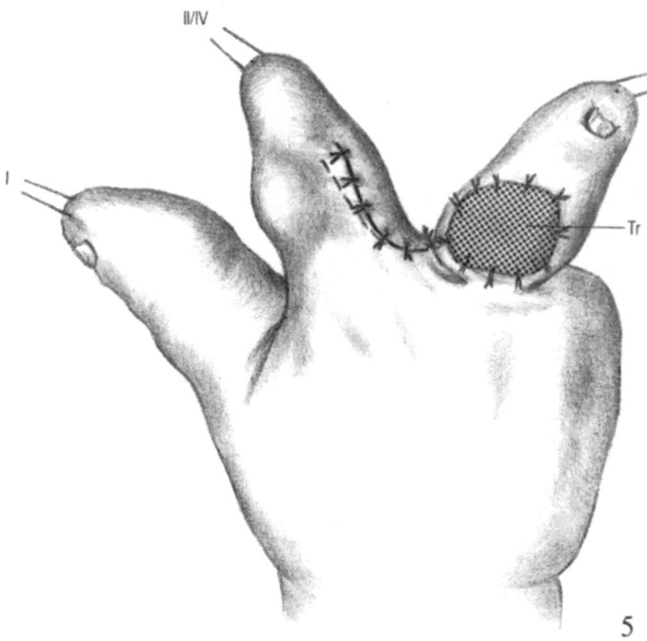

5

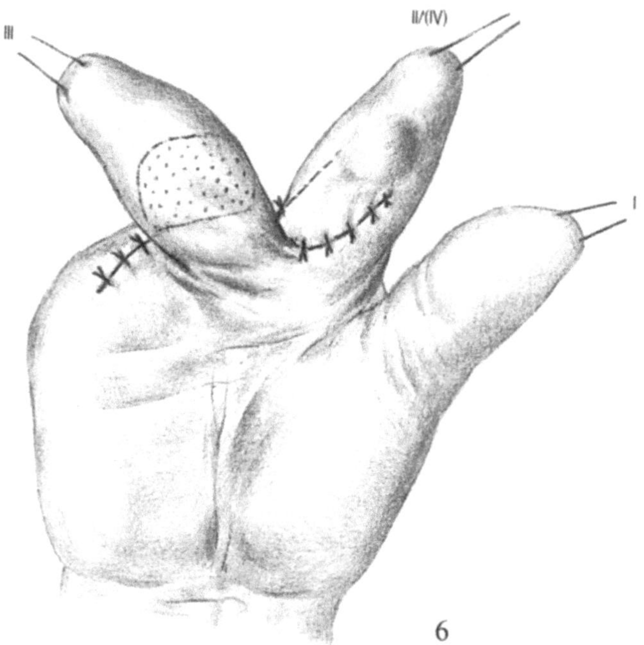

6

2nd Stage

Figs. 7, 8 Preoperative appearance and skin incision, dorsal and palmar aspects.
A very narrow distally displaced interdigital space remains between the two long fingers. The commissure will be formed by a palmar triangular flap and two dorsal swivel flaps (extension of the incisions, necessary in some cases, is marked by the *broken thick red lines*). Additional incision to remove a dorsally located excessive fat pad on the rudimentary index finger.

Fig. 9 Dorsal aspect.
The swivel flaps and the palmar triangular flap have been raised. The main veins have to be protected while removing the excessive fatty tissue. The palmar neurovascular bundles have to be visualized prior to transection of the rigid soft tissue bridge *(thick red broken line)*.

Figs. 10, 11 Postoperative appearance, apical and dorsal aspects.
Skin defects on the lateral aspects of the fingers are covered with thick-split thickness skin transplants *(Tr)*.

Postoperative Care and Errors and Their Consequences

See Sect. 2.1.2.

Remarks

It might be worthwhile to consider a deepening of the first commissure at a later date to improve function.

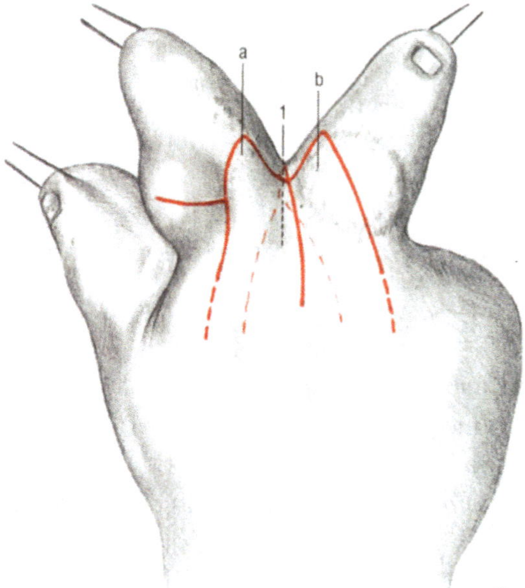

7

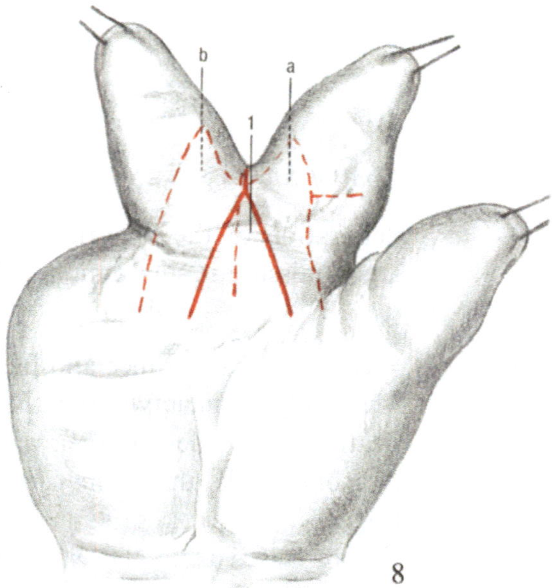

8

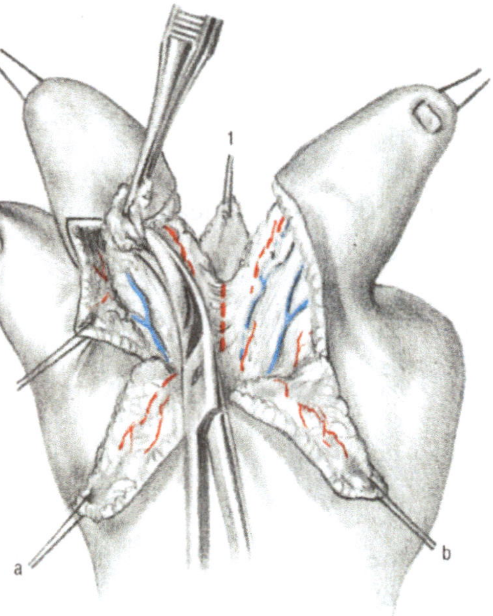

9

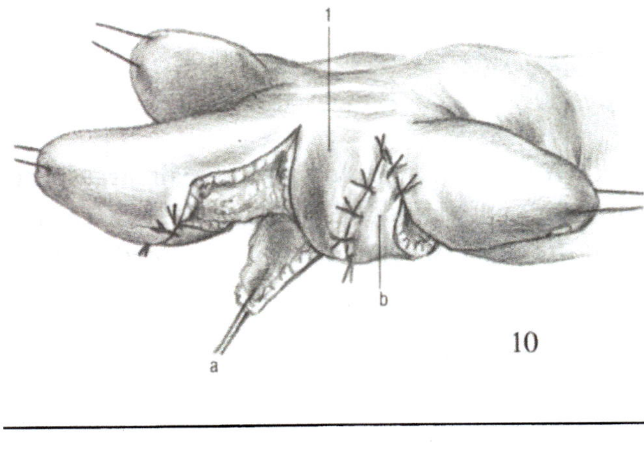

10

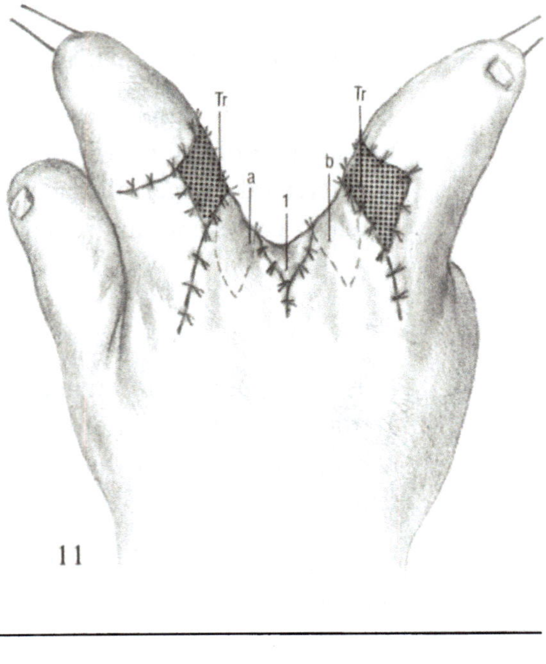

11

3.3. Interdigital Cutaneous Bridge ("Bridge Syndactyly")

Goal of Surgery

Separation of the interdigital cutaneous bridge as a preparatory step to forming a commissure in anatomic position.

Fig. 1 Preoperative apperance and incision, dorsal aspect.
The bridge syndactyly and the clinical findings on the other hand permit classification of this deformity as a peripheral hypoplasia.
A probe marks the funnel-shaped cutaneous channel between the two hypoplastic fingers.
A flap raised from the extensor surface *(a)* is based on the middle finger. The flap on the flexor surface *(1)* is nourished by vessels from the ring finger. Surgical telescopes are used while raising the flaps to protect even the smallest vessel.

Figs. 2, 3 After raising of the flaps.
Main vessels and nerves have to be protected!

Figs. 4, 5 Postoperative appearances.
Remaining skin defects are covered with thick-split thickness skin transplants *(Tr)* after suturing of the flaps without tension.

Postoperative Care

See Sect. 2.1.1.

Errors and Their Consequences

E. Particularly careful application of the pressure dressing has not been carried out in spite of the narrowness of the commissure.
C. Increased danger of maceration.
See also corresponding remarks Sect. 2.1.2.

Remarks

It is also possible to transect the skin bridge on the dorsal and palmar aspects at the level of the interdigital spaces by a longitudinal incision. It is necessary to employ thick-split thickness skin grafts if the wounds cannot be closed without tension.

Second stage: Separation of the cutaneous syndactyly proximal to the cutaneous channel and formation of a commissure at its anatomic site (see Sect. 2.1.5).

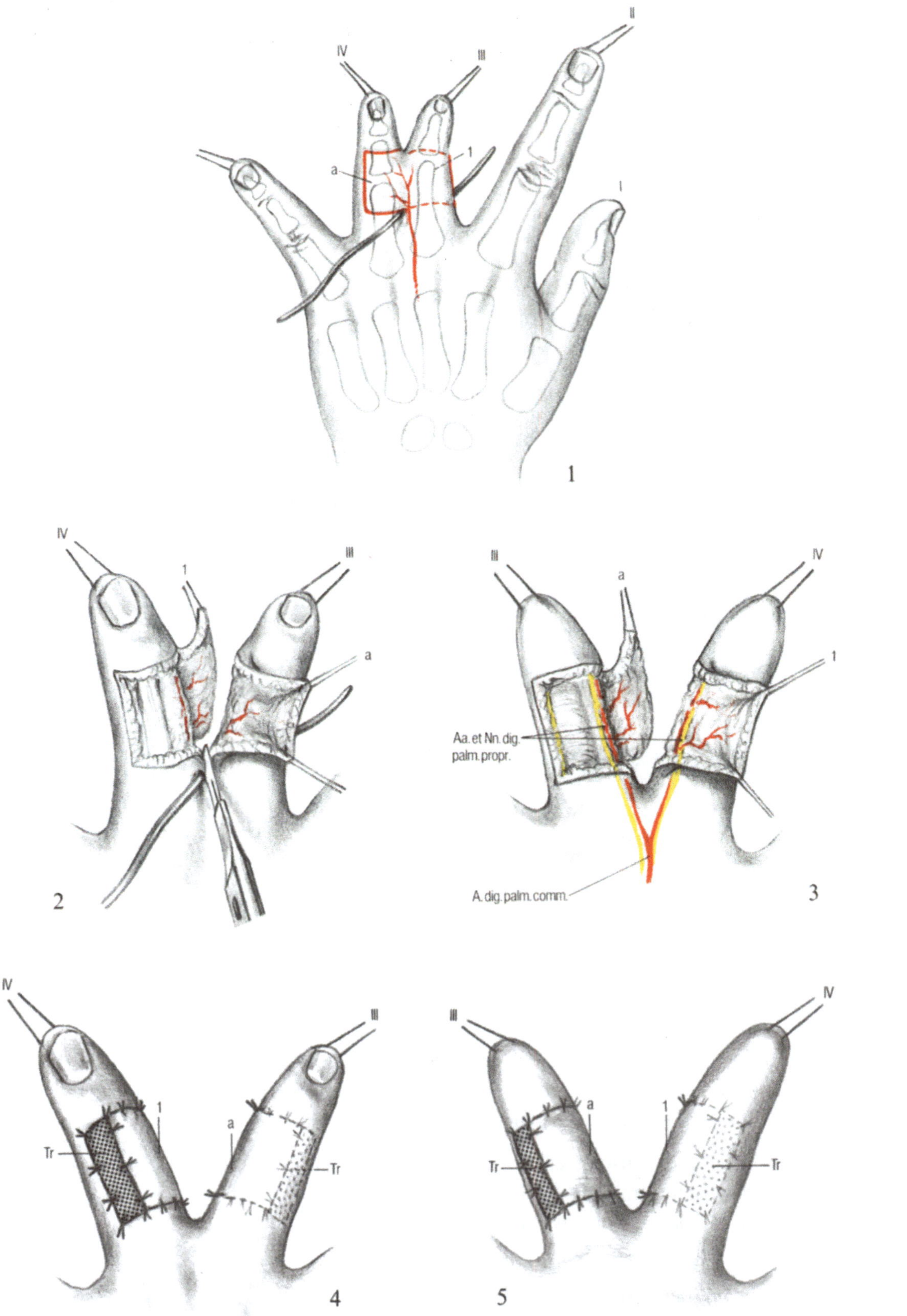

IV
III
II
I
a
1
1
IV
III
1
a
2
III
IV
a
1
Aa. et Nn. dig. palm. propr.
A. dig. palm. comm.
3
IV
III
1
a
Tr
Tr
4
III
IV
a
1
Tr
Tr
5

3.4 Partial Syndactyly Between Thumb and Index Finger

Goal of Surgery

Formation of a normal thumb commissure.

Fig. 1 Preoperative appearance and incision, dorsal aspect.
Flap *(a)* will be raised from the dorsal fascia of the hand. Afferent vessel damage has to be avoided. The *broken line* marks the incision on the volar side.

Fig. 2 Dorsal aspect after preparation of the flap.
The dorsal fascia and the m. add. poll. are sufficiently indented to permit optimal abduction of the Ist ray. An elevator is placed between the neurovascular bundle and the adductor muscle for protection.

Figs. 3, 4 Postoperative appearance.
The commissure has been formed by the swivel flap *(a)*. The Ist ray is fixed in abduction and opposition by two Kirschner wires (not shown). Suction drainage (not shown). A remaining index finger skin defect has been covered with a thick-split thickness transplant *(Tr)*.

Remarks

The figures reproduce only part of the possible width of the commissure.

Postoperative Care

The wound surfaces are covered with vaseline gauze. Long-arm plaster cast. The Kirschner wires will be removed ca. 2 weeks after surgery. A night splint is then used and exercises are instituted.

Errors and Their Consequences

E. Flap *(a)* is too narrow and too long; it has not been raised exactly from the extensor aponeuronis; the afferent main vessel has been damaged.
C. Partial or total flap necrosis.

E. The tight muscle fascia on the extensor surface has not been transected and the contracted m. add. poll. has not been incised.
C. Insufficient depth of the commissure.

E. Ligature of one of the arteries and interfascicular proximal splitting of the common nerve trunk has been omitted in the presence of a distally displaced neurovascular bifurcation (see Sect. 2.2.2. a.o.).
C. Insufficient depth of the commissure.

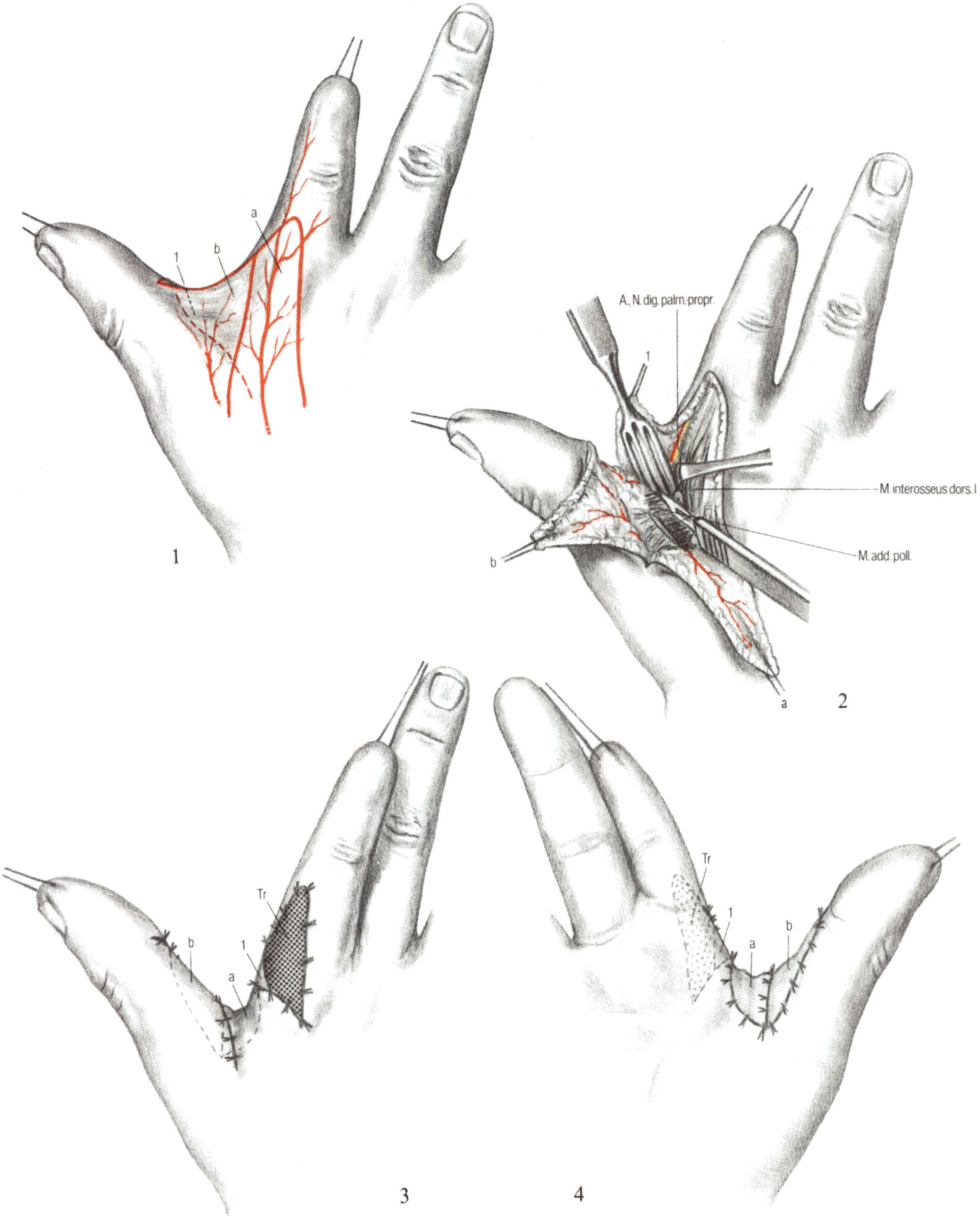
a
b
1
1
A., N. dig. palm. propr.
1
M. interosseus dors. I
M. add. poll.
b
a
2
Tr
b
1
a
Tr
1
a
b
3
4

3.5 Total Syndactyly of Rudimentary Fingers of Unequal Length

Goal of Surgery

Separation of finger stumps (phalangization) and formation of a commissure in anatomic position.

Figs. 1, 2 Preoperative appearance and incisions.

Fig. 3 After exposure of the dorsal side.
The ulnar lateral band of the rudimentary middle finger has been transected and proximally resutured (contracture). The lig. capit. transversum has been cut *(red line)*.

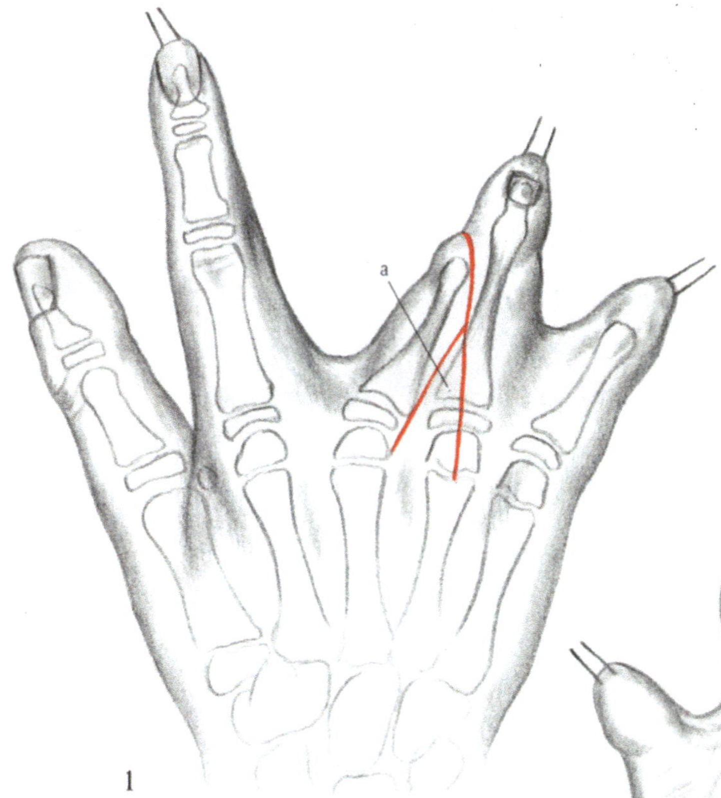
a
1

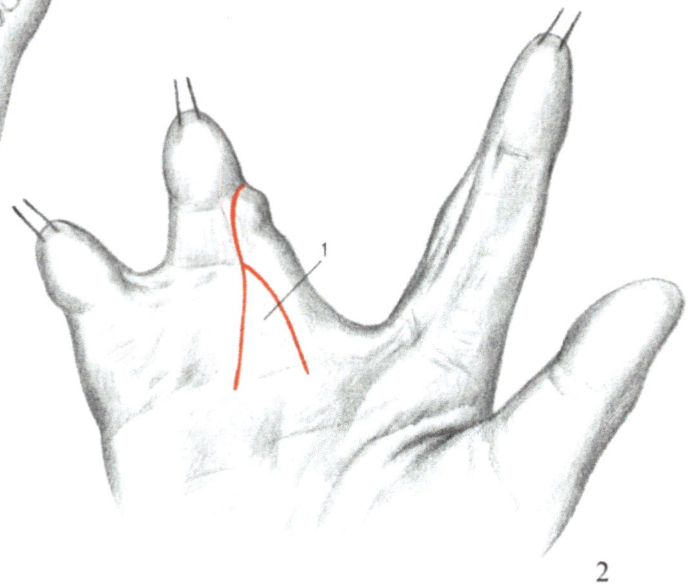
1
2

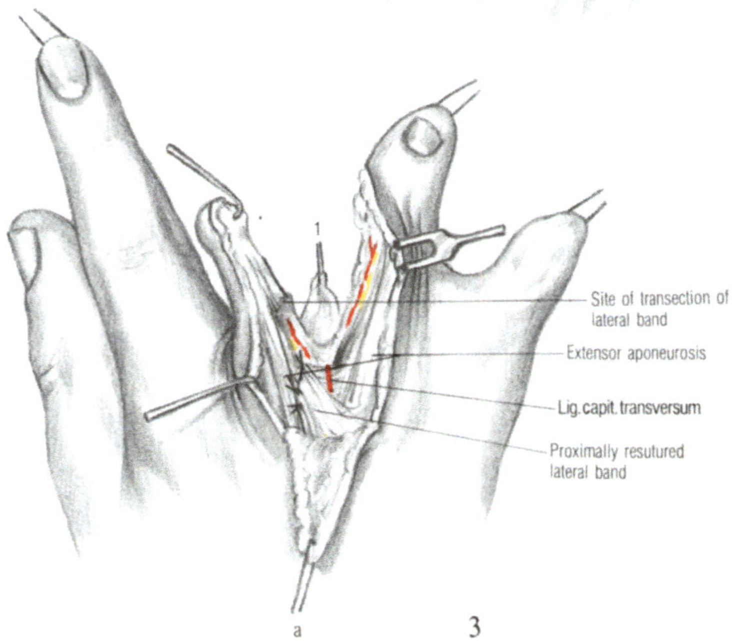
1
Site of transection of lateral band
Extensor aponeurosis
Lig. capit. transversum
Proximally resutured lateral band
a
3

Fig. 4 Dorsal aspect.
The skin on the radial side of the rudimentary middle fingers has to be displaced in a palmar direction to allow optimal coverage of the fingertip (*arrow*). It will be fixed in this position by suturing it to the subcutis.

Figs. 5, 6 Postoperative appearance.
Skin defects remaining after suturing of the flap will be covered with thick-split thickness grafts *(Tr)*.

Postoperative Care and Errors and Their Consequences

See Sect. 2.1.1 (also Sects. 2.1.3, 2.1.4 a.o.)

Remarks

Separation of the syndactyly between the hypoplastic IVth and Vth finger will be carried out in a second operation (see Sect. 2.1.6 a.o.), but not before the wound is healed and physiotherapy has been terminated.

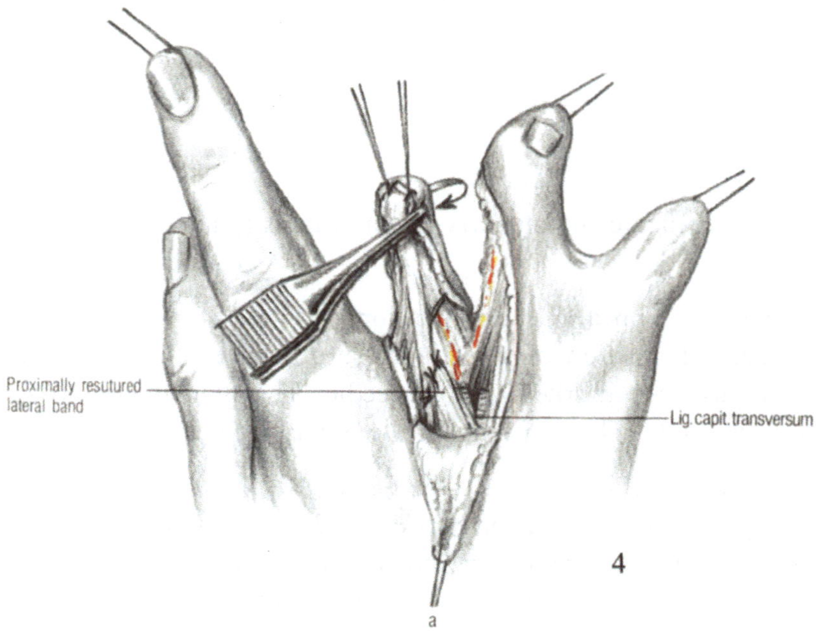
Proximally resutured
lateral band
Lig. capit. transversum
a

4

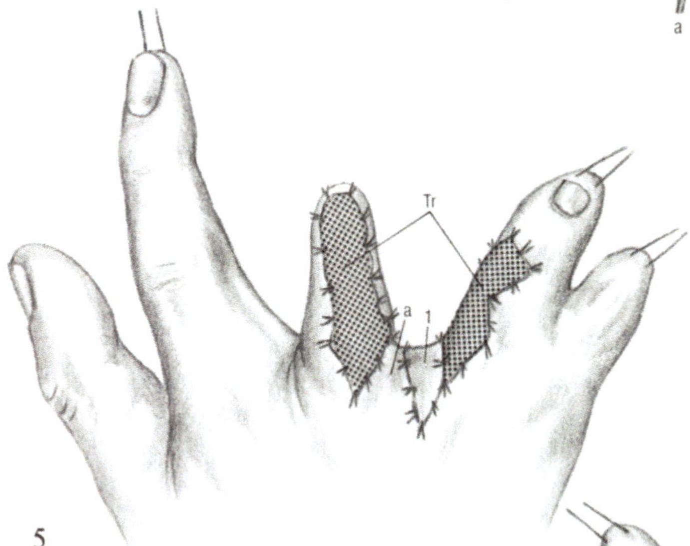
Tr
a
1

5

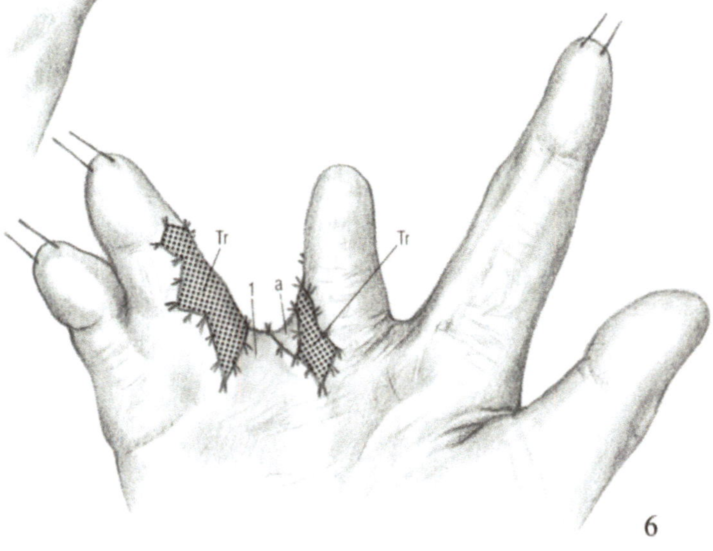
Tr
1
a
Tr

6

3.6 Total Syndactyly of Rudimentary Fingers of Equal Length

Goal of Surgery

Separation of the rudimentary finger stumps (phalangization).

Figs. 1, 2 Preoperative appearance and incision.
The desired position of the commissure between the IInd and IIIrd rudimentary finger has been marked with a needle. The palmar commissure flap extends to the dorsal side. The incisions on the other side are outlined by the *broken lines*.

Fig. 3 Dorsal aspect after raising of the flaps.
The ligamentous connection between the metacarpal heads (lig. capit. transversum) has been cut. The palmar neurovascular bundles are visible in the depth of the operative site. The vessel bifurcation is displaced distally. One artery will be ligated.

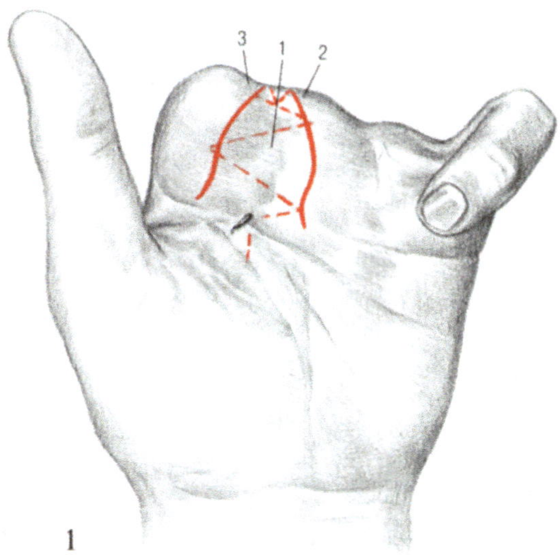
3
1
2

1

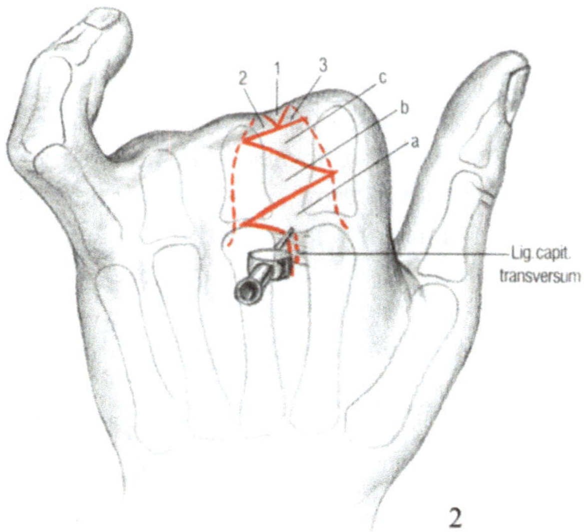
2
1
3
c
b
a
Lig. capit. transversum

2

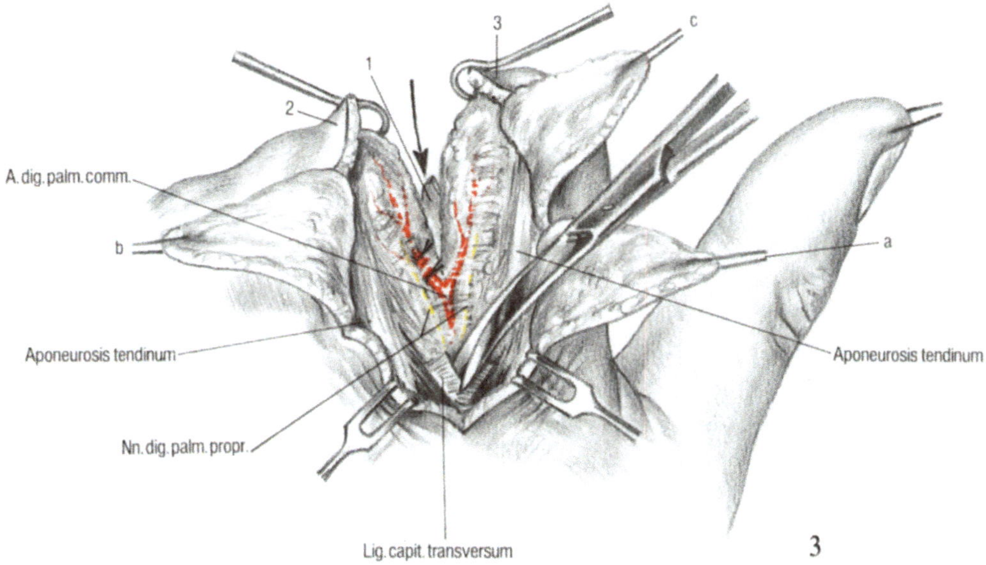
3
c
1
2
A. dig. palm. comm.
b
a
Aponeurosis tendinum
Aponeurosis tendinum
Nn. dig. palm. propr.
Lig. capit. transversum

3

Figs. 4–6 Postoperative appearance: dorsal (4), palmar (5), and apical (6) aspects.
Remaining skin defects on the lateral aspects of the fingers will be covered with thick-split thickness skin transplants.
Phalangization of the remaining rudimentary fingers can be done in a similar manner at a later date.

Postoperative Care and Errors and Their Consequences

See recommendations in Sect. 3.5 a.o.

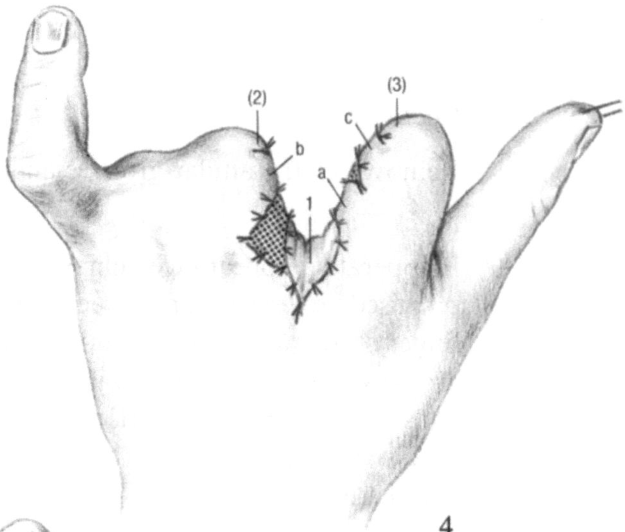

4

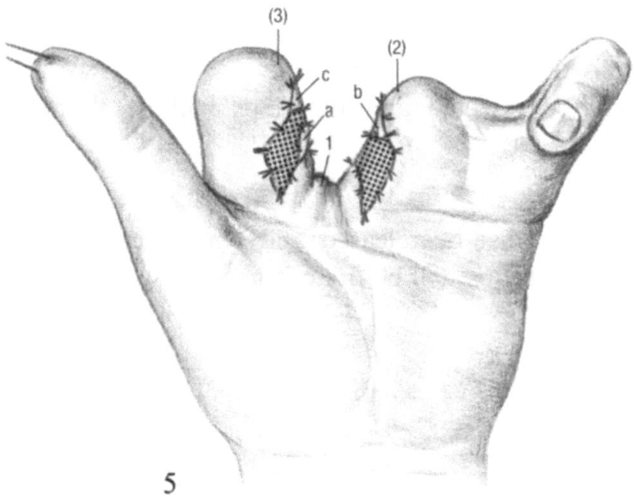

5

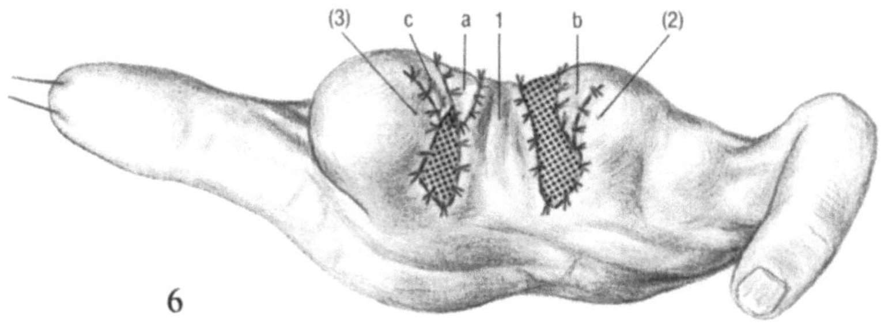

6

3.7 Anular Grooves with Excessive Dorsal Soft Tissue Finger Pads

Goal of Surgery

Removal of the anular grooves and excessive dorsal soft tissue pads.

Fig. 1 Preoperative appearance: ulnar (1 a) and dorsal (1) aspects.
A raised excessive soft tissue pad is present at the ring finger, while the index finger shows a flat pad. Semicircular incisions are employed to excise the anular grooves. The *dotted areas* will be excised after removal of the excessive soft tissue pads while forming the flaps. Additional small incisions are required to avoid excessive bulging of the flaps and to allow wound closure without tension (see Fig. 4, ring finger).

Fig. 2 The anular grooves have been excised.
Superfluous subcutaneous fat will be resected and the flaps will be shaped as marked.

Fig. 3 Trial adaptation of the swivel flap.
Prior to skin closure, the tourniquet must be released and complete hemostasis achieved. Additional shaping of the flap tips will be done if necessary.

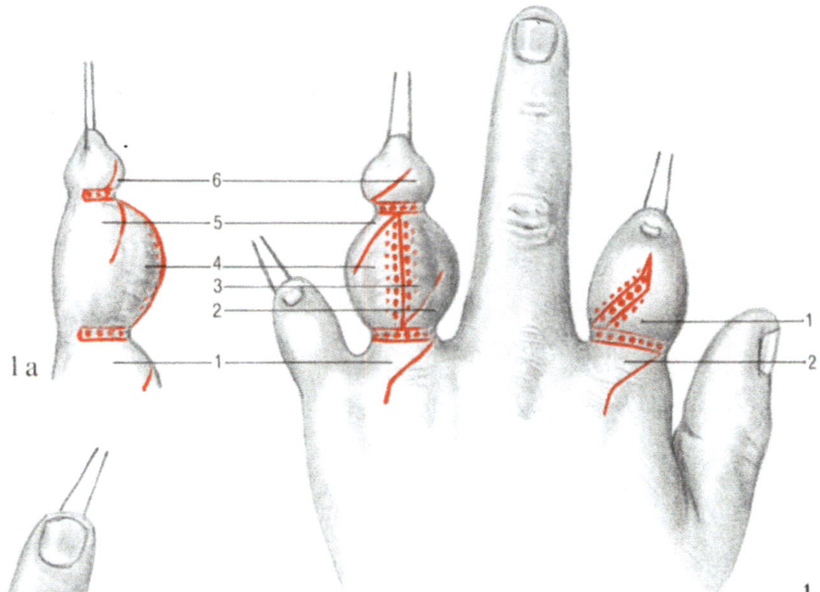
1a
6
5
4
3
2
1
1
2

1

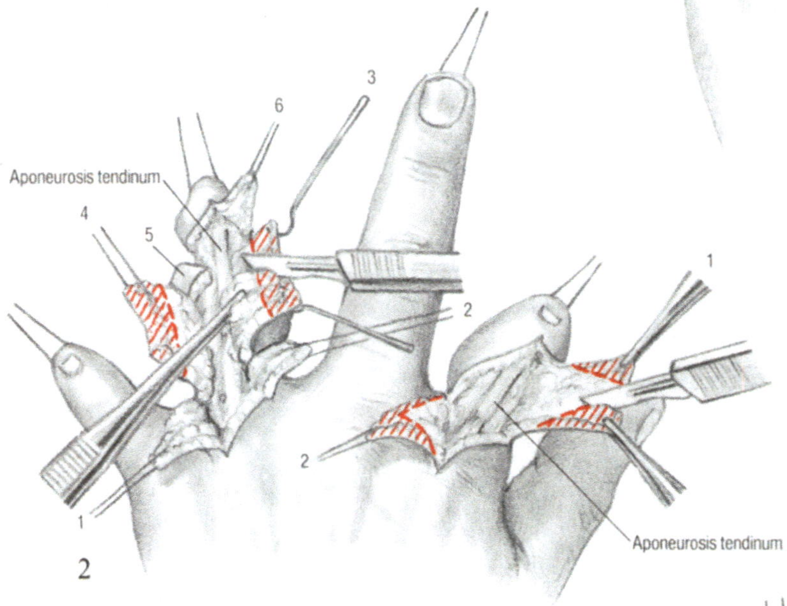
Aponeurosis tendinum
4
5
6
3
2
1
1
2
Aponeurosis tendinum

2

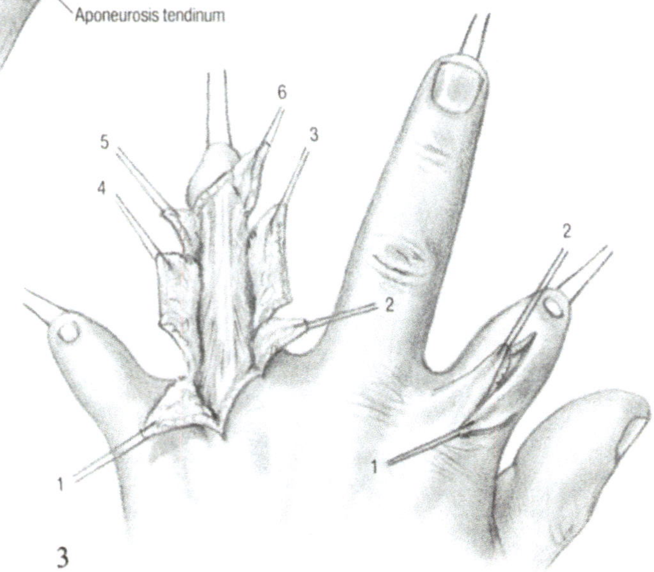
5
4
6
3
2
2
1
1

3

Fig. 4 Postoperative appearance, dorsal aspect.
Removal of the palmar sections of the anular grooves is carried out during a second operation.

Postoperative Care

Postoperative care is similar to other plastic operations involving skin only (see Sect. 2.1). Immobilization in a volar short-arm plaster splint for 8–10 days. Elevation of the involved limb and oral medication with antiphlogistics to avoid circulatory impairment.

Errors and Their Consequences

E. Removal of the excessive soft tissue finger pads has been overzealous and has not been done in several stages.
C. Skin sutures will be under tension.

E. The anular grooves have been circumferentially excised in one stage.
C. Circulatory impairment has to be expected.

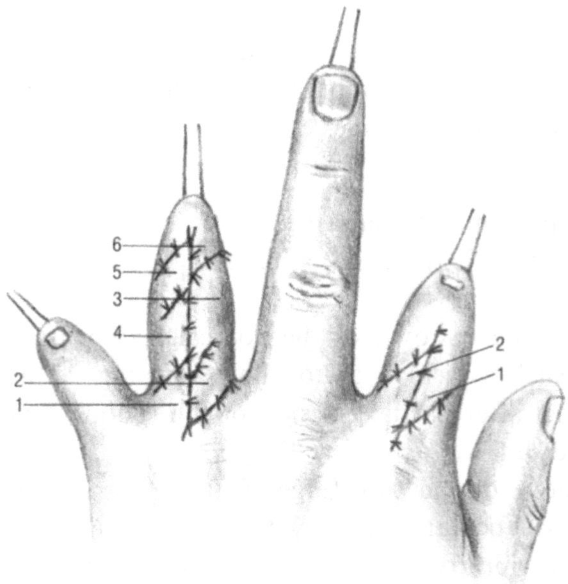

4

Goal of Surgery

Excision of the anular groove and removal of the excessive dorsal fat pad of the rudimentary ring finger; amputation of the conical rudimentary middle finger with its scant soft tissue coverage.

Fig. 1 Preoperative appearance, dorsal aspect.
The rudimentary middle finger has scant soft tissue coverage and is therefore easily vulnerable.
The incision for the removal of the conical rudiment of the middle finger has to be done in such a fashion as to allow covering of the stump with skin from the palmar aspect after partial excision of the rudimentary phalanx (*hatched area*) has been carried out.
The anular groove of the ring finger will be sparsely excised in a semicircular fashion. Surplus subcutaneous fatty tissue and the *dotted areas* of skin will be removed until tension-free skin closure is possible [modified Z-plasty can also be employed (see Sect. 3.7)].

Fig. 2 Postoperative appearance, dorsal aspect.

Postoperative Care and Errors and Their Consequences

See Sect. 3.5 a.o.

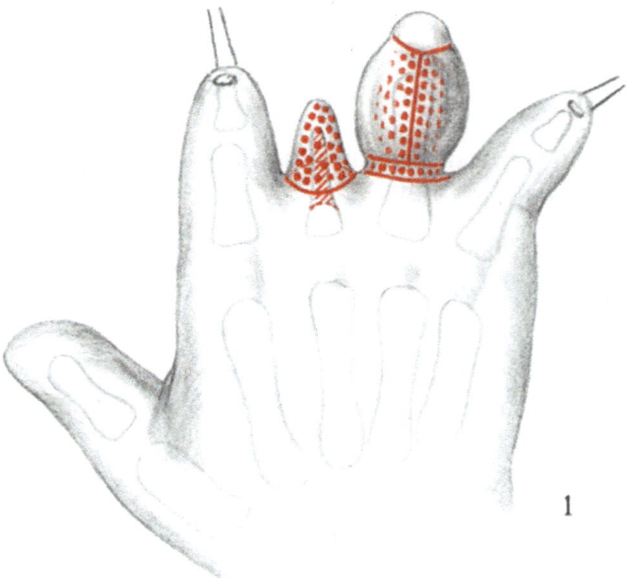

1

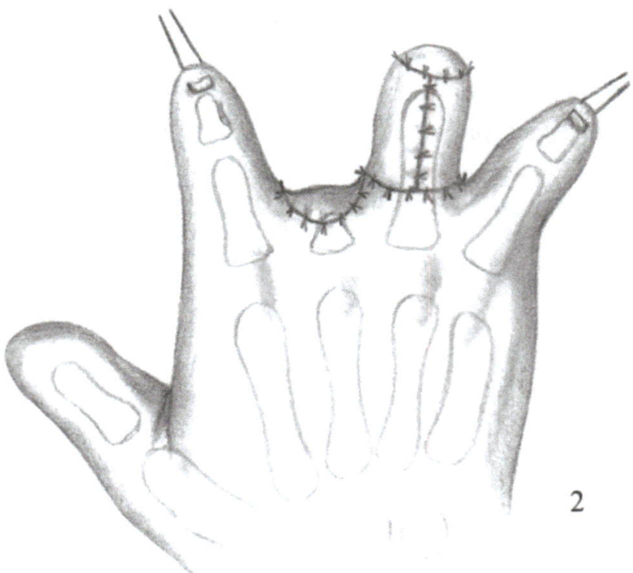

2

Goal of Surgery

Lengthening of the rudimentary thumb, removal of the soft tissue contracture at the level of the first MP joint.

Fig. 1 Preoperative appearance and incision, palmar aspect.
The nailless thumb rudiment is pulled into extension with holding sutures. The *broken black line* demonstrates the original position of the thumb at the palmar side of the hand. Four rudimentary stumps without bone represent the four long fingers.
A proximally based dorsoradial skin flap is formed; the flexor crease of the thumb is horizontally incised.

Fig. 2 Palmar aspect after formation of the flaps.
Careful removal of the fatty tissue distal to the rudimentary phalanx of the thumb is carried out to create space for an autologous bone graft. The bone graft taken from the iliac crest is prepared and implanted on the decorticated thumb rudiment. Fixation is accomplished by using a transarticular Kirschner wire *(Fig. 2b)*.
Fig. 2c depicts an alternative method in which two autologous bone grafts of equal length are employed. The grafts are fixed to a centrally placed Kirschner wire. The *hatched areas* of bone in Figs. 2b and 2c may have to be removed if circulatory embarrassment is noted after release of the tourniquet.

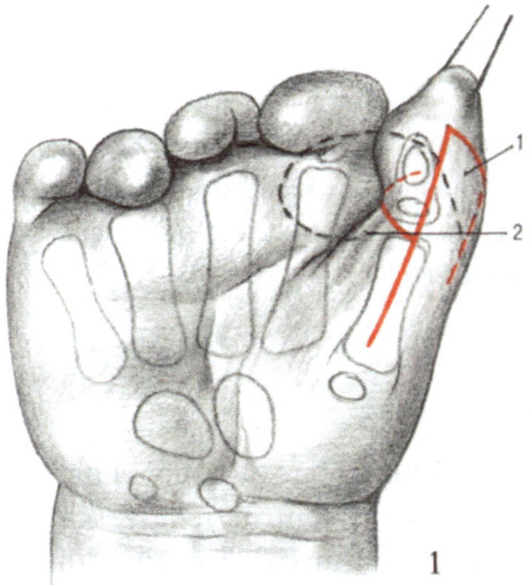

1

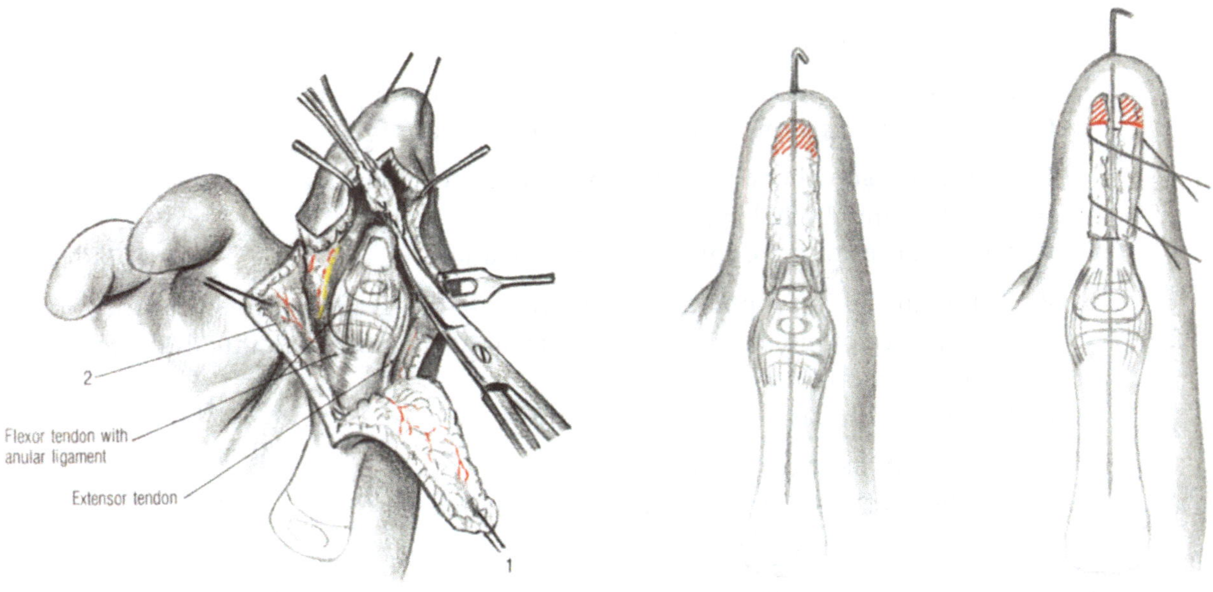

2a 2b 2c

Fig. 3 Postoperative appearance, palmar aspect.
The swivel flap *(1)* has been sutured into the flexor crease of the thumb; the defect on the extensor surface of the thumb has been covered with a thick-split thickness skin transplant *(Tr)*.

Postoperative Care

Long-arm plaster cast. Suture removal after 14 days and reapplication of the plaster cast for 6–8 weeks. Then x-ray control, removal of the Kirschner wire, and application of a tight-fitting short-arm cast for an additional 4–6 weeks. Further x-ray control; night splint after this period. Cautious exercises are begun when the graft appears to be well incorporated.

Errors and Their Consequences

E. Palmar vessels and nerves have been damaged during dissection.

E. Insufficient soft tissue removal at the distal thumb phalanx.
C. Circulatory impairment due to insufficient space for the bone graft.

E. The autologous bone graft is too thick or too long, or has not been properly fixed to the thumb phalanx.
C. Disturbances of incorporation and circulation.

E. A revision of the wound or shortening of the graft has not been performed in the presence of circulatory embarrassment at the tip of the thumb (after release of the tourniquet).
C. Fingertip necrosis.

E. The thumb has been mobilized too soon.
C. Problems of graft incorporation or circulation.

Remarks

Operations to lengthen the rudimentary fingers may be performed at a later date. The function of the thumb determines which finger should be lengthened.

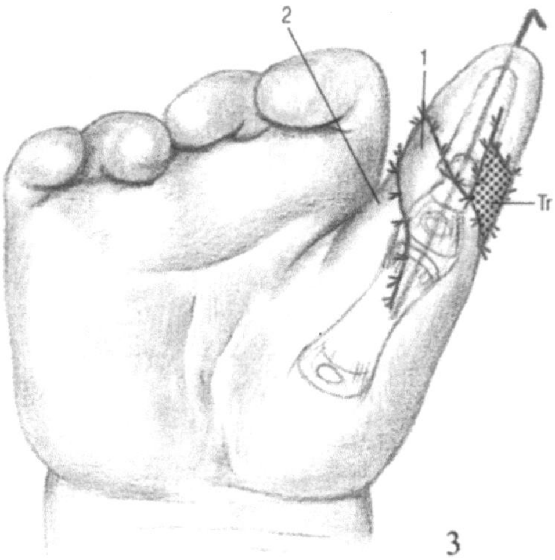

3

3.10 Anular Groove and Defect Pseudarthrosis of the Thumb

Goal of Surgery

Removal of the anular groove and the defect pseudarthrosis (operation in three stages).

First stage

Fig. 1 Preoperative appearance, dorsal aspect.
The thumb phalanges are dysplastic. A large bony defect is present in the area of the anular groove. The *dotted area* denotes skin that has to be resected and filled with a combination flap during the first stage. The dissection is carried out with surgical telescopes. Vessels and nerves of the soft tissue flap have to be protected.

Fig. 2 Thumb, dorsal aspect.
Semicircular excision of the anular groove and adjacent skin. Careful skin separation in a tangential direction. The extensor and flexor tendons are left intact. The neurovascular bundles, particularly on the palmar aspect, have to be meticulously protected.

Fig. 3 A tubed pedicle flap from the distal thorax or abdomen is sutured into the defect, beginning at the ulnar side of the thumb incision. The donor site should be closed as far as possible with interrupted sutures beginning at its distal aspect. See also Sect. 4.2.2.

Fig. 4 View of skin donor site with the hand in maximum pronation.
The free edges of the flap are sutured into the soft tissue defect of the thumb after preparation and defattening of the tubed pedicle flap. (Its edge can barely be seen on the ulnar aspect of the flap.)

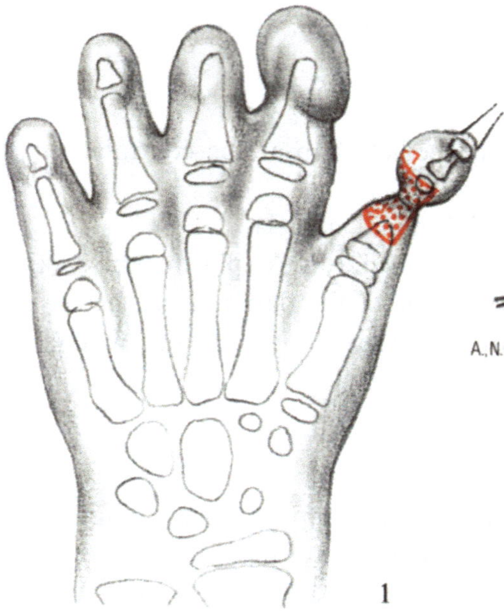

1

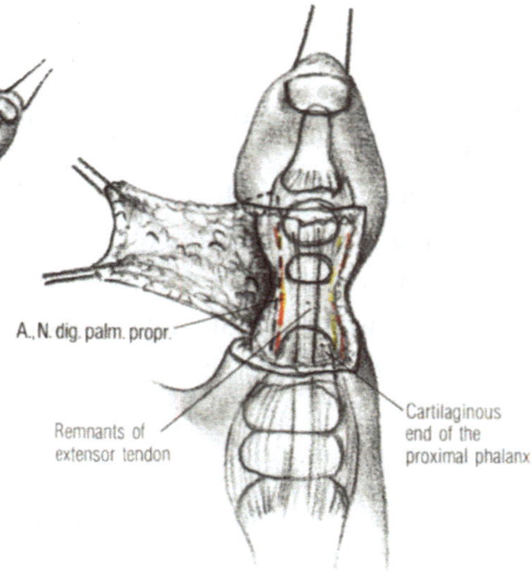

A., N. dig. palm. propr.
Remnants of extensor tendon
Cartilaginous end of the proximal phalanx

2

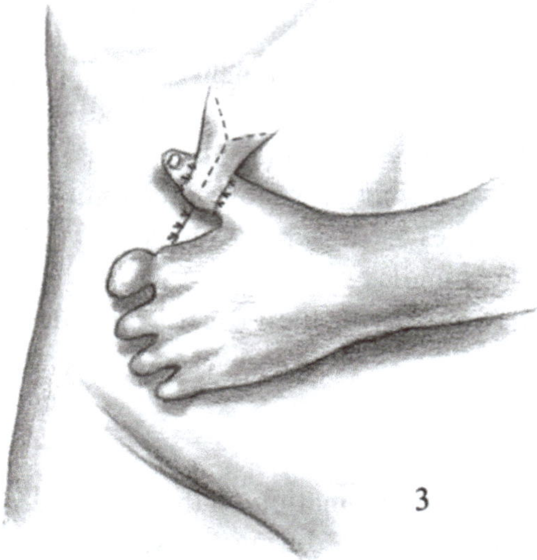

3

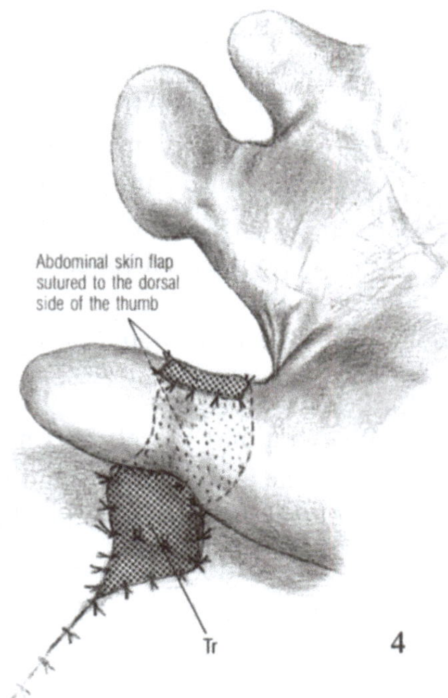

Abdominal skin flap sutured to the dorsal side of the thumb
Tr

4

Fig. 5 *Hatched area:* position of the tubed pedicle flap at the contralateral side of the thumb.
Cross section through thumb and abdominal skin flap.
The remaining defect has to be covered with a thick-split thickness skin transplant *(Tr)*. The transplant extends to the basis of the flap and has been secured, prior to the suturing of the abdominal skin flap, to the medial wound edge at the extensor surface of the thumb.

Postoperative Care

The wound is covered with vaseline gauze. Compression dressing between the full thickness skin transplant and the palmar surface of the thumb. The axilla is padded with cotton wool and the upper extremity is fixed to the torso with elastic bandages. Tension at the basis of the flap has to be avoided. The hand is fixed to the abdominal wall with a few sutures or with elastoplast. The pedicle flap should not be completely covered to allow its observation (see also Sect. 4.2.2).

Second stage (without pictures)

The pedicle flap will be removed from the abdominal wall 3–4 weeks later and the donor site will be closed. The flap wound is protected with a sterile dressing. Exsanguination of the upper limb and application of a tourniquet is carried out. After this the remaining semicircular groove including the adjacent skin on the palmar aspect of the thumb is excised. (Operation as above. Meticulous protection of the palmar neurovascular bundles.)

The skin and soft tissue defect is covered with the properly prepared free ends of the released tubed pedicle flap.

Errors and Their Consequences

First stage (excision of the anular groove and formation of the tubed pedicle flap):
E. Palmar vessels and nerves have been damaged during the semicircular excision of the anular groove and the skin areas. Surgical telescopes have not been employed, the skin areas have not been dissected superficially enough from the tissues.

E. The donor site of the tubed pedicle flap has been insufficiently covered with a thick-split thickness skin transplant that does not extend to the basis of the pedicle.
C. Increased danger of infection.

Second stage (release of the tubed pedicle flap):
E. The release is carried out too soon, i.e., prior to at least 3 weeks after the first operation.
C. Circulatory impairment of the flap.

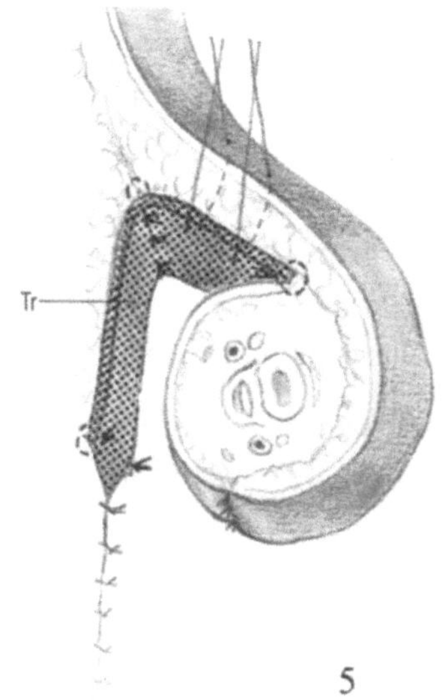

5

Third stage

Fig. 6 Partial view, dorsal aspect (after incorporation of the pedicle flap). Dorsal incision prior to insertion of the bone graft.

Fig. 7 The extensor tendon has been exposed and retracted. Both rudimentary phalanges have been decorticated. The graft site is prepared by removal of fatty and connective tissue. Vessels and nerves have to be protected, surgical telescopes are necessary. The ends of the phalanges are properly prepared.

Fig. 8 A Kirschner wire is first inserted in a distal direction into the distal phalanx. Its proximal end should be level with the proximal end of the distal phalanx. A properly shaped autologous bone graft taken from the iliac crest is then inserted with slight distraction of the fragments. The Kirschner wire is then advanced through the graft and the rudimentary proximal phalanx into the first metacarpal.
The tourniquet is released and circulation is checked. The graft may have to be shortened if circulation at the tip of the thumb appears to be impaired due to excessive soft tissue tension.

Fig. 9 Postoperative appearance.
Fixation of the graft with a second Kirschner wire. Skin closure.

Postoperative Care

Long-arm plaster cast. The tip of the thumb remains uncovered to permit observation of circulation. Suture removal is carried out 2 weeks later and a new long-arm cast is applied. X-ray control of the thumb 6–8 weeks after surgery, depending on the patient's age and the length of the bone graft. The graft is usually incorporated at that time and the longitudinal Kirschner wire can be safely removed. Application of a tight-fitting short-arm cast for another 4 weeks. After this, removal of the second Kirschner wire, x-ray control, and introduction of carefully supervised exercises. Regular reevaluation at 4–6 week intervals.

Errors and Their Consequences

Third stage (bone bridge plasty):
E. Excessive fatty tissue has not been removed.
C. Insufficient space for the bone graft, resulting in circulatory impairment.

E. The ends of the phalanges have not been sufficiently decorticated or the bone graft not properly prepared or secured.
C. Impaired incorporation of the bone graft.

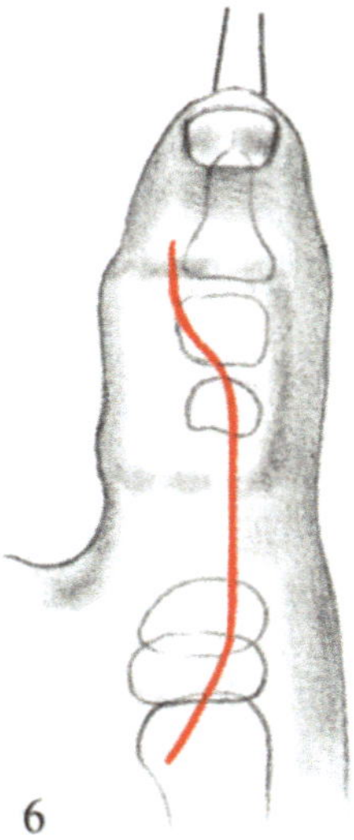

6

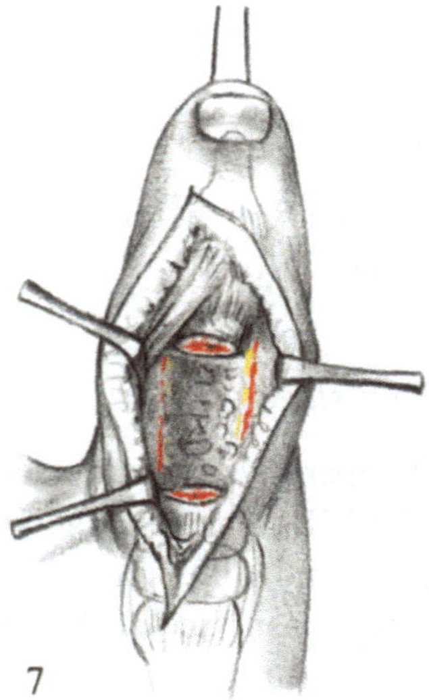

7

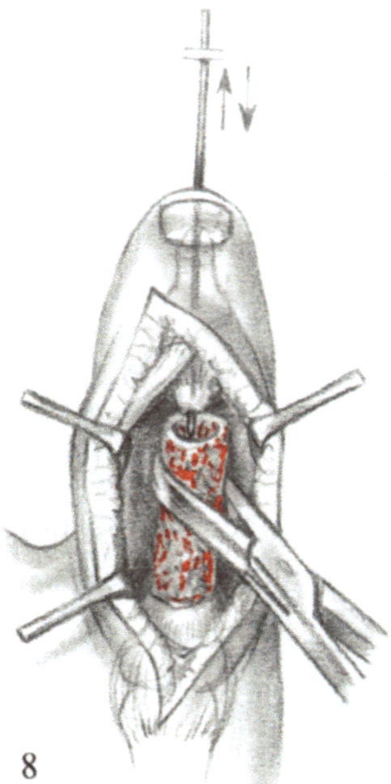

8

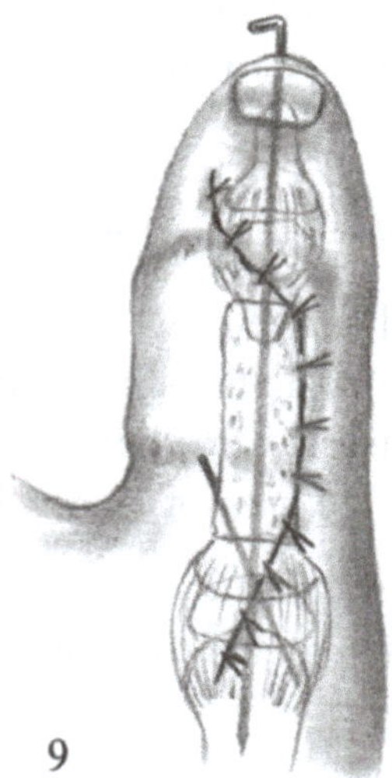

9

3.11 Rudimentary Index Finger with Excessive Soft Tissue and Anular Groove

Goal of Surgery

Removal of the anular groove and lengthening of the index finger phalanx (three stages).

First stage

Fig. 1 Preoperative appearance, dorsal aspect.
The PIP joint has a good range of motion.
Formation of a cross finger flap according to TEMPEST, originating from the extensor surface of the neighboring digit. Great care has to be taken not to damage the dorsal radial finger artery. The area of implantation at the index finger is outlined by the *broken line*.

Fig. 2 Palmar-radial aspect.
Careful excision of an area of skin at the grooved section of the index finger which corresponds in length and width with the outline of the pedicle flap. The flap is approximated without tension.

Fig. 3 Picture after the cross flap has been sutured in place. The donor site has been covered with a thick-split thickness skin transplant *(Tr)*.

Second stage (ca. 3 weeks later)

Fig. 4 Dorsal aspect.
The interdigital skin bridge (including the thick-split thickness skin transplant) is transected at the ulnar border of the index finger on its dorsal aspect. The *red dotted area* of skin will be excised during wound closure.

Fig. 5 Palmar aspect.
Release of the cross finger flap from the donor digit.

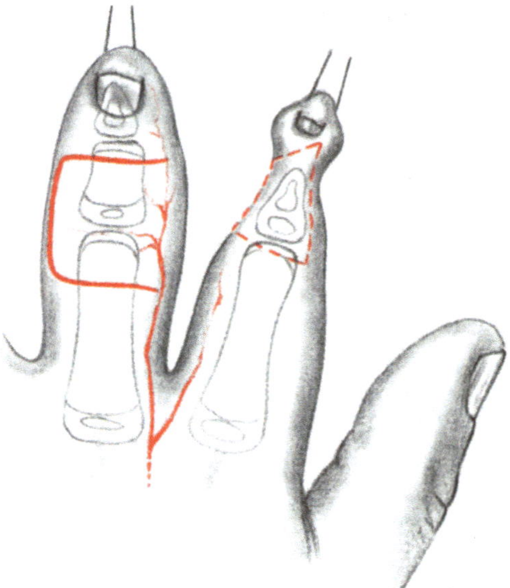

1

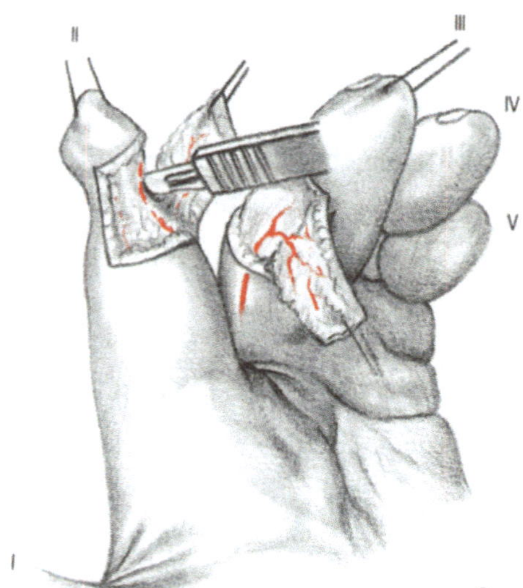

2

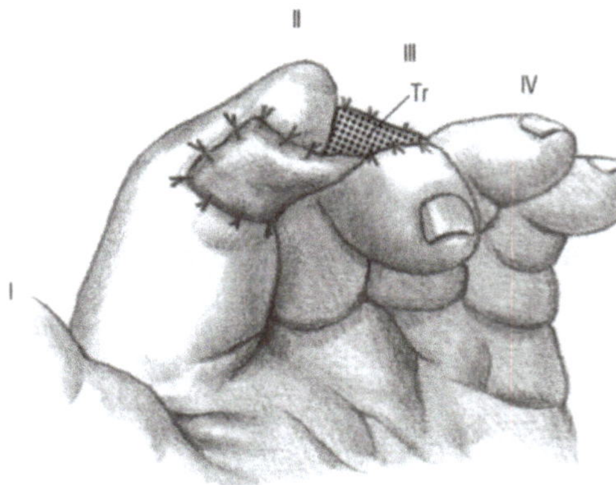

3

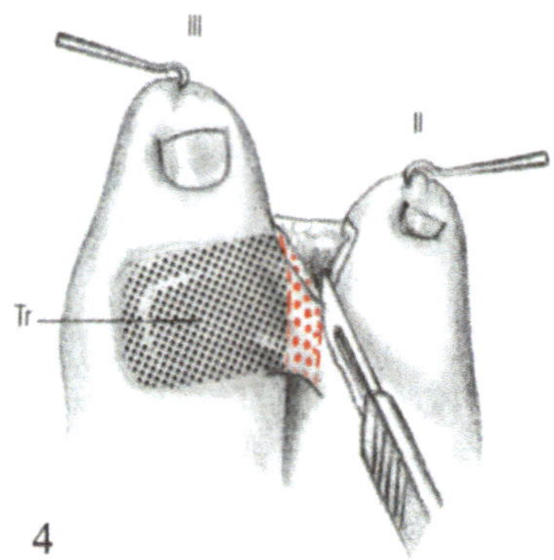

4

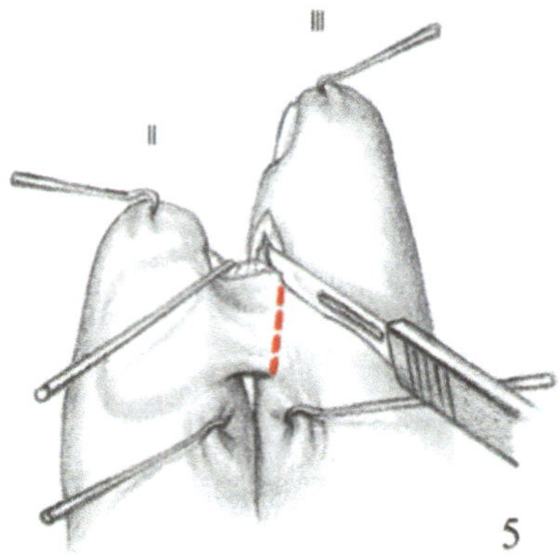

5

Fig. 6 Postoperative appearance.
Skin closure after proper preparation of the flaps.

Third stage (after 6 weeks)

Fig. 7 Preoperative appearance and incision for the bone graft implantation.
The incorporated skin flap is still recognizable by the irregularities of its contour.

Fig. 8 The phalangeal rudiment has been exposed and decorticated.
Creating a bed for the bone graft, parts of the fatty tissues are excised by carefully spreading the soft tissues of the fingertip.

Fig. 9 The extensor tendon (aponeurosis) has been retracted. A Kischner wire is introduced through the open wound past the fingertip. After this it is advanced proximally and centrally into the proximal phalanx of the index finger.

Fig. 10 Two properly shaped autologous bone grafts are placed around the Kirschner wire and secured with cerclage sutures. (A solitary cancellous bone graft can also be employed, see Sect. 3.10).

Fig. 11 Postoperative appearance after wound closure.

Postoperative Care and Errors and Their Consequences

See Sects. 3.10 and 3.9

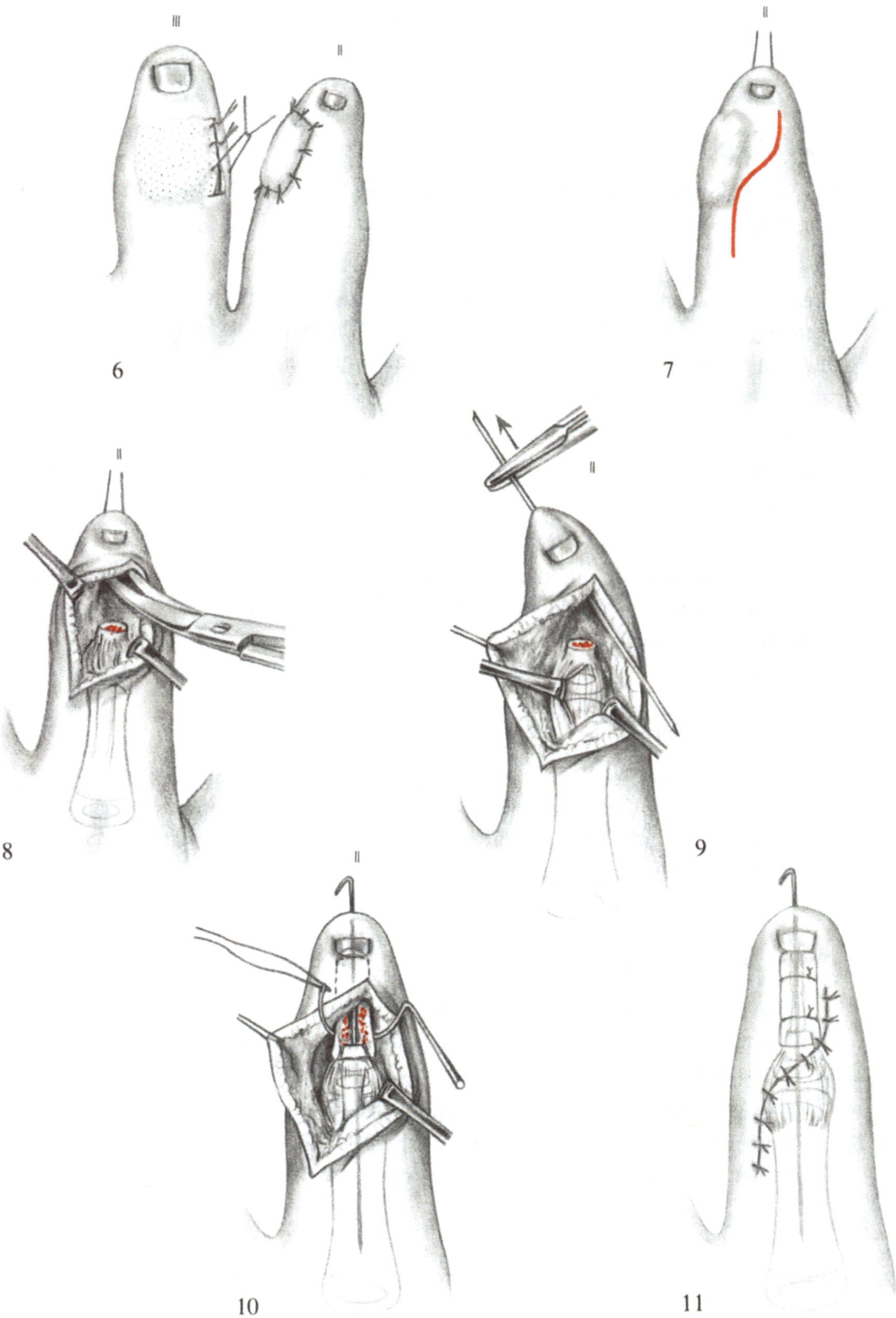

III
II
6
II
7
II
8
II
9
II
10
11

Goal of Surgery

Removal of the anular groove including the fascia antebrachii. Bridging of the soft tissue defect with local swivel flaps (two stages).

Fig. 1 Preoperative appearance and incision, palmar aspect of the right forearm. Semicircular removal of the anular groove on the palmar side. Its excision requires surgical telescopes and careful and parsimonious resection, as vessels and nerves can be easily damaged during this step.

Fig. 2 Careful excision of the fascia antebrachii is carried out after the skin flaps have been raised. Some skin flaps will require additional shaping (*dotted areas*) prior to wound closure.

Fig. 3 Postoperative appearance.
Slight indentations of the skin that are still visible laterally, disappear after the second operation, in which the dorsal anular groove is removed using the same technique (ca. 6 weeks later).

Postoperative Caree

The wound is covered with vaseline gauze and loosely applied fluffs. An elastic bandage with *slight* compression has to be loosened 1–2 h after surgery. Elevation of the involved limb. Immobilization with a padded long-arm cast for ca. 2 weeks, followed by suture removal.

Errors and Their Consequences

E. The fascia antebrachii has not been excised or only insufficiently removed. (Only the complete excision of the fascia antebrachii results in a "decompression" of vessels, nerves, tendons, and muscles.)

E. The dressing has been applied with too much compression, elastic bandages have not been loosened approximately 2 h after surgery.
C. Impaired wound healing, flap necrosis etc.

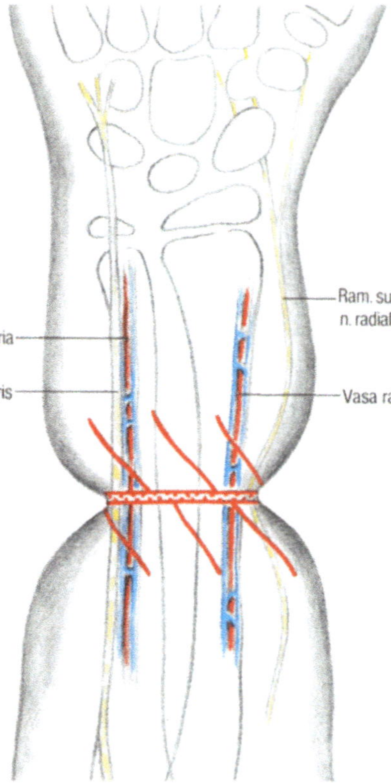

Ram. superfic.
n. radialis
Vasa ulnaria
N. ulnaris
Vasa radialia

1

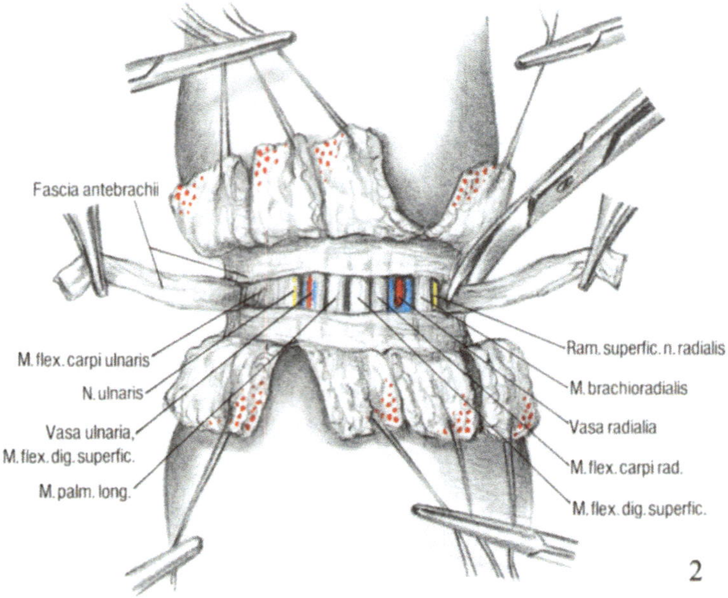

Fascia antebrachii
M. flex. carpi ulnaris
N. ulnaris
Vasa ulnaria,
M. flex. dig. superfic.
M. palm. long.
Ram. superfic. n. radialis
M. brachioradialis
Vasa radialia
M. flex. carpi rad.
M. flex. dig. superfic.

2

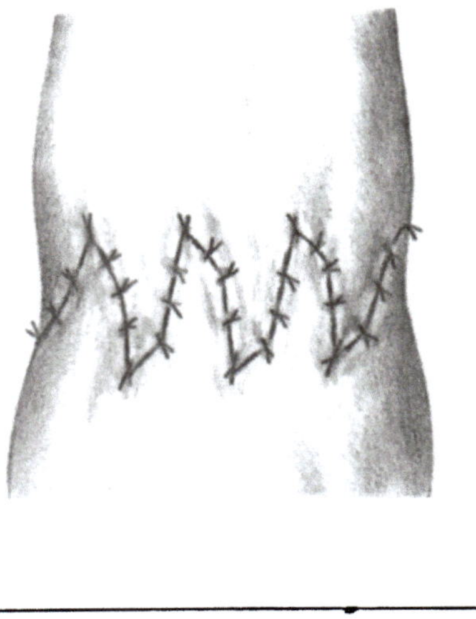

3

4 Numerical Variations

4.1 Introduction

4.1.1 General Remarks

The concept of "numerical variations" encompasses deformities that differ from the normal development of five independent finger rays. They occur as plus or minus variations. A large number of these poly- or oligodactylies can be deduced from *an overextensive or incomplete differentiation in width;* consequently they appear as partial or total "partitions" or "fusions" of single skeletal rays. W. MÜLLER (1937) demonstrated the mutuality in morphological appearance for these plus or minus variations, using the picture of the more or less peripherally opening "prong". Identical forms within a single ray (in poly- and oligodactylies) can be present. The difference between such recessive and excessive forms lays only in the direction of the deformity. When systematized from a teratologic point in view, one notices in *oligodactylies* a line of progression by lack of differentiation in width (fushion, proximal skeletal aplasia) from central to distal segments; in *polydactylies,* on the other hand, excessive differentiation (partitioning) occurs from distal to central segments.

The least-developed *minus* variations present only as a proximal coalescence of contiguous metacarpal bones or as a diminution in size or partial aplasia (suppression) of one of these bones. The most pronounced minus variants result in a complete fusion even of the distal rays, ending in the picture of "total aplasia" of the rays. The *plus* forms range from partial, forklike duplications of the distal phalanx to the formation of two complete, mirrorlike finger rays.

The deformities have a great variability. Their appearance can be influenced by concomitant cutaneous syndactylies, by dislocations, hypoplasias, and aplasias of single skeletal parts (metric variations), or even by hypersegmentations. As a rule one can expect an unequal size of the partners forming a bifurcation.

4.1.1.1 Polydactylies

Polydactylies are one of the most common forms of hand deformity [blacks are affected ten times more than whites (MELLIN 1963)]. The border rays are most commonly involved.

In mild cases the distal phalanx of the *thumb* may show an enlargement in width and circumference. Sometimes two nails are present, sometimes a common nail band with some segmentation. More pronounced deformities result in bifurcations of the distal or proximal phalanges. Severe types may present as two thumbs with their own metacarpals. In these cases one often finds one of them to be hypoplastic or to have three phalanges. Triple thumbs with syndactylies and (occasionally) triphalangy have also been described.

A similar line of progression can be noted at the *ulnar border ray*. These forms of excessive proliferation are probably just as common as the medial ray deformities. Some of them consist solely of a soft tissue appendage, which is found on the ulnar side at the level of the MP joint. It contains one or two hypoplastic phalanges or no bone at all and has no bony contact with the normally shaped little finger. Striking changes can be observed if the duplication extends to the metacarpal bone, e.g., the border ray on the ulnar side can deviate at a right angle from the common metacarpal. In these instances we found the bases of both proximal phalanges in a common joint capsule. They articulate with the metacarpal bone on two separate articular surfaces. In other cases one finds prong-shaped metacarpal bones. The ulnar duplication of the little finger frequently contains only two phalanges. Extensor and flexor tendons branch off from a "common" tendon at the basis of the prong, as do nerves and vessels. This also pertains to the thumb rays. The thenar and hypothenar musculature, which is frequently atrophic, inserts at the lateral aspect of the finger bifurcation. Combined duplications of radial and ulnar border rays are not infrequently found.

Duplication processes of the *central rays* are in principle similar; they frequently occur in association with syndactylies and are therefore "hidden."

Polydactylies may be facultative or obligatory traits of other *deformity syndromes* (Bardet-Biedl syndrome, Ellis-van Creveld syndrome, Carpenter syndrome a.o.).

Incomplete or complete duplications of the hand (dicheiria, diplocheiria, mirror hand) constitute a separate entity, also in their formal genesis. These extremely rare defects are seen in ulnar duplications (frequently associated with radius aplasia). They are always mirrorlike duplications of ulnar parts (see BONOLA and MORELLI 1972).

4.1.1.2 Oligodactylies

Regressive forms of numerical variations are of greatest importance if the *thumb* is involved, as they result in severe functional impairment. The different deformities can be grouped within a line of teratologic progression, based on practical functional considerations according to the degree of involvement (W. MÜLLER 1937; BLAUTH 1967). Regressive deformities of the thumb ray require classification in a special category. In such cases – contrary to similar changes of the long fingers which result in coalitions with the contiguous ray – one finds a progressive hypo- or aplasia of skeletal and soft tissue elements from central to distal segments as a sign of suppression. It seems to be caused by the early separation of the thumb from the common hand plate.

First-degree hypoplasias present as a slimness of the thumb ray with hypoplasias of the mm. abd. poll. brev. and opp. poll. The function of the hand is not impaired at all, or only barely so.

Second-degree hypoplasias are characterized by more pronounced changes of form and function. The thenar musculature is poorly developed. The loss of function is determined by adduction contracture of the thumb ray, tightness of the thumb commissure, and occasionally quite pronounced laxity of the first MP joint. The surgeon will always encounter anomalies of the muscles, nerves, and vessels as well as joint dysplasias.

We classify cases of partial aplasias of the first metacarpal bone as *third-degree hypoplasias*. The atrophy and instability of the Ist ray is striking. The thenar musculature is nearly completely absent; nerves and muscles show severe anomalies.

The metacarpal bone is completely absent in cases of *fourth-degree thumb hypoplasia*. The thumblet is loosely connected to the hand by a simple soft tissue tube that contains some vessels and nerves (so-called floating thumb, *Pendeldaumen, pouce flottant*), or it originates from the proximal phalanx of the index finger on its radial side.

The degree of regression ends with a *complete aplasia of the thumb*. Four-finger hands have a considerable number of anomalies as far as muscles and tendons are concerned. The course of finger nerves and vessels can also be nonanatomic, These facts are of great importance if surgery (pollicization) is considered. We refer to "nerve loops" which frequently cling to or encircle metacarpal arteries (Sect. 4.5.7, Fig. 5 a.o.). Such nerve loops have also been described in normal hands (see BLAUTH 1972).

Involution of the thumb ray is frequently observed in connection with *radius dysplasia* (Chap. 10), which was more often seen in thalidomide embryopathies. Oligodactylies due to *aplasias of the IVth and Vth ray*, rarely of the Vth ray alone, are frequently associated with *ulnar dysplasias*. The remaining (border) middle finger ray usually has more or less pronounced bifurcations. These variations of external form correspond with Müller's classification.

The bifurcation anomalies of *plus* variations are repeated at the long fingers if recessive processes are present and if ulnar dysplasia is absent. *Oligodactylies of the central rays* are extremely rare (except in cleft hand deformities, see Chap. 9).

Oligodactylous spoon-shaped hands are a *separate entity*. In such cases one observes total syndactylies of all long fingers with multiple bony coalitions of contiguous skeletal parts of the finger rays. They are frequently seen in connection with aplasia of the Ist ray. Their origin is supposed to be a primary defect of the soft tissue blastema and secondary interference of skeletal differentiation due to soft tissue deficiency.

4.1.2 Timing of Surgery

The optimal time for surgical intervention depends on the extent of disturbances of form and function. This axiom is also relevant in the presence of oligo- or polydactylies. In general it is our aim to perform surgery between the 3rd and 5th year of life and to finish therapy prior to the patient entering school. This recommendation is particularly important in all cases of hypo- or aplasia of the thumb and in most cases of partial or complete duplication of thumb or of little fingers. In some circumstances children with more severe oligosyndactylies in the form of spoon hands or children with functionless finger rudiments should be operated on between the 1st and 2nd year of life. In contrast, surgery to achieve the fusion of two fingers should be postponed as far as is possible until the end of the first decade or to the second decade of life, if complicated techniques involving a danger of damage to the epiphyses must be employed.

4.1.3 General Surgical Directives

In the presence of *higher-degree hypoplasias of the thumb ray* only *pollicization of the index finger* will give good results (Sects. 4.2.4–4.2.6) (Buck-Gramcko 1966, 1968; Blauth 1967, 1969, 1970, 1972). Only first-degree and mild second-degree hypoplasias are suited for operations to improve function while at the same time preserving the thumb. In such cases some prior surgical interventions, i.e., increasing the depth and width of the thumb commissure (Sects. 4.2.1, 4.2.2), should precede an opponens plasty (Sect. 4.2.3) or stabilization of the first MP joint (Sect. 4.2.3).

In general, treatment of patients with *oligosyndactylies* is the same as for syndactylies. *Acrosynostoses* with a common nail band require not only proportional splitting of the nail but also resection of the lateral borders of the nail matrix to prevent future nail deformities (Sects. 4.3.1–4.3.3).

Patients with *oligodactylies combined with pronounced spoon hand* can expect functional improvement if removal of interposed skeletal parts is carried out, if necessary even into the metacarpal area (Sects. 4.3.2, 4.3.3).

Surgical fusion of two fingers is a very complicated operation and requires extremely careful dissection. Preoperative diagrams add to the precise knowledge of the size of the fragments and the correct osteotomy sites. Future deterioration in joint function has to be expected if joint segments have to be partially or completely resected (Sects. 4.3.4, 4.3.5, 4.4.3). These joints are usually already dysplastic or more or less immobile. Joints most frequently affected are the PIP and DIP joints. Therefore, one does not have to worry too much about their loss of function after surgery.

Similar points of view are applicable for cases of *polydactyly*. No satisfactory result can be expected if in the presence of hypoplastic partners of *similar size* only one of them is removed. The discrepancy of the remaining part in comparison to the size of the other fingers will be intensified after amputation. Fusion of the hypoplastic partners is a better, but more difficult procedure (Sect. 4.4.1).

In the presence of partners of *unequal size* one should not amputate the smaller one before careful dissection of the palmar vessels and nerves (Sects. 4.4.2, 4.4.4, 4.4.5, 4.4.7, 4.5.2, 4.5.3). Impairment of the neurovascular bundles of the partner finger can occur if this step has been omitted.

A defect in the *common joint capsule* and a *widening of the head* remain after amputation of a partner when the bifurcation occurs at the level of the MP or PIP joint. The size of the head has to be diminished and the capsular defect has to be closed (Sects. 4.4.4, 4.4.7, 4.5.2; also 4.4.2). Neglecting to reshape the head results in a steadily increasing enlargement of this structure.

Careful smoothing of the resection site below the level of the diaphysis is indicated if the bifurcation occurs at the metacarpal head (Sect. 4.4.2).

Amputation of a *supernumerary central ray* may require an additional partial resection and corrective osteotomy of the (common) metacarpal bone and a tethering operation to the contiguous metacarpal (Sect. 4.5.4).

4.1.4 Postoperative Care

The general principles of hand surgery apply to all operations for the correction of oligo- or polydactylies. Some procedures do, however, require alterations (i.e., pollicization: see Sect. 4.2.4).

The duration of immobilization of the involved limb depends on specific circumstances. In general one can assume that cutaneous operations require ca. 2 weeks, soft tissue surgery involving joints and joint capsules ca. 3–4 weeks, and bony operations ca. 4–6 weeks of immobilization.

4.2 Thumb Hypo- and Aplasias

4.2.1 Partial Syndactyly Combined with Second-Degree Thumb Hypoplasia

Goal of Surgery

Creation of a wide, smooth web space between thumb and index finger formed from local swivel flaps.

Fig. 1 Preoperative appearance and incision, dorsal aspect.
The incision on the palmar side and the indentation of the m. add. poll. are demonstrated by the *broken line,* as are possible enlargements of the skin incisions. In most cases it will be necessary to extend the swivel flap on the extensor surface of the index finger (*b*) distally in order to create a web space of sufficient depth and width.
Indentation of the muscle is required if insufficient abduction persists after preparation of the skin flaps and partial incision of the dorsal and palmar fascia, and if present, of the lig. capit. transvers. I/II. This lack of abduction is caused by a shortening of the muscle fibers.
For particulars in regard to the following steps and the respective figures see Sect. 3.4 a.o.

Fig. 2 Postoperative appearance, dorsal aspect.
The remaining skin defect on the index finger has to be covered with a thick-split thickness skin graft *(Tr)* after the skin flaps have been sutured in place. The first metacarpal bone should be temporarily fixed in position of function with two crossed Kirschner wires (not shown). *Broken line:* border of the palmar skin flap.

Fig. 3 Postoperative appearance, palmar aspect.
Position of the dorsal skin flaps is outlined by the *broken line.*

Postoperative Care

The wound is covered with vaseline gauze, properly shaped compresses, and a small elastic bandage. A padded long-arm cast that has to be split open down to the elastic bandage. First dressing change after 8–10 days and application of a short-arm splint. Suture removal after 10–12 days, removal of the Kirschner wires after 15–20 days. After this, institution of active exercises. A splint in the position of abduction and opposition is initially worn between exercises. Later this splint is employed only a night for a total period of approximately 4 months.

Additional operations, if necessary (see Sect. 4.2.3 a.o.), should not be performed before 4–6 weeks have elapsed.

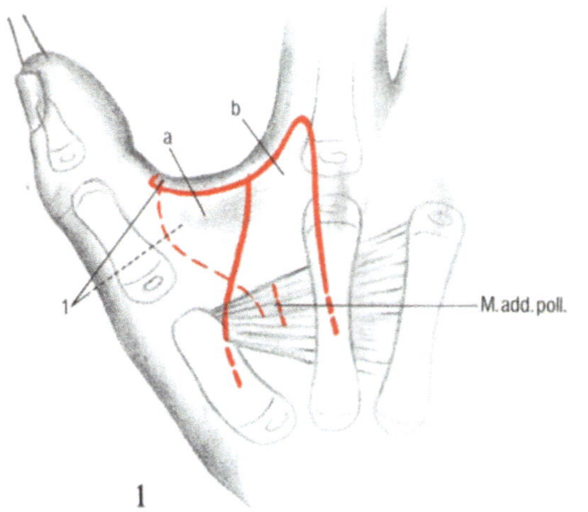

1

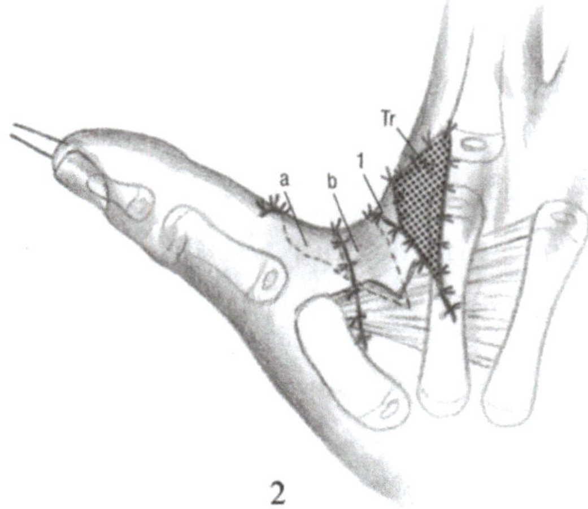

2

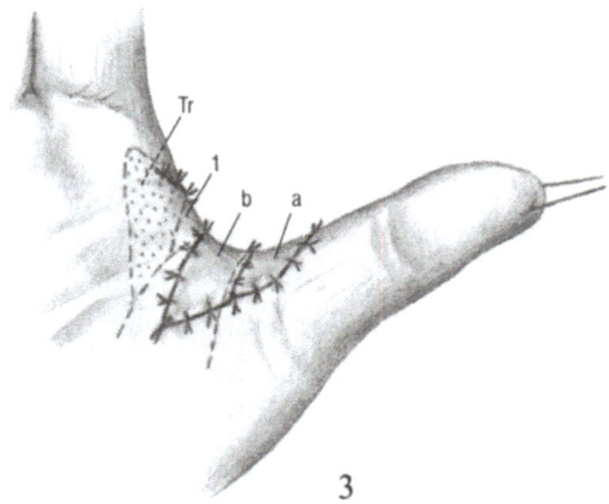

3

Errors and Their Consequences

E. A Z-plasty has been employed to create the web space. It is nearly always impossible to form a web space of sufficient depth and width without swivel flaps. In the presence of an extremely tight web space it may even be necessary to use a tubed pedicle graft (Sect. 4.2.2).

E. The dorsal swivel flap is too short.

C. Depth and width of the web space remains unsatisfactory. Skin tension and circulatory problems may develop.

E. Indentation of the fascia and/or the m. abd. poll. has been omitted.

C. Abduction of the Ist ray will be insufficient. A tight capsule of the first carpometacarpal joint can limit abduction in spite of sufficient fasciotomy and muscle indentation. The joint capsule can be incised through a separate skin incision.

See "Remarks" in Sects. 3.4 and 2.2.3 and Sect. 2.1.1.

4.2.2 Partial Syndactyly Combined with Second-Degree Thumb Hypoplasia and a Tight Web Space

Goal of Surgery

Separation of the Ist ray and alignment of the thumb in a position of function. Formation of a web space by employing a tubed pedicle graft (three stages).

First stage

A two-tailed tubed pedicle graft is raised from the contra- or ipsilateral abdominal wall according to BUNNELL's method (1959). In general we prefer the contralateral wall as the donor site. Occasionally it is necessary to form the tubed graft on the ipsilateral abdominal wall if contractures of the joints of the upper limb are present. A groin flap (McGREGOR and JACKSON 1972) can also be employed (Sect. 1.3).

Fig. 1 Skin incisions (right abdominal wall).
The main incisions are directed obliquely from laterocranial to mediocaudal. They have to be outlined with a marking pen. The ratio of width to length of the tubed flap should be 1:2.5. One has to consider its shrinkage (BUNNELL suggested that its diameter should be 25% larger than the area to be covered), the thickness of the subcutaneous fatty tissue at the donor site (sufficient width of the tube for its closure without tension), and the expected size of the skin defect at the site of implantation (according to the required width of the web space and the size of the hand). It has been our experience that in children the length of the tubed flap has to be 12–18 cm and its width 5–8 cm.
Two pointed tips (1, 2) are formed at the caudal skin incision by employing two additional incisions. This step enables us to place the skin sutures of the abdominal wall lateral to the closing suture of the tube (see Fig. 2a). The same reason necessitates making the caudal skin incision somewhat larger. Skin (with subcutaneous tissues) is mobilized very generously down to the muscle fascia, in particular vertical to the skin incisions. Undermining of the tissues is carried out from the linea alba to the lateral caudal aspect of the iliac crest. Without this step it is usually impossible to close the defect of the abdominal wall without tension after the tubed graft has been raised. Closed suction drainages are then inserted; they have to be placed into the deepest parts of the undermined skin, particularly caudally (not shown).

Fig. 2 Skin suture lines at the cranial part of the tube pedicle flap (a mirror image of the appearance in the caudal part of the flap). The two tips (1, 2) are sutured into the corners of the upper incision. This is followed by closing the interposed skin and by trimming excessive fat from the wound edges, particularly at the future tails of the tube. The tube is then formed and closed by sutures. Great care has to be taken while closing the skin of the tails, as soft tissue tension

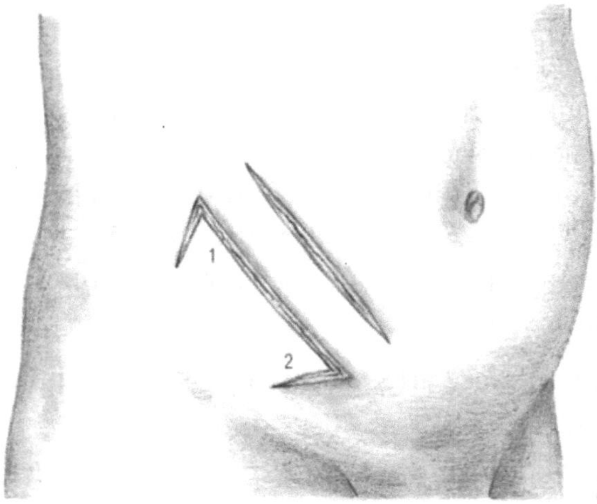

1

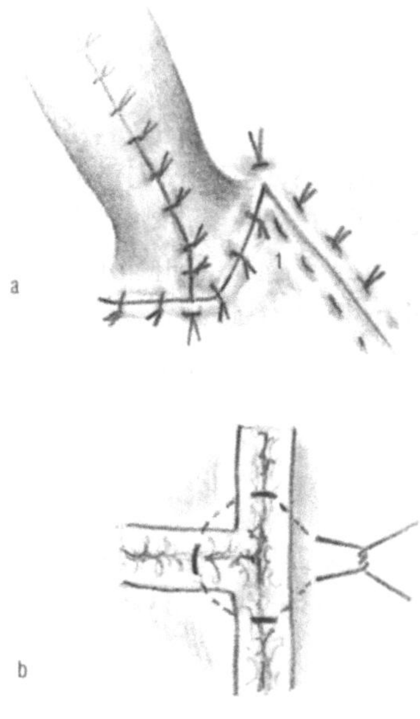

2

can easily ensue. We have found it helpful to begin the suture at the upper border of the tubed graft with the lateral border of the skin tips (1) and (2). In this way it is possible to place the longitudinal suture of the tubed graft far enough away from the suture of the abdominal wall and in a slightly ventral position.
For details, see *Fig. 2a.* (The tubed pedicle flap has been lifted to demonstrate its undersurface and the position of the abdominal sutures. *Figure 2b* shows the technique of the angle sutures).

Fig. 3 Postoperative appearance after closure of all skin sutures.

Postoperative Care

The wound is covered with vaseline gauze; the tubed pedicle graft is separated from the abdominal wall by a thin layer of fluffs. Torsion and tension of the tube has to be avoided. A thick layer of fluffs is placed on each side of the tube and the area is covered with a protective dressing, windowed over the tubed graft for exposure.

Positioning the patient in bed has to avoid tension on the abdominal wall; he should be placed in semi-Fowler's position. Pressure caused, for example, by a coverlet is to be avoided.

First dressing change after 5 days. All sutures are removed after 2 weeks. After 3 weeks, intermittent clamping of the tube stem to be released first for several minutes until no circulatory embarrassment of the tube is noted.

Errors and Their Consequences

E. Oblique positioning of the graft (in correspondence with the vessels of the abdominal wall) has not been observed; the ratio of its length to its width is larger than 3:1.
C. Great danger of impaired circulation.

E. The middle section of the tubed graft has been sutured prior to its bases.
C. Danger of strangulating afferent vessels.

E. The skin contiguous to the tubed graft has not been widely enough undermined.
C. The tube is under tension; wound dehiscences, infections, skin necrosis etc. may occur.

E. The borders of the tubed pedicle graft have been excessively or insufficiently defatted.
C. The tubed flap sutures may develop tension (graft necrosis); formation of subcutaneous hematoma in the tube is possible.

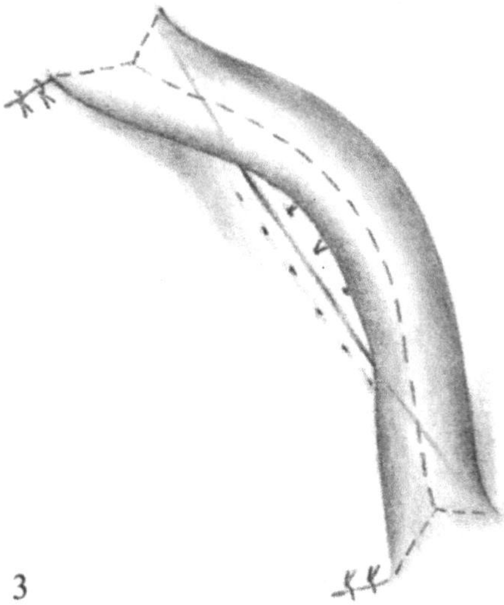

3

E. Insufficient or excessive pressure of the dressing, particularly under the stems of the tubed graft.
C. Macerations followed by infection or circulatory impairment etc.

E. The stem has not been clamped and/or intervals between the different stages have been too short.
C. Graft necrosis.

Second stage

Release of the tubed pedicle graft and its insertion into the dorsum of the hand.

Fig. 4 Preoperative appearance and skin incision.
The separated end of the tubed pedicle graft will be inserted into the space between the first and second metacarpal. The ventral tip of the graft will be placed dorsally and proximally (see Fig. 6).

Fig. 5 Dorsal aspect, skin incision (skeletal parts outlined).
Second-degree hypoplasia of the thumb and second-degree brachydactyly are noted. The Vth ray is aplastic; its absence diminishes function minimally.
An oval area of skin extending into the web space will be excised between the first and second metacarpal on the dorsal aspect *(hatched area)*. The incision is extended into the palmar area. This allows a slight but insufficient improvement of abduction of the Ist ray. Fascial and ligamentous tissues (lig. cap. transversum) are incised and removed.
Next, fixation of the Ist ray in optimal abduction and opposition. The position is held with two Kirschner wires (see Figs. 10 and 11) and the defatted end of the tubed graft is sutured into the defect (not demonstrated).

Fig. 6 Postoperative appearance.
The tubed pedicle graft has been sutured in place.

Postoperative Care

This is the same as outlined for *stage 1*. The arm is fixed to the body with elastic bandages; plaster fixation may have to be employed. Children who are very restless may require a few fixation sutures holding their hand to the abdominal wall. First dressing change after 5 days. Bed rest for 2 weeks to avoid tension at the abdominal suture line. The sutures can be removed after 2 weeks. *Stage 3* should be scheduled 4 weeks after *stage 2*.

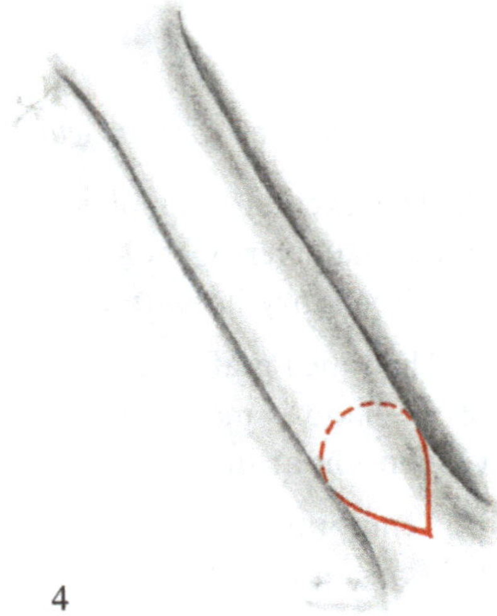

4

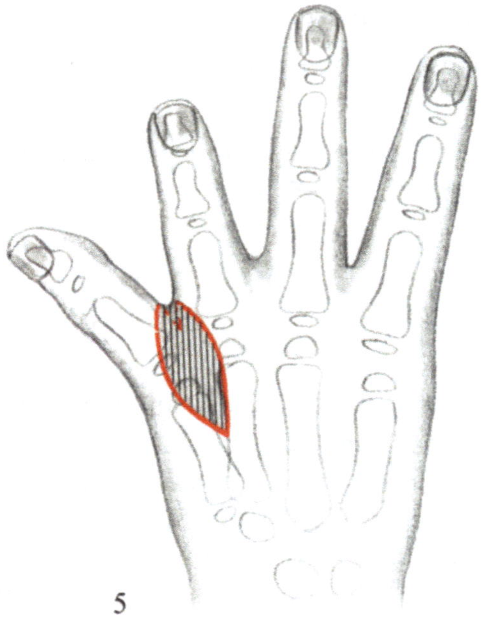

5

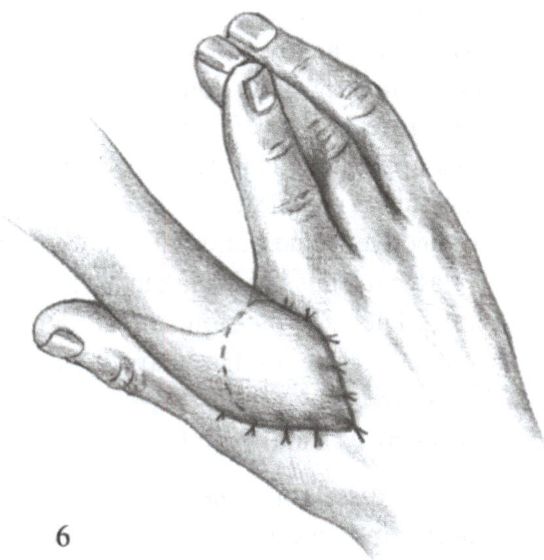

6

Errors and Their Consequences

E. The excised area of skin at the dorsum of the hand is too small compared to the diameter of the tubed graft.
C. Circulatory impairment.

E. The tubed graft becomes twisted and/or has been sutured under tension; fixation of the hand is inadequate.
C. Tension at the tubed pedicle graft resulting in circulatory impairment.

E. Temporary fixation of the first and second metacarpals has been omitted.
C. Tension at the skin sutures.

E. Position and circulation of the tubed pedicle flap has been inspected inadequately, particularly during the early postoperative phase.

Third stage

Fig. 7 Palmar radial aspect.
The tubed pedicle graft has been released from the abdominal wall and the abdominal wound has been closed (not demonstrated). It may be advantageous to leave the remaining graft connected to the abdominal wall if it becomes apparent that the entire length of the graft may not be required for the web space formation. This appendage can be used in the future if complications develop.
The tubed pedicle graft is then incised along its old scar to its center. A whitish connective tissue band acts as a guiding structure.
Great care has to be taken not to damage important vessels at the basis of the graft. The skin incision on the palmar aspect of the hand follows the skin crease and has to be wedge shaped *(hatched area)*. Appropriate width of the area to be excised is required to permit insertion of the tip of the flap, and to guarantee sufficient vascular supply.

Fig. 8 Palmar vessels and nerves are exposed after splitting of the palmar aponeurosis. Fascial and tendinous structures between the metacarpal heads have been transected during *stage 2*. The (deep?) flexor tendons of the thumb and index finger are fused at the level of the web space. They should be separated as far proximal as possible *(black broken line)*. A common nerve bundle has to be split interfascicularly *(broken line)*.

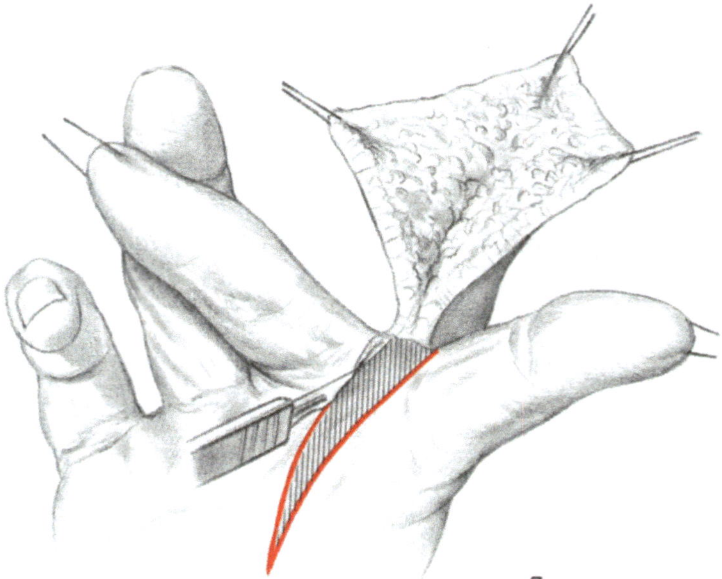

7

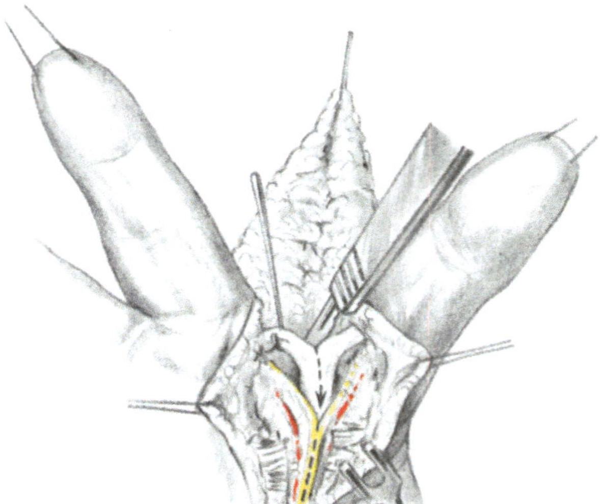

8

4.2.2 Partial Syndactyly Combined with Second-Degree Thumb Hypoplasia and a Tight Web Space

Fig. 9 The m. add. poll. is indented; its vessels and nerves have to be carefully protected. The tubed pedicle graft is then shaped and sutured into the defect.

Figs. 10, 11 Postoperative appearance.
The position of the thumb in abduction and opposition is protected with Kirschner wires.

Postoperative Care

Long-arm cast for 2–$2^1/_2$ weeks, leaving the interphalangeal (I.P.) joints of the thumb and index finger free. During this time, bed rest to prevent widening of cutaneous scars on the stomach. Early active mobilization of the joints to avoid adhesion of the separated flexor tendon is imperative! Closed suction drainage is removed after 48 h and the Kirschner wires after $2^1/_2$ weeks. A plantar splint in position of function, to be used as a night splint only during the later stages, should be applied and employed for 4–6 months.

A derotation osteotomy of the first metacarpal may have to be performed as a *fourth stage* if optimal functional position of the Ist ray has not yet been obtained.

Errors and Their Consequences

E. The tubed pedicle graft diameter is too small or too large, it has not been sufficiently defatted.
C. Web space is not smooth, its width and depth is insufficient, circulatory impairment may occur.

E. The tubed pedicle graft has not been inserted far enough proximally.
C. Abduction of the Ist ray is suboptimal and the appearance of the hand will be cosmetically unsatisfactory.

E. The IP joints of the thumb and index finger have not been mobilized early enough.
C. Adhesions of the separated flexor tendon, impaired function.

E. A night splint has not been employed.
C. Scar tissue will diminish the width of the web space.

Other errors and consequences, see above and Sect. 4.2.1 a.o.

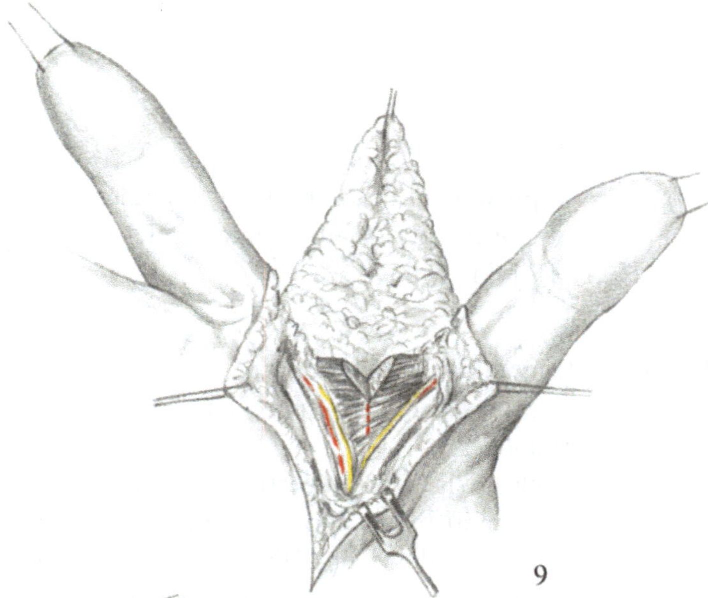

9

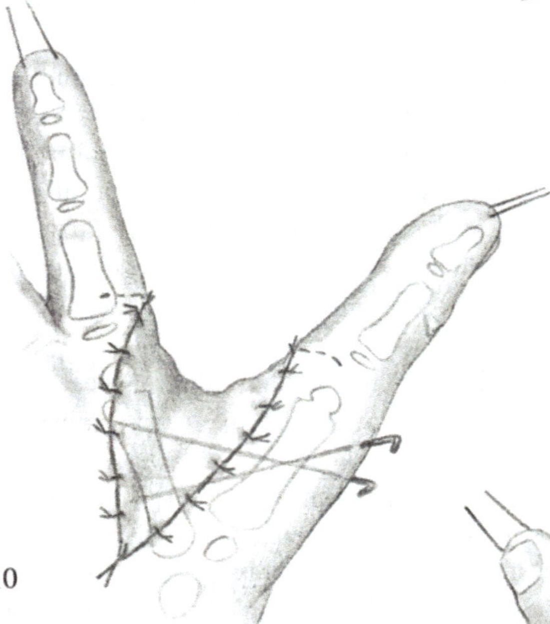

10

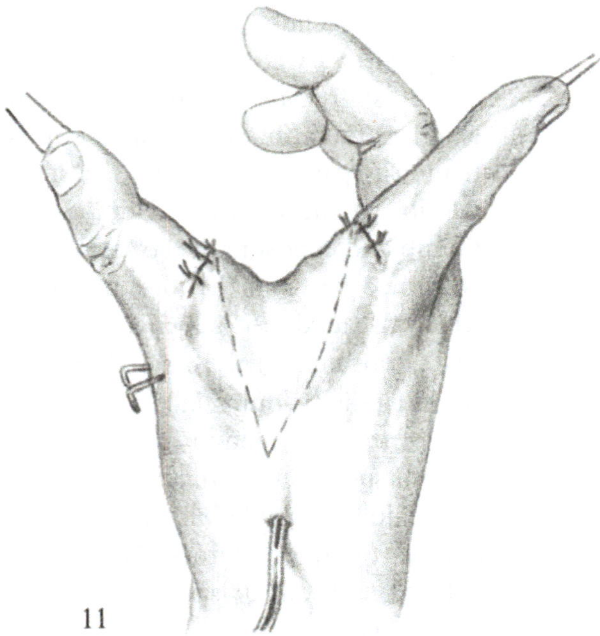

11

4.2.3 Second-Degree Thumb Hypoplasia with Dysplasia of the First Metacarpophalangeal Joint and Hypo- or Aplasia of M. Opponens

Goal of Surgery

Improvement of the rotatory alignment of the Ist ray and the m. opponens function (opponens plasty modified after THOMPSON and BUNNELL), stabilization of the first MP joint.

Fig. 1 General view and incision.

A satisfactory web space has been formed during previous surgery (Sects. 4.2.1 and 4.2.2).

Each leash of the superficial flexor tendon is transected through a small transverse incision at the level of the middle flexor crease of the ring finger. A second palmar incision at the level of the fourth metacarpal head allows its retraction. The tendon leashes should not be transected too close or too far from their point of insertion. In the first instance hyperextension at the PIP joint due to joint capsule weakness has to be expected. A flexion contracture of this joint may occur in the second instance, as the excessively long tendon stumps have a tendency to scar down (joint in flexion!)

A third curvilinear incision is made over the palmar–ulnar aspect of the wrist joint. The tendon is identified, pulled through the lig. carp. transversum, and wrapped in a wet sponge.

A distally based portion of the tendon of the m. flexor carpi ulnaris of 2–2.5 cm length is then obtained and a loop is formed through which the ring finger flexor tendon is passed. It is then directed toward the Ist ray. Closure of the transverse incision at the IVth ray. Next, S-shaped incision over the extensor surface of the thumb and exposure of the soft tissues at the first MP joint. A subcutaneous tunnel is formed between the loop at the pisiform bone and the first MP joint, through which the tendon is advanced.

The periosteum of the distal diaphysis of the first metacarpal bone is then removed. A drill hole 3–4 mm in diameter is made in the frontal plane of the bone. One half of the split tendon is passed from radial to ulnar. The thumb is then brought into its position of function, and the tendon part is sutured to the ulnar side of the joint capsule which may have to be reefed. The other half of the tendon courses obliquely across the extensor aponeurosis to the ulnar side of the first MP joint. There it is sutured to the joint capsule and the extensor tendon after an orange-slice shaped segment has been excised from the capsule (see Fig. 2). The joint capsule is closed with the thinnest atraumatic suture material.

The Ist ray is fixed in a position of function with thin Kirschner wires and the wounds are closed.

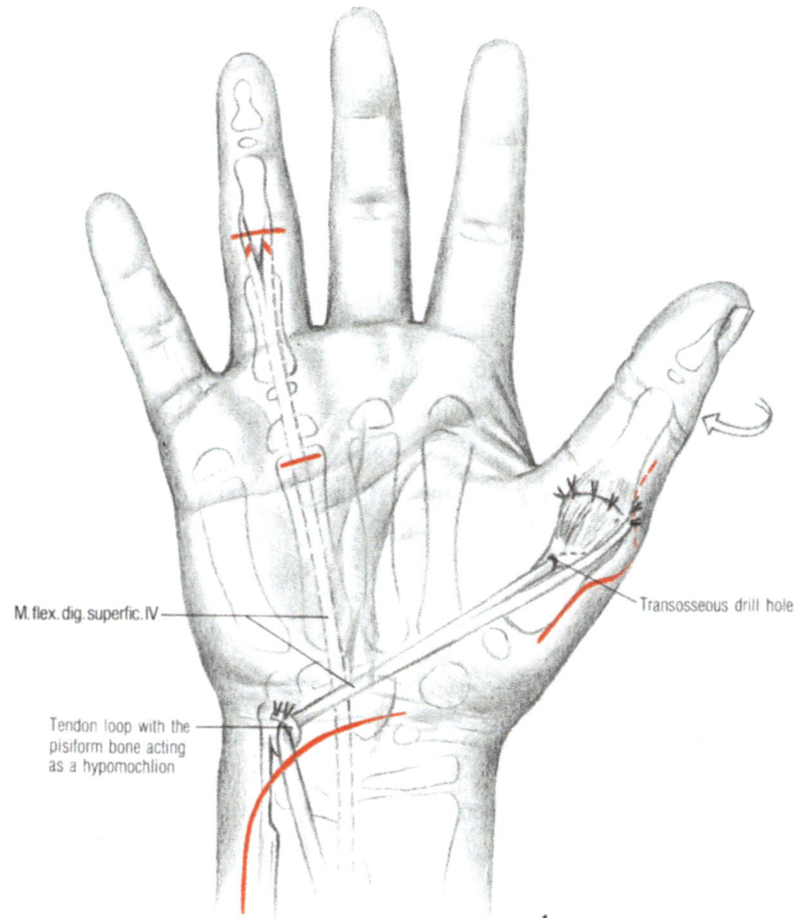
M. flex. dig. superfic. IV
Transosseous drill hole
Tendon loop with the pisiform bone acting as a hypomochlion

1

Fig. 2 Enlarged view of the first MP joint after suture of the tendon parts, dorsal aspect.

Fig. 3 Same aspect.
Alternative method without transosseous fixation in young children where the bone diameter is too small.

Remarks

The following methods may be required to stabilize the first MP joint:
Reinforcement of the radial collateral ligament with a free tendon graft or by transplanting one half of the mobilized ring finger flexor tendon. The method can also be used for reinforcing the ulnar collateral ligament.
Formation of a second drill hole distal to the epiphyseal plate of the proximal phalanx for repassage of part of the tendon.
Arthrodesis after growth has ceased.

Postoperative Care

Long-arm cast for 3 weeks with the thumb in abduction and opposition and the MP joint in minimal flexion. Cast change after 2 weeks. After 3 weeks, institution of cautious exercise therapy, protection with an opponens splint at night and during nonexercise periods.

Movements of the first MP joint have to be avoided initially. Increasing activities 8 weeks after surgery (i.e., pinch exercise).

Errors and Their Consequences

E. The epiphyseal plate has been damaged while drilling the bone.
C. Growth disturbance.

E. The radial part of the tendon courses distal to the first MP joint.
C. Flexion deformity may develop.

E. One tendon segment has been sutured to the extensor aponeurosis.
C. Extension deformity of the first MP joint is possible.

E. The first MP joint has been inadequately immobilized.
C. Instability persists.

E. The method has been employed in the presence of a more pronounced dysplasia of the joint.
C. Reinforcement plasty of the lig. coll. uln. is unsuccessful.

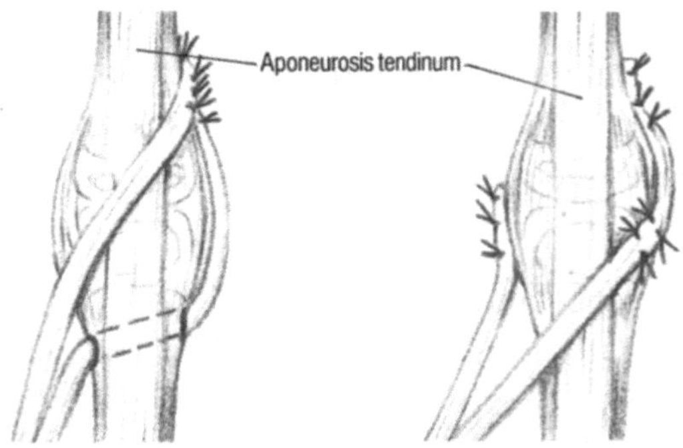

2 3

E. The transposed flexor tendon has been sutured with insufficient or excessive tension.

C. Opposition is insufficient, movement of the first metacarpal is limited.

E. The flexor tendon leashes of the IVth ray have been transected too long or too short.

C. Distal tendon stumps scar down and limit motion; a hyperextension deformity of the PIP joint can develop.

4.2.4 Second/Third-Degree Thumb Hypoplasia (Index Finger Pollicization; Incision According to Blauth)

Goal of Surgery

Amputation of the thumb with insufficient function. Transposition of the shortened index finger with its neurovascular supply as a thumb substitute, formation of a smooth web space (see also Sect. 4.5.7).

Figs. 1,2 Preoperative appearance and incision.
The *dotted areas* of flaps *(2)* and *(3)* will be excised later, as will the *hatched bony elements*. Flap *(1)* has to be of sufficient size: the distance between the tip and the basis of the flap has to be *at least* as long as the length of the incision on the extensor surface of the index finger.
[Lately we have placed the semicircular incision on the palmar side of the index finger even further distal, approximately equidistant from the flexor creases at the MP and PIP joints (not shown, see Sect. 4.5.7). The cosmetic results are even better.]

Fig. 3 Dorsoradial aspect after preparation of the skin flaps.
The main veins of the index finger have to be spared, including those on the dorsal side! Larger vessels should be ligated and not coagulated (see figure). The tendons of the hypoplastic thumb should be transected in such a manner as to permit their use at a later stage.

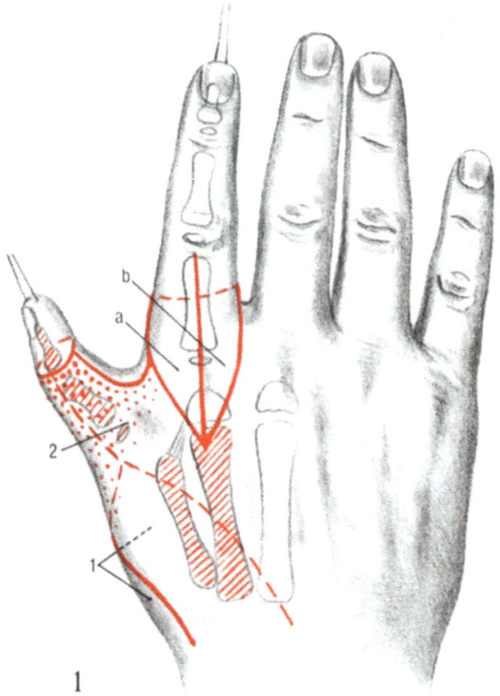
b
a
2
1

1

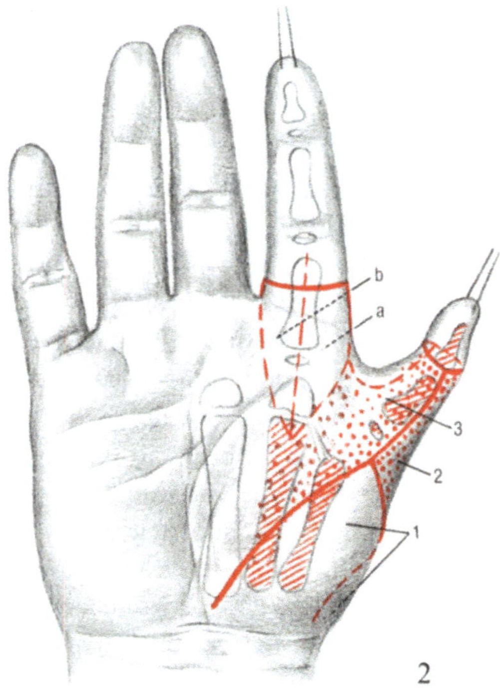
b
a
3
2
1

2

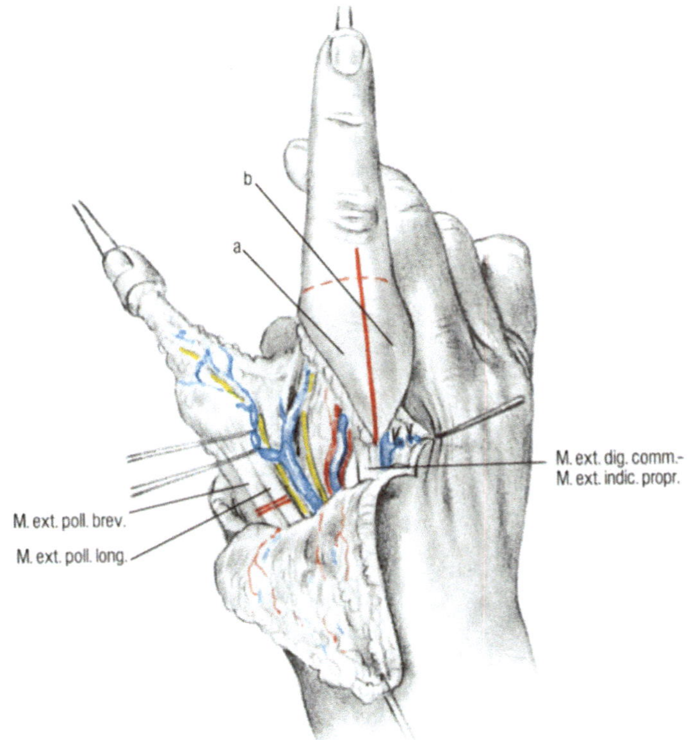
b
a
M. ext. dig. comm.-
M. ext. indic. propr.
M. ext. poll. brev.
M. ext. poll. long.

3

Fig. 4 Palmar aspect after preparation of the flaps and visualization of the neurovascular bundles.

After the large skin flap *(3)* at the palm of the hand has been raised, one continues to dissect strictly at the palmar aponeurosis. The vessels and nerves are exposed step by step. The branches of the two palmar arteries of the index finger coursing to the middle finger and the hypoplastic thumb are ligated. Interfascicular splitting of the common nerve trunk or transection of its ramus to the thumb slightly distal to its bifurcation. Surgical telescopes have to be used during this step.

Possible insertion anomalies of the short muscles of the hand have to be expected. (The figure shows a broad muscle which courses from the tendon of the m. flex. poll. long. to the radial lateral band of the index finger: m. lumbr. II?)

Skin flap *(1)* has to be carefully mobilized proximally beyond its base. Its afferent and efferent vessels have to be spared. If this important step is omitted the flap will kink easily after the index finger has been transplanted (see Figs. 7 and 8). Impaired circulation will result.

Fig. 5 After amputation of the thumb and its metacarpal bone.

The tendons of the mm. interossei have been transected. After dissecting the lateral bands from the extensor aponeurosis (not demonstrated) to the level of the PIP joint, one transects the two extensor tendons proximal to the MP joint of the index finger, and their proximal stumps are separated.

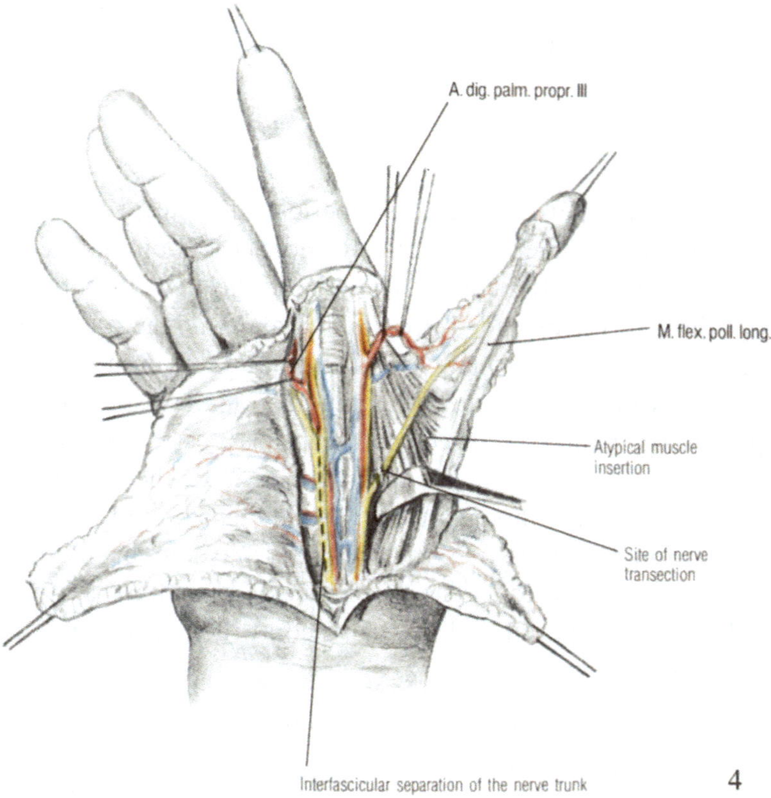
A. dig. palm. propr. III
M. flex. poll. long.
Atypical muscle insertion
Site of nerve transection
Interfascicular separation of the nerve trunk

4

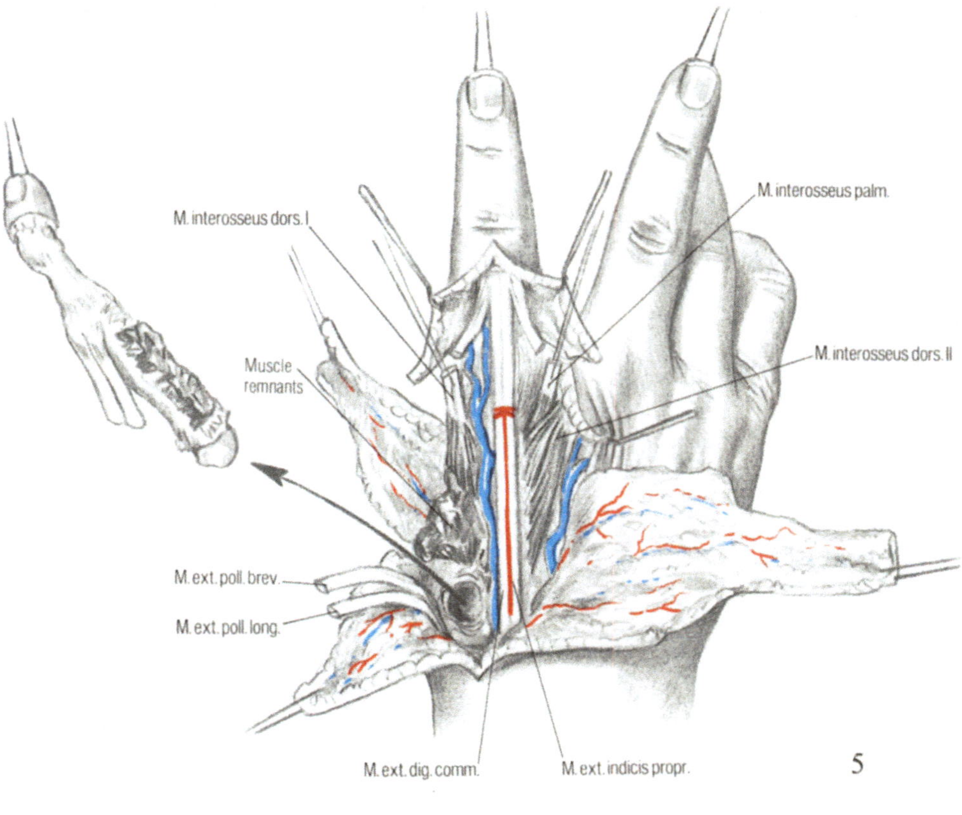
M. interosseus dors. I
M. interosseus palm.
Muscle remnants
M. interosseus dors. II
M. ext. poll. brev.
M. ext. poll. long.
M. ext. dig. comm.
M. ext. indicis propr.

5

4.2.4 Second/Third-Degree Thumb Hypoplasia (Index Finger Pollicization; Incision According to Blauth)

Fig. 6 The second metacarpal is resected subperiosteally except for its head. (If the phalanges of the index finger are relatively short, parts of the metacarpal bone close to its basis may be left behind. The tip of the new thumb should be opposite the distal third of the extended proximal phalanx of the middle finger.)

The remaining epiphyseal plate is curetted and the mm. interossei are carefully mobilized proximally without damaging the small vessels and nerves. Next, the lig. capit. transversum is transected. Now it is possible to move the index finger away from the IIIrd ray and to approximate it to the carpal bones. During this step it is particularly important to observe tension on the palmar vessels and nerves: additional soft tissue structures may have to be mobilized or transected to avoid abnormal tension. The radial distal carpal bones (ossa trapezium and trapezoideum) are exposed and decorticated at their distal ends to create a proper bed for the bone implantation.

Figs. 7a,b Prior to the transposition of the index finger it is advisable to extend the head of the second metacarpal in its joint capsule dorsally as far as possible. It is held in this position with a small one-pronged hook and is fixed with a fine transarticular Kirschner wire (Fig. 7b). In this way one avoids unsightly hyperextension deformities of the future first carpometacarpal joint (Buck-Gramcko 1966, 1968, 1971).

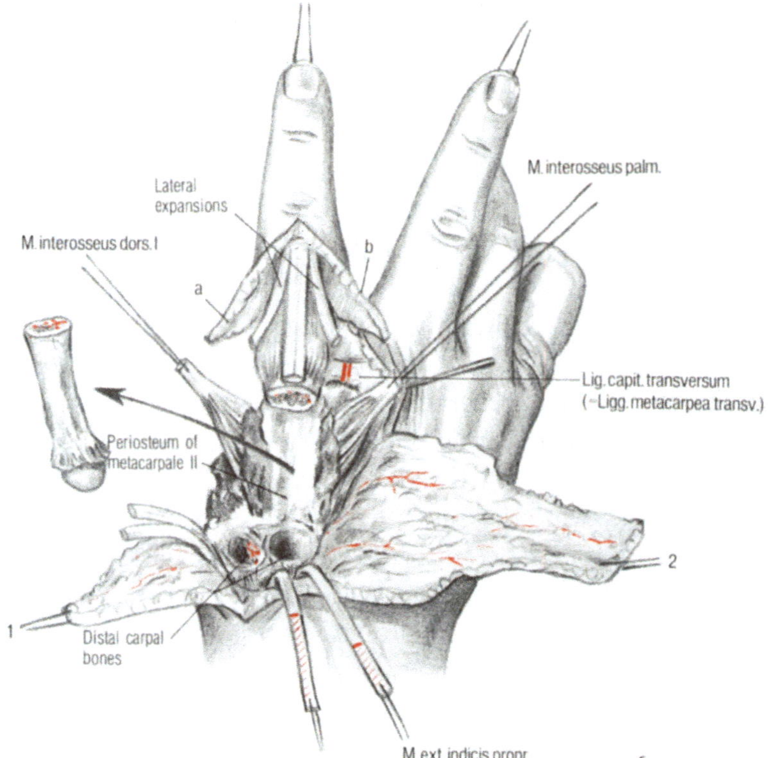

Lateral expansions
M. interosseus palm.
M. interosseus dors. I
b
a
Lig. capit. transversum
(=Ligg. metacarpea transv.)
Periosteum of metacarpale II
2
1
Distal carpal bones
M. ext. dig. comm.
M. ext. indicis propr.

6

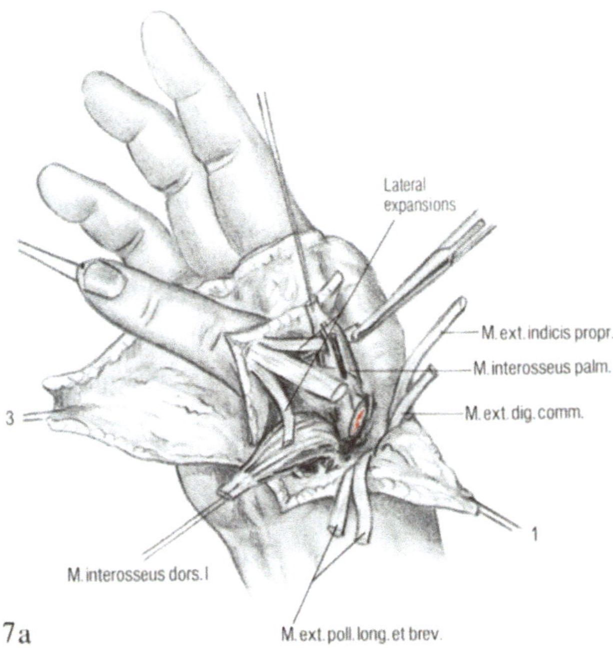

Lateral expansions
M. ext. indicis propr.
M. interosseus palm.
3
M. ext. dig. comm.
1
M. interosseus dors. I
M. ext. poll. long. et brev.

7a

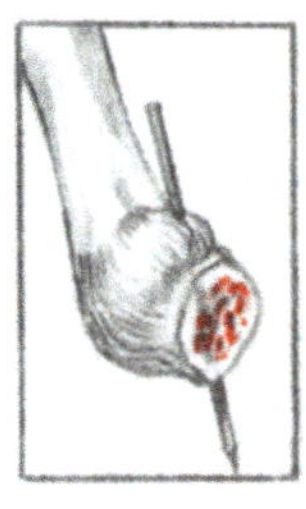

7b

Fig. 8 Position after transposition of the index finger.

The index finger is fixed on the decorticated carpal bones in 130–140° rotation and 25–30° abduction. The transarticular Kirschner wire is advanced proximally into the carpal bones. A second Kirschner wire may have to be employed after final adjustment of the position of the finger. (The position and length of the wires should allow their easy removal at a later date.) The mobilized lateral expansions are sutured to their respective interosseous muscles. This is accomplished by pulling the tendinous expansions through the muscle bellies and suturing them into themselves. Excessive musculature is carefully removed. The *m. interosseus dorsalis I* connected with the radial tendinous expansion acts as an opponens; the *m. interosseus palmaris I* connected to the ulnar expansion acts as the adductor of the future thumb (Buck-Gramcko 1966, 1969, 1971). The tendon of the *m. ext. ind. propr.* is sutured under proper tension (distal phalanx extended) into the extensor aponeurosis of the index finger. The tendon of the *m. ext. dig. comm.* of the index finger will act as an abductor. It will be properly sutured to the thumb ray, as will the two extensor tendons of the amputated thumb. It is unnecessary to shorten the flexor tendons as they will adapt to the new length of the finger within a few weeks.

The tourniquet is released and all bleeding is carefully stopped. The status of circulation will determine whether flap (*2*) or (*3*) is to be used for formation of the web space. Flap (*1*) is sutured in place, the other flaps are properly shaped, closed suction drainage is employed (and the wound edges are closed).

Figs. 9, 10 Postoperative appearance after skin closure.

In this case the commissure is formed by the (properly shaped) dorsal flap (*2*). For demonstration purposes the thumb has not been positioned in optimal functional alignment.

Postoperative Care

The palm and web space are loosely packed with fluffs and a small (5 cm) elastic bandage is applied. The hand is elevated in a well-padded long-arm cast. The dressing is split to the skin 1–2 h after surgery. The first dressing change is made after 6–8 days. Application of a long-arm cast which incorporates the IP joint of the thumb (which opposes the distal phalanx of the ring finger) after swelling has subsided (and sutures have been removed). This may have to be done under anesthesia to permit slight positional adjustments. About $2^1/_2$ weeks after surgery the cast should be reduced to allow exercise of the IP joint. The cast should be removed 4–5 weeks after surgery, depending on the x-ray evaluation. The Kirschner wires are removed at that time and a removable short-arm splint with the

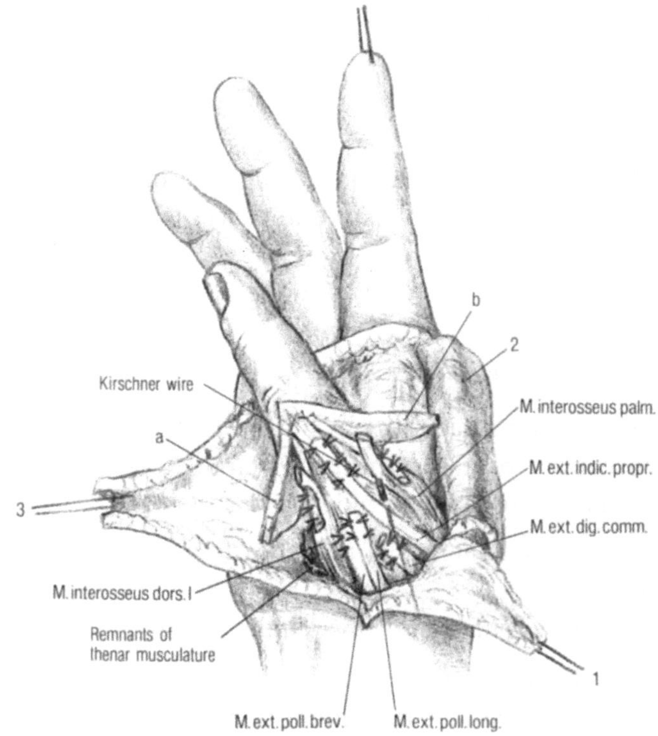
b
2
Kirschner wire
M. interosseus palm.
a
M. ext. indic. propr.
3
M. ext. dig. comm.
M. interosseus dors. I
Remnants of
thenar musculature
1
M. ext. poll. brev.
M. ext. poll. long.

8

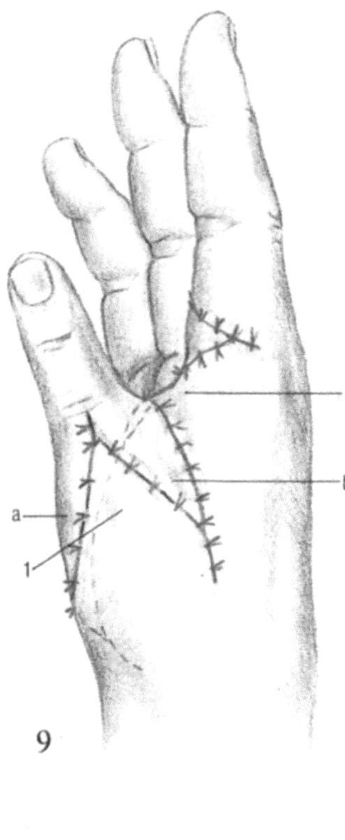
2
b
a
1

9

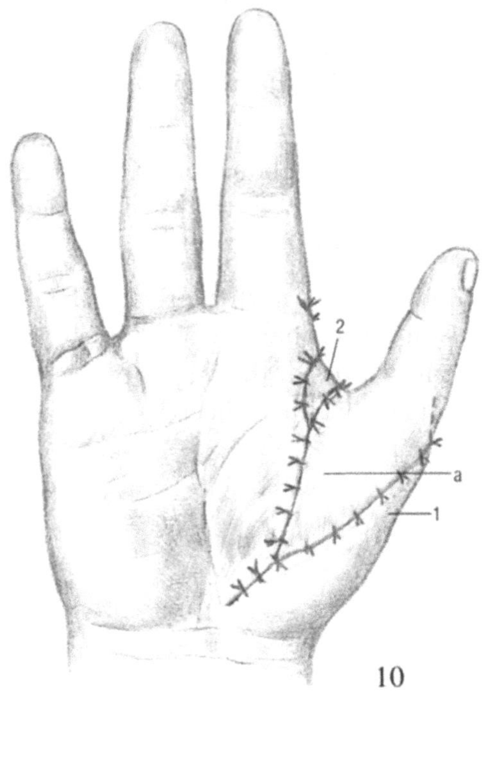
2
a
1

10

thumb in the position of function is applied. In- and out-patient physiotherapy for several weeks. An exercise instruction sheet is given to the patient or his parents (see below).

Errors and Their Consequences

E. The proximal triangular flap has not been undermined beyond its basis.
C. The flap cannot be raised properly, circulatory impairment may develop, the transposed mm. interossei may bulge under the skin.

E. The volar vessels and nerves of the index finger have been damaged, strangulated, or stretched.
C. Sensibility and circulation of the "index finger thumb" is impaired.

E. Tendons have been sutured under improper tension.
C. Muscular imbalance and functional impairment. Malposition will subsequently occur.

E. The distal growth plate has not been curetted.
C. The second metacarpal bone is not short enough.

E. The angulation of the metatarsal head of the MP joint has been omitted.
C. An unsightly hyperextension deformity of the first carpometacarpal joint remains or will develop.

E. Rotation and abduction of the thumb ray is insufficient.
C. Secondary corrective surgical procedures to improve position and function will become necessary.

E. Skin sutures, particularly of the proximal triangular flap, are under tension. The skin sutures have not been removed and resutured without tension (on occasion with an additional thick-split thickness skin-transplant).
C. Skin necrosis (even in cases of slight tension), infections, and scar tissue formation may occur.

Instruction sheet for index finger-thumb exercises (see Blauth 1969, Fig. 2).

1. Your new thumb says "hello" to each finger one by one. Keep your fingers as straight as possible. Mother will help you if you can't do it yet. She will hold the fingers straight and help the thumb to move. Exercise slowly and carefully. The thumb has to be fully straightened and placed in a hitchhiker's position each time.
2. Turn your hand so you can see your palm. Try to bring your thumb as close as possible to the index finger and then push it as far away as you can.
3. Put your hand on the table. Try to bring your thumb as close as possible to the index finger (forefinger) and then push it as far away as you can.
4. Make a fist; press your thumb as tightly as you can against your index finger. Shake your fist so that your whole arm begins to shake.
5. Take a big glob of Play-dough in your hand. Try to press your thumb and fingers into it until they disappear.
6. Take a small piece of Play-dough and make a ball with it between your thumb and index finger.
7. Grab a bottle or bowling pin between thumb and index finger and swing it, but don't let go.
8. Play with a tennis ball. Throw it to the ground and catch it. Throw it into the air and catch it.
9. Take a broomstick. Put it upright on the floor, let go, and catch it with your new hand before it falls. Clap your hands once and catch it. Can you clap your hands twice or several times and catch it?

Advice for mothers (and physiotherapists).

Each exercise should be repeated several times in succession. Children will tire easily with repetitive exercises and their concentration diminishes quickly. Repetition and exercise time depend on this fact. Exercises should be performed several times daily. A play situation will enhance the will to exercise and the child's concentration. Encouragement and praise are important.

4.2.5 Thumb Aplasia (and Fourth-Degree Thumb Hypoplasia) (Index Finger Pollicization; Incision According to Blauth)

Goal of Surgery

Transposition of the index finger with its neurovascular supply as a thumb substitute and formation of a supple web space.

Figs. 1, 2 Preoperative appearance and incision.
The *dotted areas* of skin will be removed prior to skin closure. A rudimentary thumb should be removed through an additional incision (see also Sect. 4.4.7); afferent thumb vessels have to be ligated. A large portion of the skin of the rudimentary thumb can be removed at the end of the operation. The rest of the operation is similar to the descriptions given in Sects. 4.2.4 and 4.5.7 (see above all text to Fig. 1, Sect. 4.2.4!).

Figs. 3, 4 Postoperative appearance after pollicization.
In this particular case the thumb commissure had been formed with a palmar flap.

Remarks

Fixation of the first metacarpal to the carpal bone can be done by using a transosseous suture with absorbable suture material instead of Kirschner wires. Advantage: no foreign material has to be removed.

Postoperative Care and Errors and Their Consequences

See Sects. 4.2.4, 4.5.7 a.o.

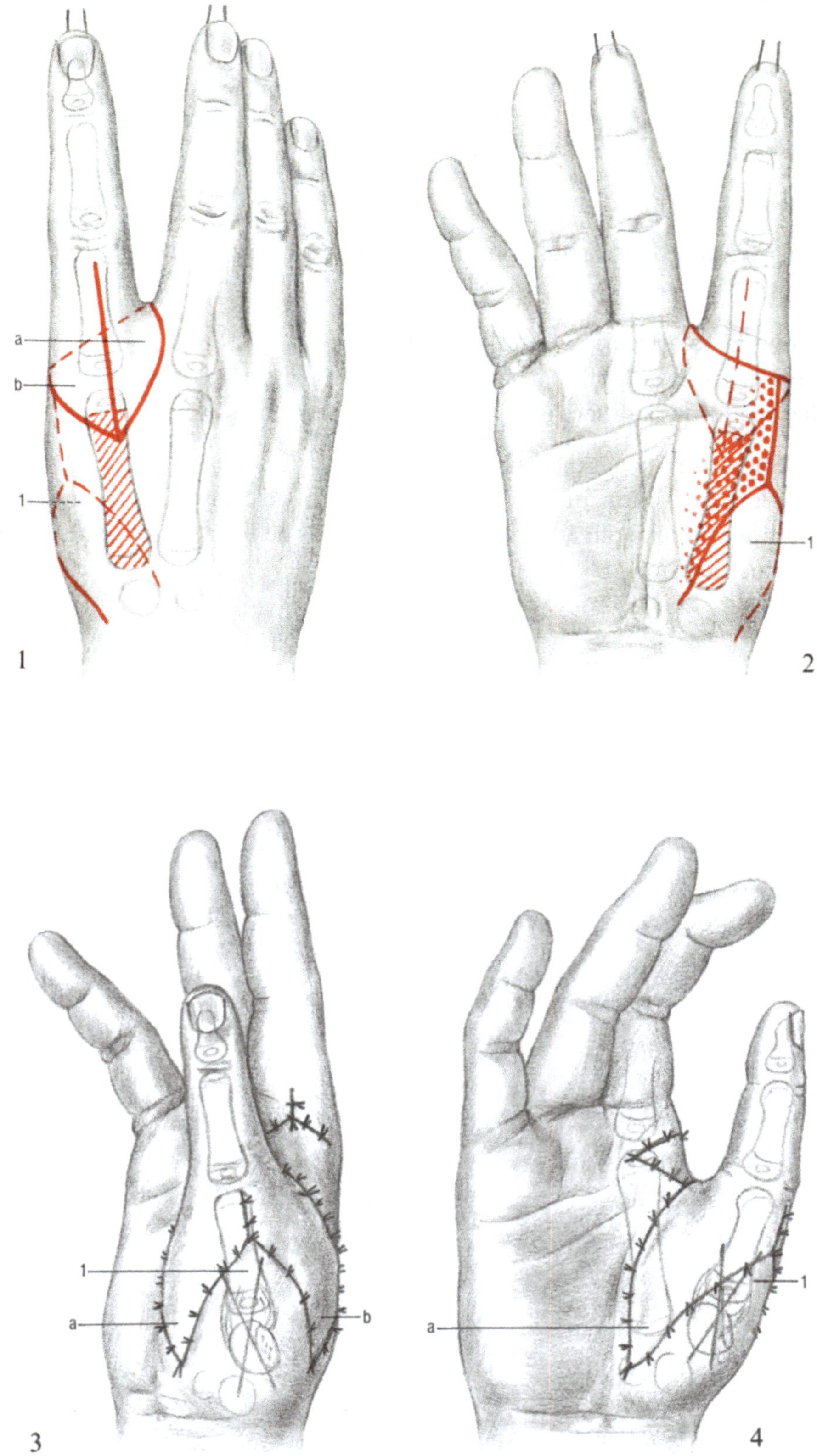
a
b
1
1
2
1
a
b
3
a
1
4

4.2.6 Thumb Aplasia (Index Finger Pollicization; Incision According to Buck-Gramcko)

Goal of Surgery

Transposition of the index finger with its neurovascular supply to create a thumb.

Figs. 1, 2 Preoperative appearance and incision.
The *hatched area* of the metacarpal bone with its epiphyseal plate will be removed. The operation is otherwise similar to that described in Sect. 4.2.4.

Figs. 3, 4 Postoperative appearance after pollicization.
The flexed position of the metacarpal head held by Kirschner wires is visible. Additional thick-split thickness grafts have to be used if the skin sutures are under too much tension.

Postoperative Care and Errors and Their Consequences

See Sects. 4.2.4, 4.2.7 a.o.

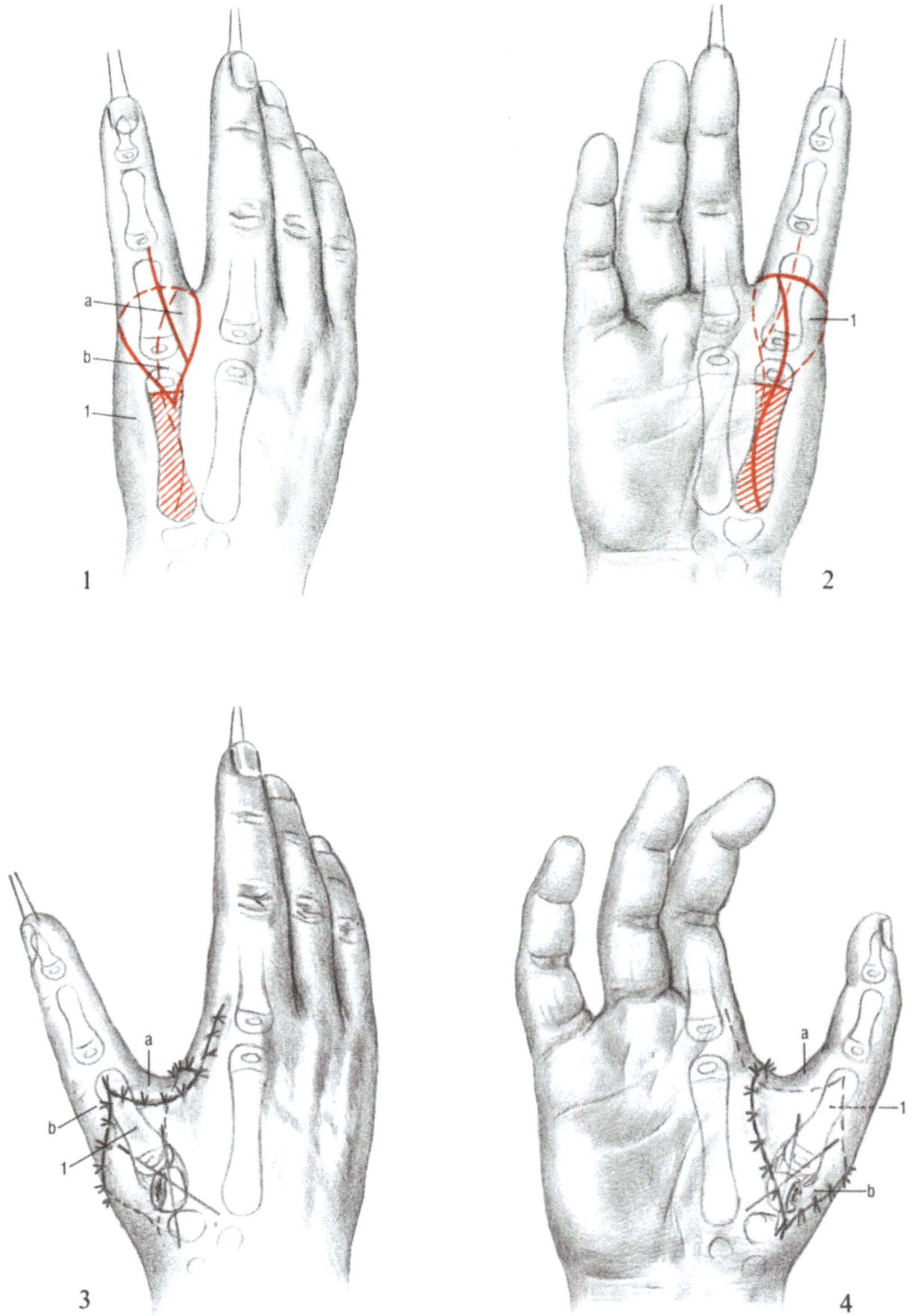
a
b
1
1
2
3
4

4.3 Long Finger Oligodactylies

4.3.1 Oligosyndactyly with Acrosynostosis

Goal of Surgery

Separation of the cutano-osseous syndactyly, excision of the rudimentary middle finger, formation of a web space by employing a dorsal swivel pedicle flap.

Fig. 1 Preoperative appearance and skin incision, dorsal view.
A common nail band from the index to the ring finger is present. The peripherally located skeletal rudiment of the middle finger is fused to the distal phalanx of the ring finger.
The zig-zag incisions have to reach the midline of the dorsal aspect of the index and ring finger. The middle section including the nail bed has to be excised from the nail band (*black hatched area*). The synostosis between the distal phalanges III and IV is osteotomized with a narrow osteotome or a Luer rongeur after it has been exposed subperiosteally. The resection site will be covered with a periosteal graft (from the excised middle finger rudiment) and, if possible, with subcutaneous tissue. The dorsal two-tailed swivel pedicle flap (*a*) extends distally past the midsection of the proximal phalanges.

Fig. 2 Preoperative appearance and incision, palmar view.
Zig-zag incisions are also employed to separate the interdigital space. In this manner one raises skin flaps *(5, 6, 7)* whose tips lay approximately at the same level as the dorsal flaps *(c, d, e)*. The most proximal skin flap *(1)* is located at the palmar aspect of the future web space and will be sutured to the dorsal swivel flap *(a)* (see Fig. 4).

Figs. 3, 4 Postoperative appearance.
The skin flaps are sutured without tension. Thick-split thickness skin transplants *(Tr)* cover the remaining skin defects.

Postoperative Care

See Sect. 2.1.1.4.

Errors and Their Consequences

E. The epiphyseal plate of the distal phalanx of the ring finger has been damaged during the excision of the middle finger rudiment.

E. The bony rudiments of the middle finger have not been exposed subperiosteally.

E. The DIP joint of the ring finger may have been unintentionally entered.
C. The joint may become unstable.
For other errors and their consequences, see Sects. 2.1.2, 2.2.4 a.o.

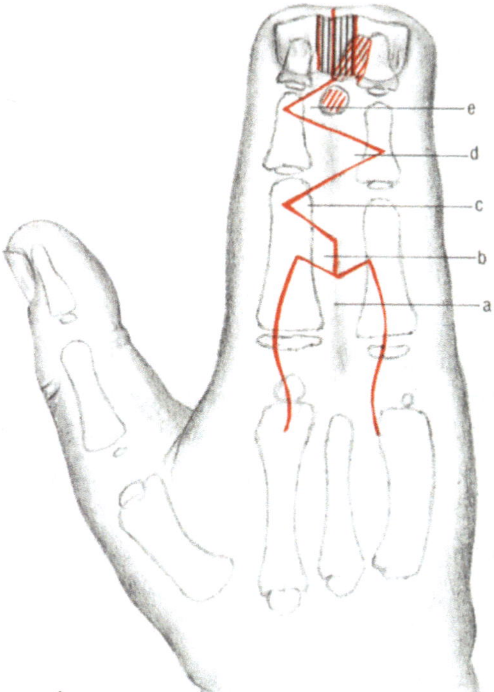
e
d
c
b
a

1

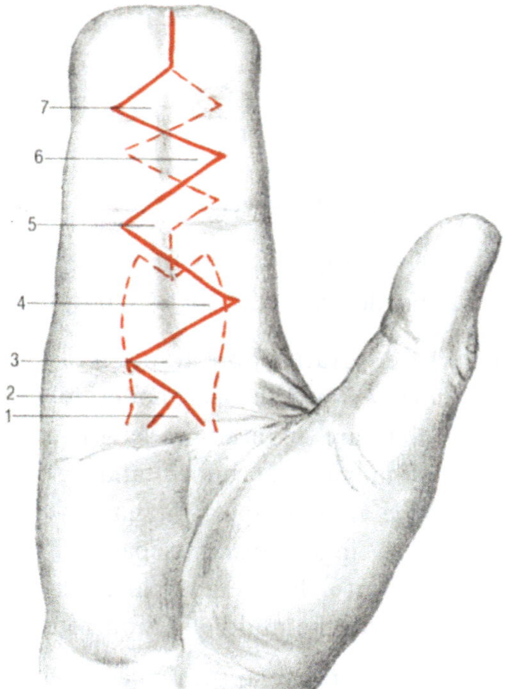
7
6
5
4
3
2
1

2

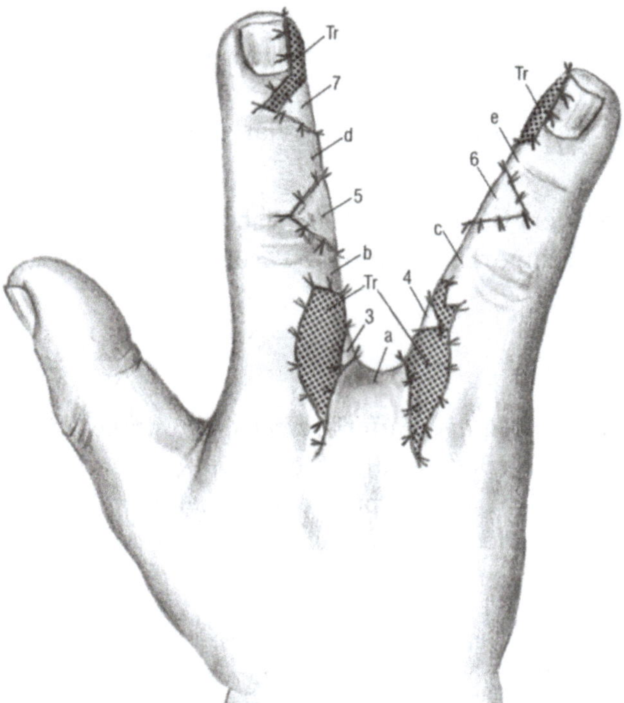
Tr
7
d
5
b
Tr
3
a
4
c
6
e
Tr

3

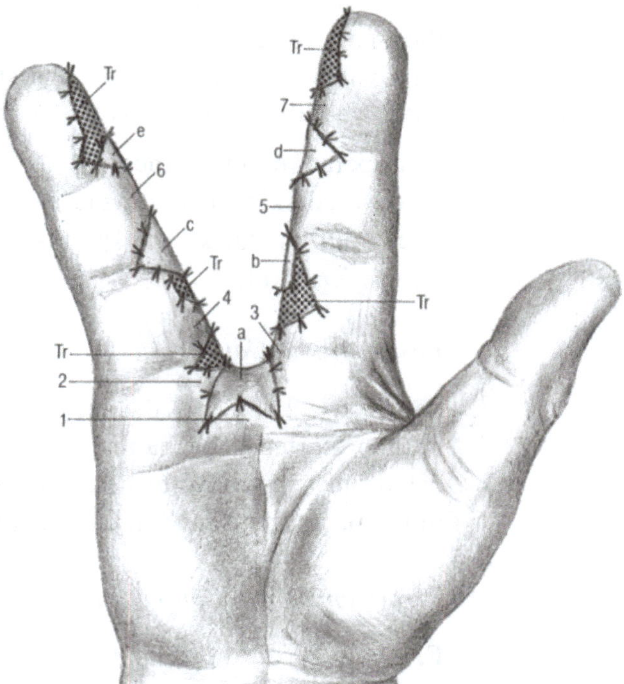
Tr
e
6
c
Tr
4
Tr
2
1
a
3
b
Tr
5
d
7
Tr

4

4.3.2 Oligodactyly with Total Syndactylies ("Spoon Hand")

Goal of Surgery

Creation of a two finger hand to permit pincer movements by separation of the border rays and metacarpolysis

Fig. 1 Preoperative appearance and incision, dorsal view.
This is a case of a moderately severe oligosyndactyly with four recognizable rays that are reduced in length and partially conjoined (so-called spoon hand). To obtain a better understanding of the vascular topography we recommend a preoperative angiogram of the hand.
The finger rays are separated by employing zig-zag incisions extending proximally far into the metacarpal area. The *hatched areas* of bone will have to be excised, as will the middle section of the nail band including its matrix (*dotted area*).

Fig. 2 Preoperative appearance and incision, palmar view.
The interdigital space will be formed from a palmar leaf flap *(1)*. The skin incision ends distally midway between the conjoined fingertips. This leaves enough local skin to cover the distal phalanges. Flaps *(c)* and *(3)* require additional shaping prior to wound closure. The dorsal skin incision is demonstrated by the *broken line*. While dissecting the palmar side, care has to be taken to avoid damage to the main vessels and nerves. We do not show an interoperative picture as it is impossible to give general suggestions due to the great variety of possible soft tissue changes. For details we refer to previous sections, particularly Sect. 2.2.4.

Figs. 3, 4 Postoperative appearance.
Uncovered skin areas on the lateral borders of the fingers have been closed with thick-split thickness transplants *(Tr)*. Temporary fixation is accomplished with Kirschner wires.

Postoperative Care

See Sect. 2.2.4. The Kirschner wires will be removed after 4 weeks. Physiotherapy is then started. The hand is protected by a splint at all other times. A rotatory osteotomy may have to be considered at a later date if pincer movements are suboptimal, as this function cannot always be adequately predicted prior to surgery.

Errors and Their Consequences

E. Damage of the epiphyseal plates of the border rays during excision of the middle rays.
C. Abnormal bony development.

E. No temporary postoperative fixation with Kirschner wires.
C. Instability of the remaining finger joints a.o.

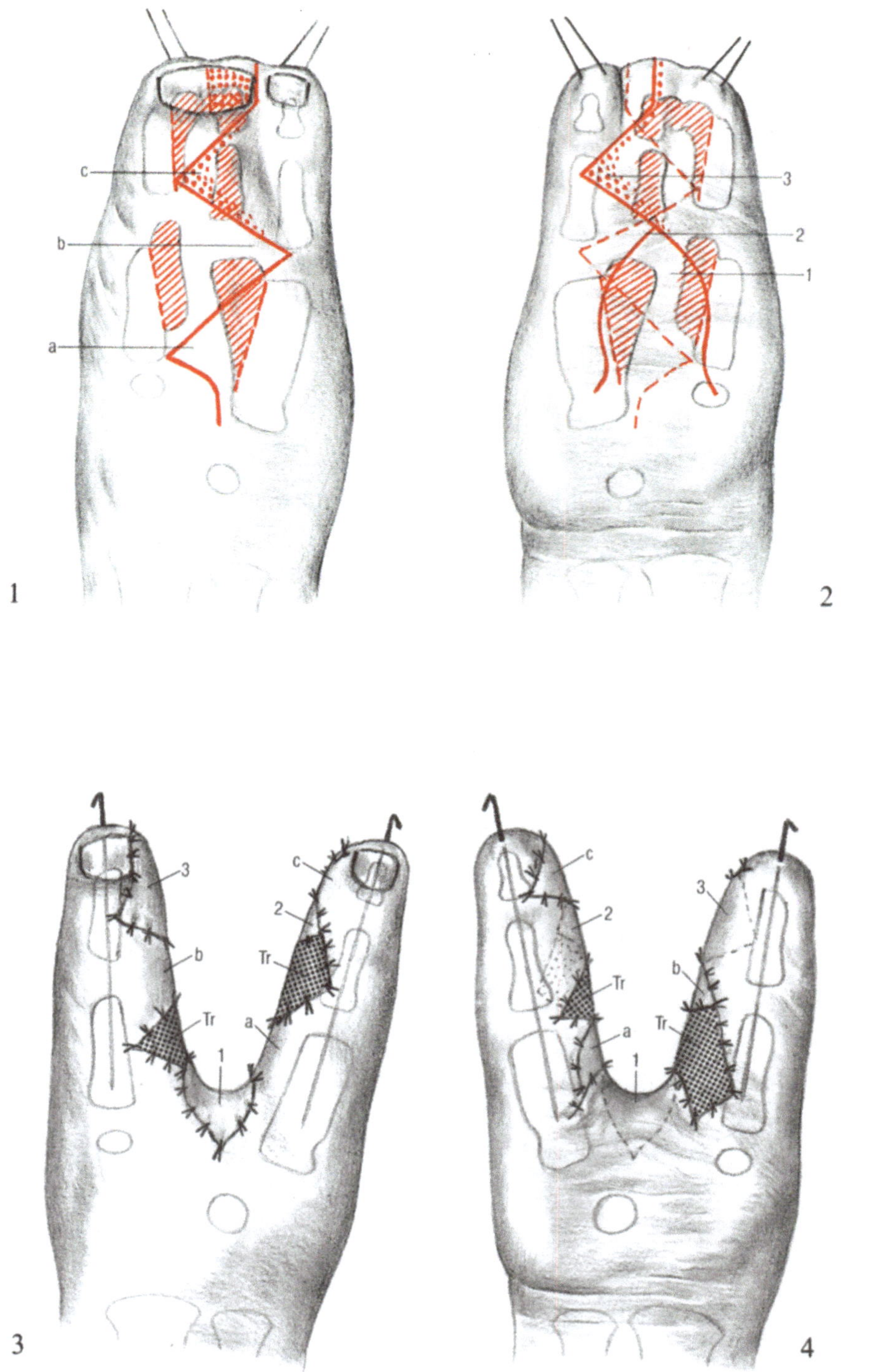
1
c
b
a
2
3
2
1
3
3
b
Tr
1
c
2
Tr
a
4
c
2
Tr
a
1
3
b
Tr

4.3.3 Oligodactyly with Total Syndactyly of the Long Fingers and Acrosynostosis

Goal of Surgery

Separation of the syndactyly by excising the rudimentary middle finger parts. Creation of a wide, supple web space between the remaining long fingers.

Fig. 1 Preoperative appearance and incision, dorsal aspect.
The long finger area is distally cone shaped. Radiologic findings consist of a plump IInd ray, a bifurcation of the ulnar border ray, and fusion of the long fingers at their distal phalangeal areas.
The interdigital space is exposed with a zig-zag incision. The *hatched areas* of bone and, if necessary, medial portions of the common nail band, including the matrix, will later be resected (see Fig. 3).

Fig. 2 Preoperative appearance and incision, palmar aspect.
The web space will be formed with a proximally based palmar swivel pedicle flap *(1)*. The *dotted* radial and ulnar triangles of skin will be excised prior to wound closure to avoid scar formation along the longitudinal axis of the fingers.

Fig. 3 Excision of the dysplastic middle finger rudiment. This is followed by transection of the soft tissue bridge from distal to proximal. The fingers are gradually spread apart during this step. Palmar vessels and nerves have been exposed prior to this (not shown in the figure).

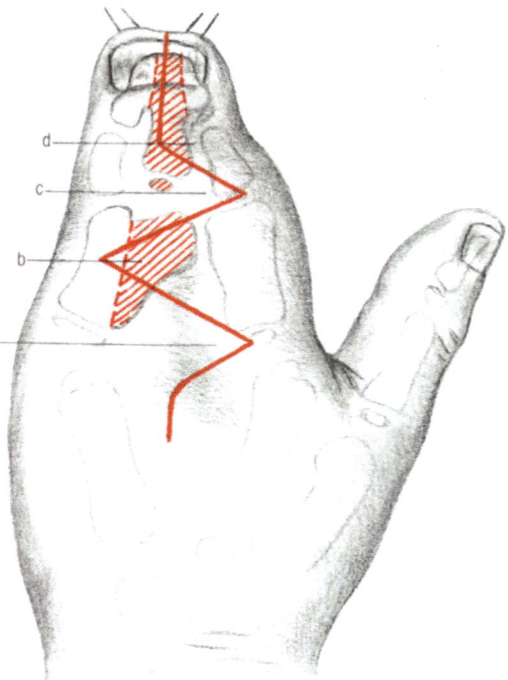

1

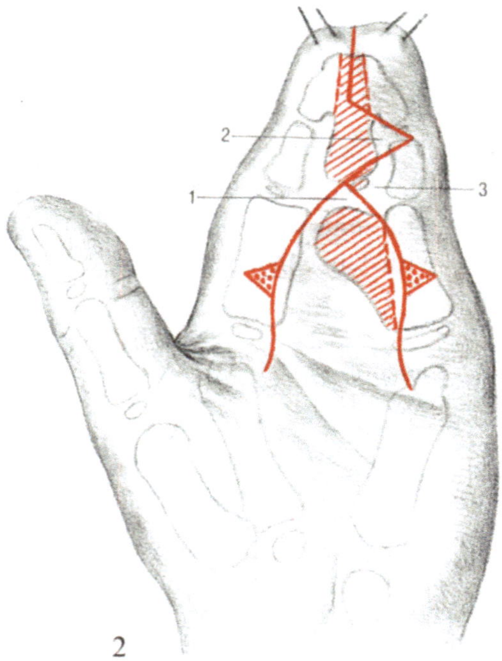

2

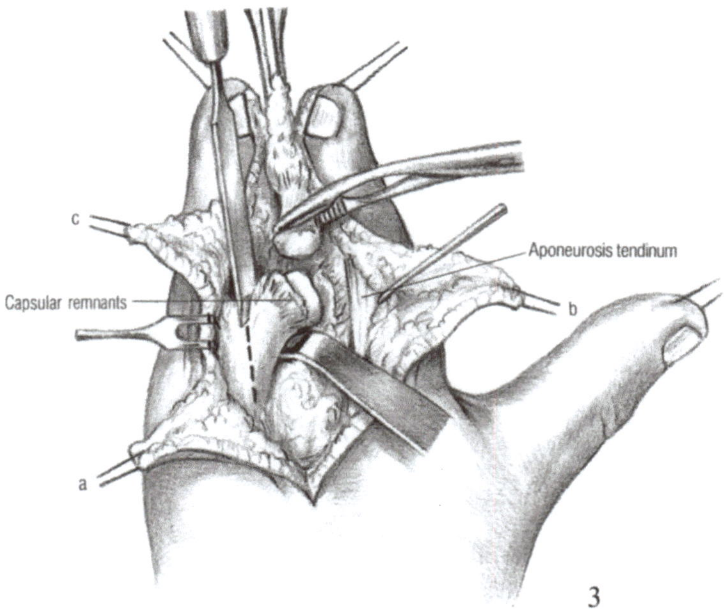

3

Figs. 4,5 Postoperative appearance.
The skin flaps have been sutured. The remaining skin defects have been covered with thick-split thickness skin transplants *(Tr)*. Temporary fixation of the IP joints with Kirschner wires.

Postoperative Care

See Sect. 4.3.2.

Errors and Their Consequences

See Sects. 4.3.2, 2.2.4 a.o.

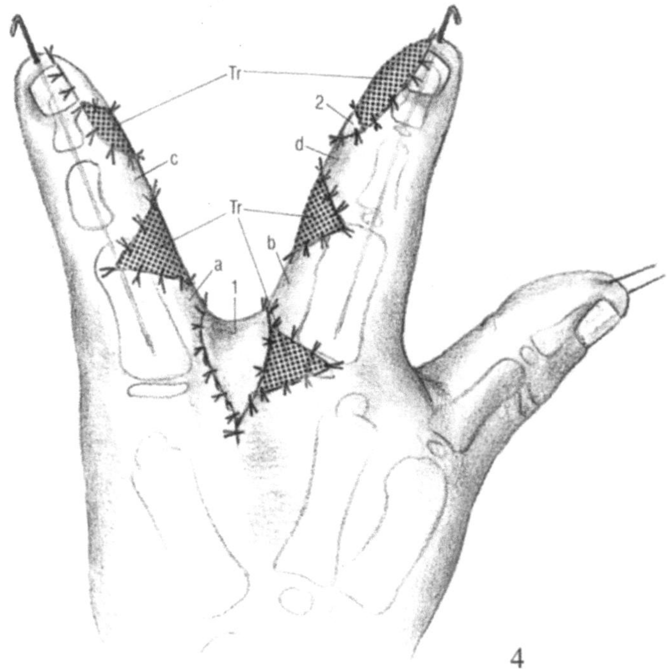

4

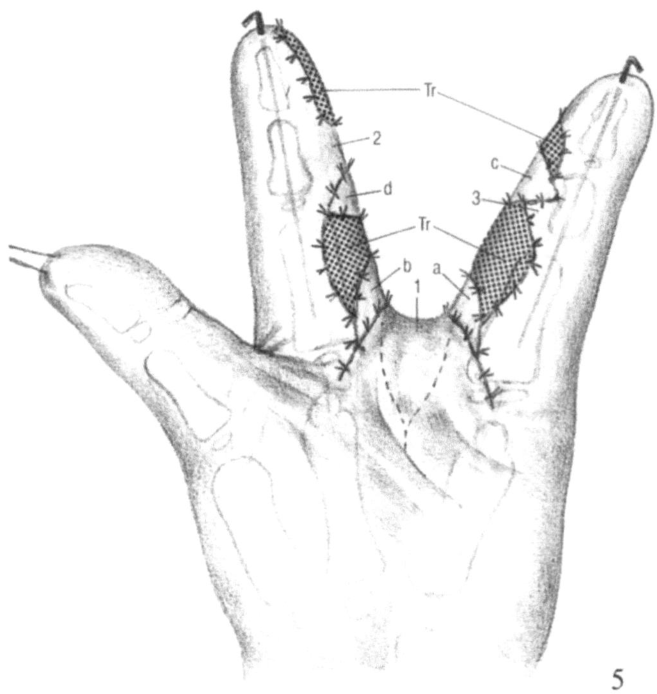

5

4.3.4 Oligodactyly with "Duplication" of a Middle and Distal Phalanx (and Acrosynostosis)

Goal of Surgery

Fusion of the duplicated middle phalanx of the IIIrd finger and excision of one dysplastic distal phalanx.

Fig. 1 Preoperative appearance, dorsal aspect.
Only minimal motion is present at the DIP and PIP joints of the IIIrd finger. *Hatched areas* of bone will have to be resected.

Fig. 2 Skin incision, dorsal aspect of the IIIrd finger.
The *hatched areas* of skin and nail will be excised. Additional trimming of the *dotted area* will be necessary prior to skin closure.

Fig. 3 Long fingers, palmar aspect.
The ulnar skin flap has been raised in a palmar direction. The two flexor tendons are tethered to the middle phalanges by a wide ringlike band. The ulnar neurovascular bundle (a. and n. dig. palm. propr.) remains in the flap.
The hypoplastic flexor tendon of the ulnar bony duplication will be transected (*red line*).

Fig. 4 Dorsal aspect.
One of the extensor tendons has been severed from the ulnar element. The ulnar distal phalanx has been freed. The common capsule of the PIP joint will be opened, the *hatched areas* of bone will be excised.

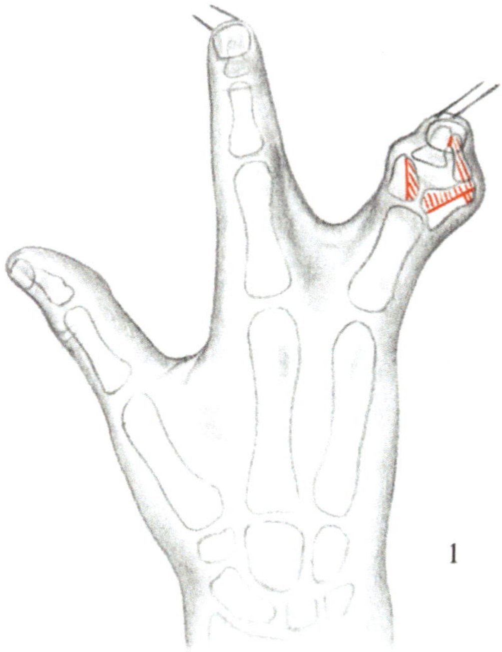

1

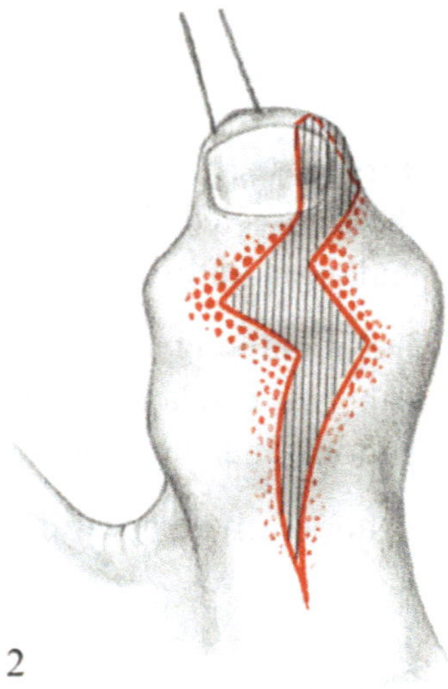

2

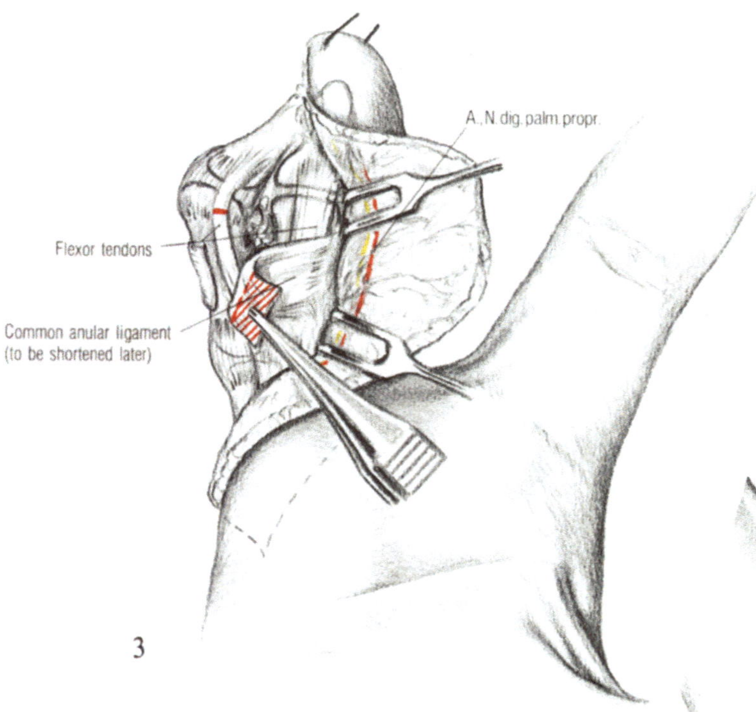
A., N. dig. palm. propr.
Flexor tendons
Common anular ligament
(to be shortened later)

3

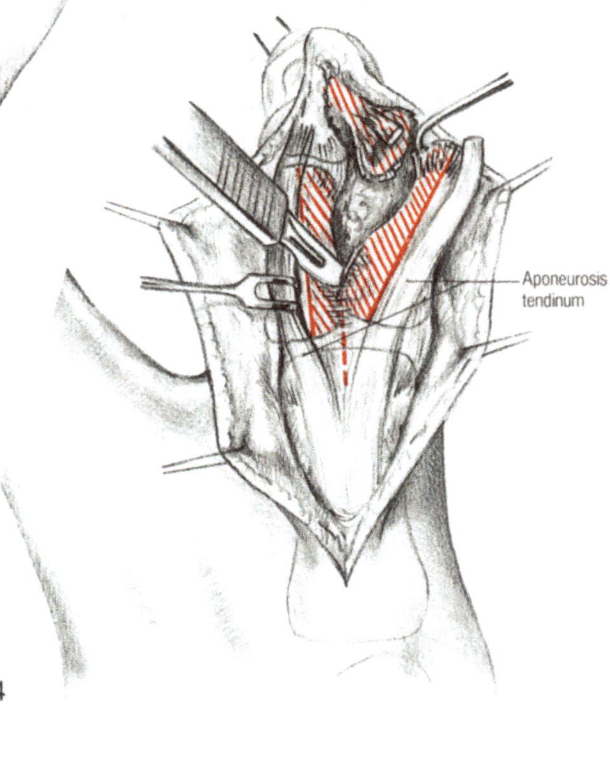
Aponeurosis
tendinum

4

4.3.4 Oligodactyly with "Duplication" of a Middle and Distal Phalanx (and Acrosynostosis)

Fig. 5 Dorsal aspect.
The transected flexor tendon (see *Fig. 3*) is visible. The facing halves of the middle phalanges and the ulnar distal phalanx will be excised.

Fig. 6 The remaining halves of the phalanges are carefully adapted and held together with two cerclage sutures. After this, closure of the capsule and suturing of the tendons and the ring band.

Fig. 7 Postoperative appearance, dorsal aspect.

Postoperative Care

The partial cutaneous syndactyly of the remaining long fingers will be treated at a later date (see Sect. 2.1). A volar short-arm plaster splint in position of function will be worn for (3–) 4–6 weeks.

Errors and Their Consequences

E. The operation is performed long before cessation of bone growth.
C. Crooked growth and reduction in length.

E. Palmar vessels and nerves have been damaged during surgery.

E. The osteotomy sites of the middle phalanx do not fit smoothly.
C. Bony union is unnecessarily delayed.

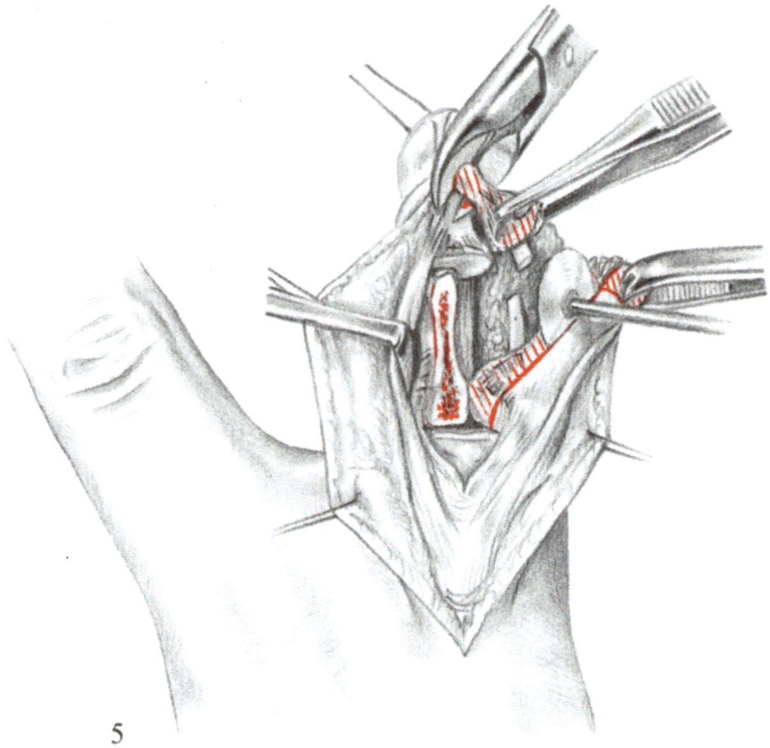

5

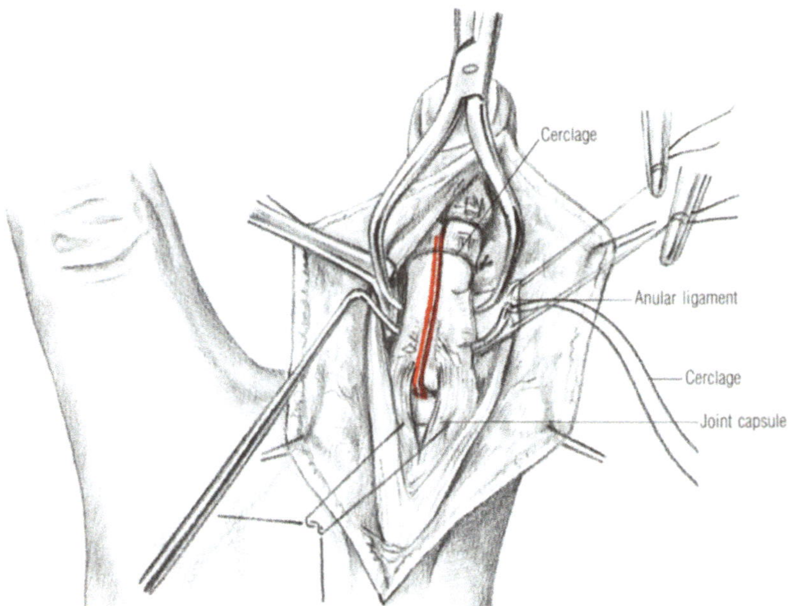

6

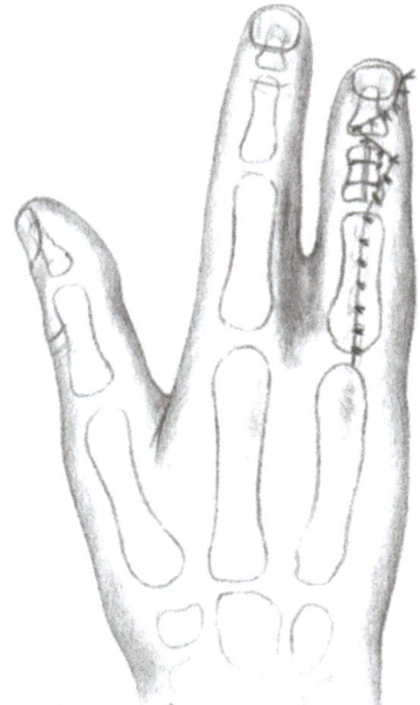

7

4.3.5 Oligodactyly with Synostosis of the Proximal Phalanges

Goal of Surgery

Partial resection and fusion of fingers (modified after BILHAUT-CLOQUET).

Figs. 1,2 Preoperative appearance and incision, dorsal and palmar aspects.
The *hatched areas* of bone will be resected. In this patient marked limitation of motion was present in the IP joints.

Fig. 3 Palmar aspect.
The excess skin will be removed. Vessels and nerves have to be carefully protected during this stage. The dorsal surplus skin will be removed in a similar manner.

Fig. 4 Dorsal aspect.
Removal of the middle portions of bone (see *Fig. 1*) by using a saw and narrow osteotomes. Bennett retractors protect palmar vessels and nerves.

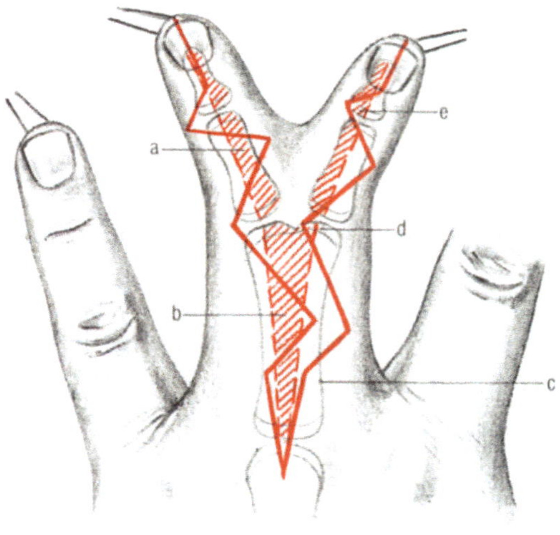

1

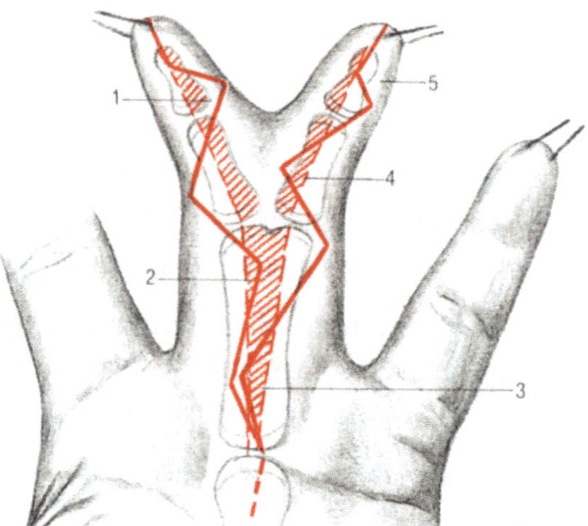

2

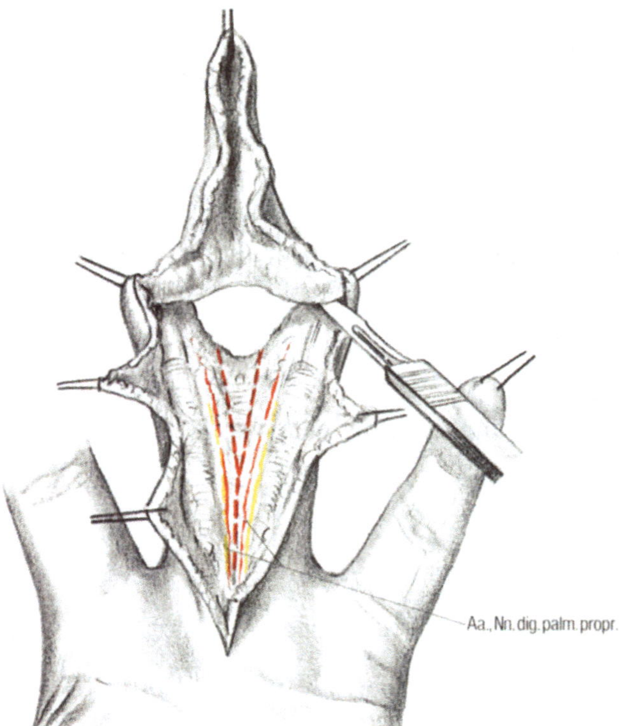

3

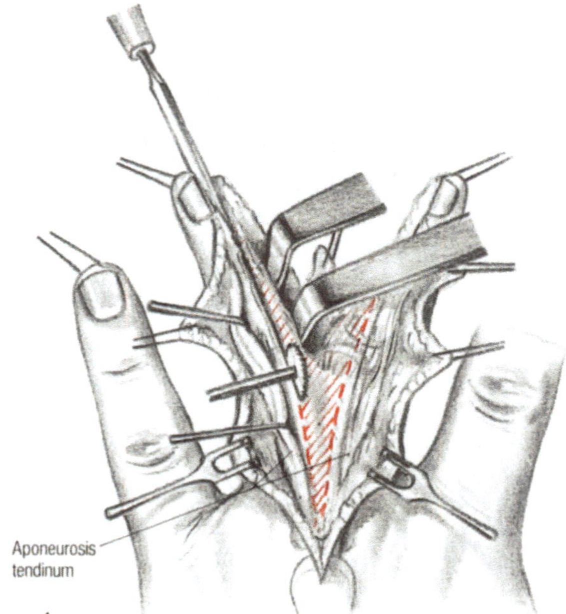

4

Fig. 5 Radial aspect.
The medial sections of the distal and middle phalanges and a central wedge of the proximal phalanx have been removed.

Fig. 6 The remaining phalangeal parts have been adapted. They are held together with a transverse Kirschner wire and cerclages. (Do not employ *wire* cerclages!) Capsule and extensor apparatus is closed with atraumatic suture material.

Figs. 7, 8 Postoperative appearance, palmar and dorsal aspects.

Postoperative Care

Long-arm plaster cast for 3–4 weeks, followed by x-ray control and removal of the Kirschner wire. Physiotherapy is then instituted (active flexion exercises). With this procedure, reduced motion in the IP joints is to be expected.

Errors and Their Consequences

E. Vessels and nerves have been damaged during dissection of the skin flaps and phalanges.

E. Tendons have been damaged.

E. The resected areas of bone are uneven.
C. Adaptation is insufficient, bony union is unnecessarily delayed.

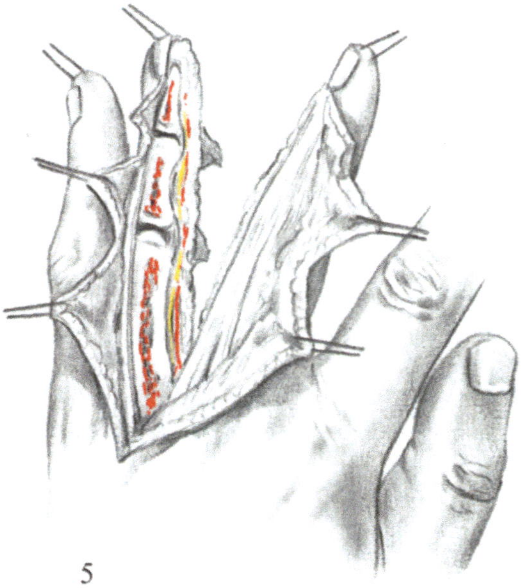

5

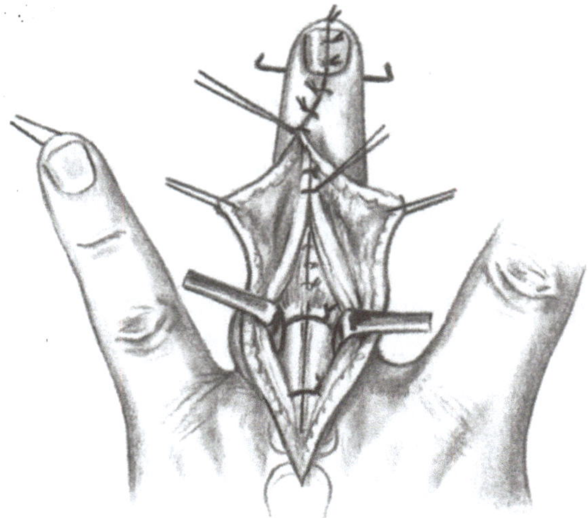

6

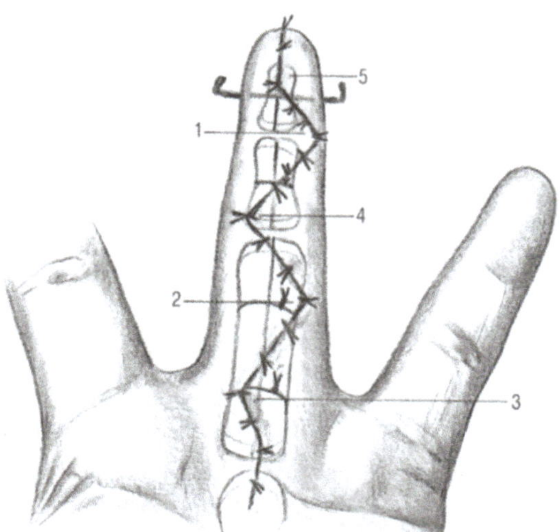

7

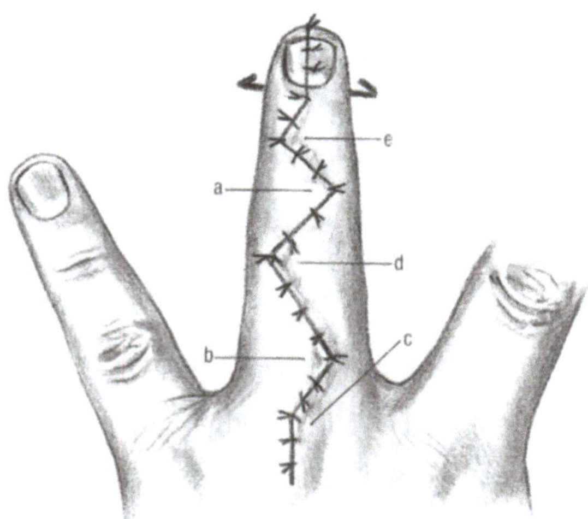

8

4.4 Thumb Duplication

4.4.1 Incomplete Duplication of the Distal Phalanx of the Thumb

Goal of Surgery

Creation of a normally shaped distal phalanx of the thumb by means of a wedge resection according to BILHAUT-CLOQUET.

Fig. 1 Preoperative appearance and incision, dorsal aspect.
So-called butt thumb. The *hatched area* of the synostosis will be excised.

Fig. 2 Wedge excision of the dorsal and palmar skin and of the middle portion of the nail band. Similar excision of the tendon insertion and of the capsule of the common DIP joint.

Fig. 3 The joint capsule has been opened.
Wedge resection of a medial bony segment, using thinnest osteotomes.

Fig. 4 The DIP joint is widely opened. Parts of the flexor tendon are visible. On a trial basis, the cut bony surfaces are placed together. They will then be carefully adapted and smoothed off.

Fig. 5 Postoperative appearance.
The bone fragments have been adapted. They are held together by two small transcutaneous Kirschner wires. Capsule, tendon, and skin have been sutured.

Postoperative Care

Long-arm plaster cast for 4 weeks, followed by x-ray control, removal of the Kirschner wires, and active exercises.

Errors and Their Consequences

E. The bony wedge resection has been performed with inadequate instruments (size of saw or osteotome too large).
C. Bony adaptation is insufficient, infractions may occur.

E. Bones and soft tissues have not been adapted with utmost care.
C. Malposition due to bone growth, scar contractures a.o.

Remarks

It is practically impossible to avoid longitudinal scarring of the nail and irregularities of the paronychia, even with optimal surgical technique. Partial loss of motion of the DIP joint has to be expected.

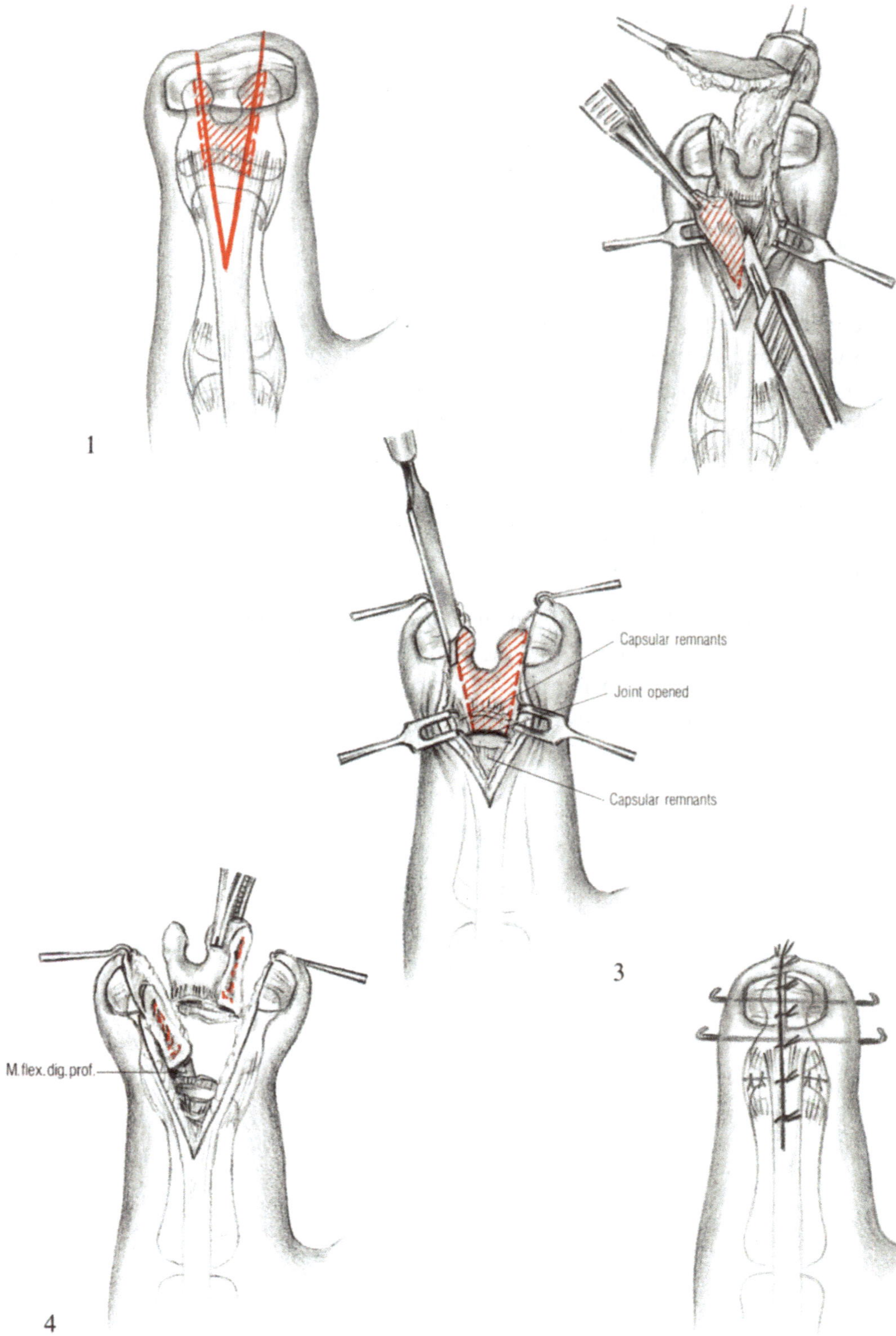
1
2
Capsular remnants
Joint opened
Capsular remnants
3
M.flex.dig.prof.
4
5

4.4.2 Mirrorlike Duplication of the Distal Phalanx of the Thumb (with Widening of Its Proximal Phalanx)

Goal of Surgery

Creation of a normal-appearing thumb by wedge resection (according to BILHAUT-CLOQUET).

Fig. 1 Preoperative appearance and incision, dorsal aspect.
Only minimal mobility is present in the IP joint of the thumb. Therefore in this situation one can, as an exception, employ the outlined incision, which will result in a longitudinal scar along the finger axis past the IP joint. *Hatched areas* of bone will be excised.

Fig. 2 A triangular area of skin has been excised on the dorsal and palmar side.
The extensor aponeurosis has been incised longitudinally and pushed off laterally. The IP joint has been opened.

Fig. 3 The width of the thumb is diminished by partial excision of the distal phalanges and by a wedge resection from the common proximal phalanx. The palmar soft tissues are protected by a Bennett retractor.
Narrow osteotomes and saws with thin blades have to be used for the osteotomy.

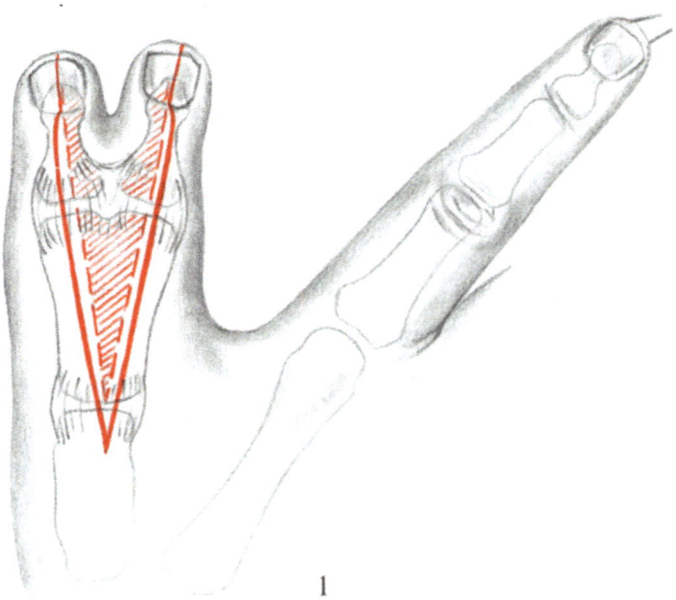

1

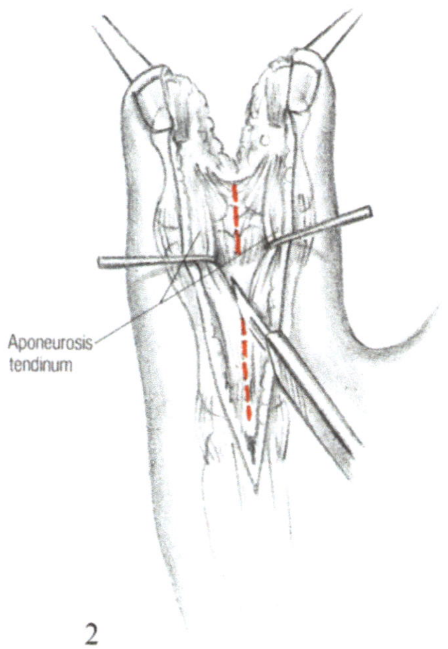

2

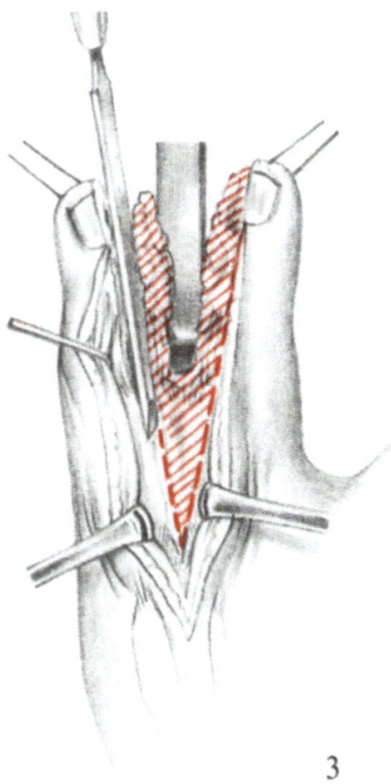

3

4.4.2 Mirrorlike Duplication of the Distal Phalanx of the Thumb (with Widening of Its Proximal Phalanx)

Fig. 4 The joint surface (*) of the first metacarpal bone is visible in the depth of the wound. A cerclage is placed subperiosteally around the halves of the proximal phalanx (the figure shows a wire cerclage, but we generally prefer *plastic* suture material, which does not have to be removed at a later date).

Fig. 5 The resected areas are held together by employing transverse transcutaneous Kirschner wires (at the proximal phalanx, near the cerclage). The capsules and the extensor aponeurosis are closed. Careful alignment of the nail segments and skin closure are the last steps of the operation.

Fig. 6 Postoperative appearance.

Postoperative Care and Errors and Their Consequences

See Sect. 4.4.1.

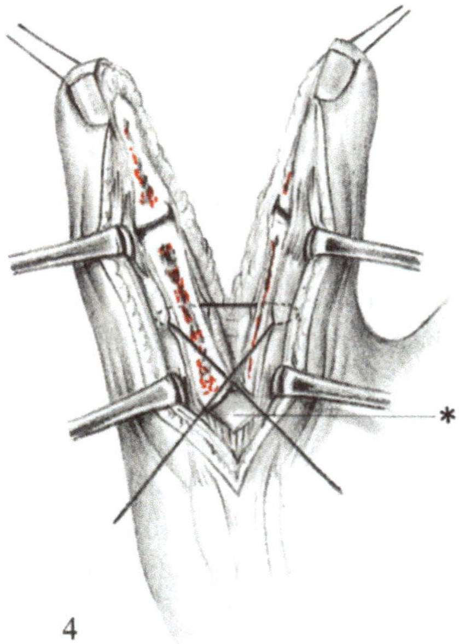

4

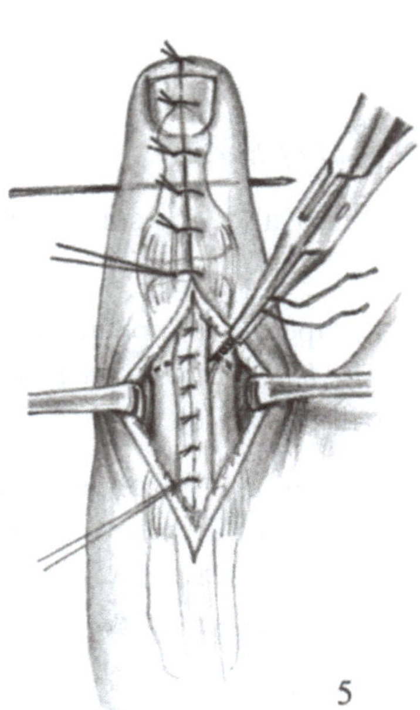

5

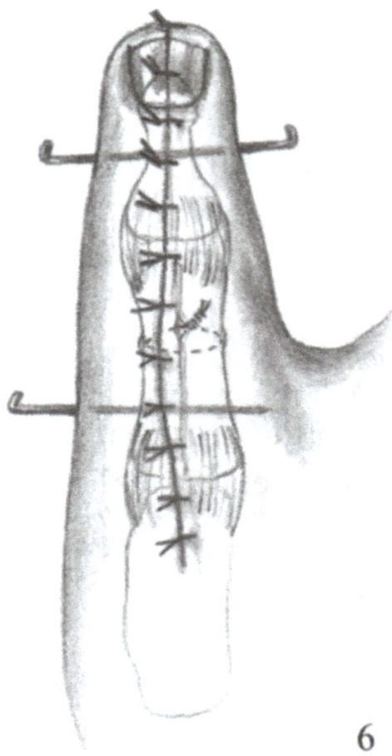

6

4.4.3 Duplication of the Distal Phalanx of the Thumb with a Smaller Radial Element

Goal of Surgery

Removal of the smaller element.

Fig. 1 Preoperative appearance and incision, dorsal aspect.
The *hatched bony areas* will be removed, the extensor tendon of the smaller element will be excised.

Fig. 2 Nerves and tendons have been transected (* distal stump of flexor poll. long. tendon) and blood vessels, ligated. Amputation of the element at the IP joint. Subperiosteal resection of the prominent portion of the common proximal phalanx. The IP joint is entered during this step. The resection area has to be smoothed.

Fig. 3 Postoperative appearance.
The capsule of the IP joint has been closed with interrupted sutures. The distal phalanx is stabilized with a transarticular Kirschner wire. Skin suture.

Postoperative Care

Slightly padded short-arm cast for 3 weeks. Removal of the Kirschner wire 2 weeks postoperatively.

Errors and Their Consequences

E. Intracapsular approach to the proximal phalanx.
C. Danger of impairment of its epiphyseal plate.

E. Kirschner wire fixation has been omitted.
C. Joint instability possible.

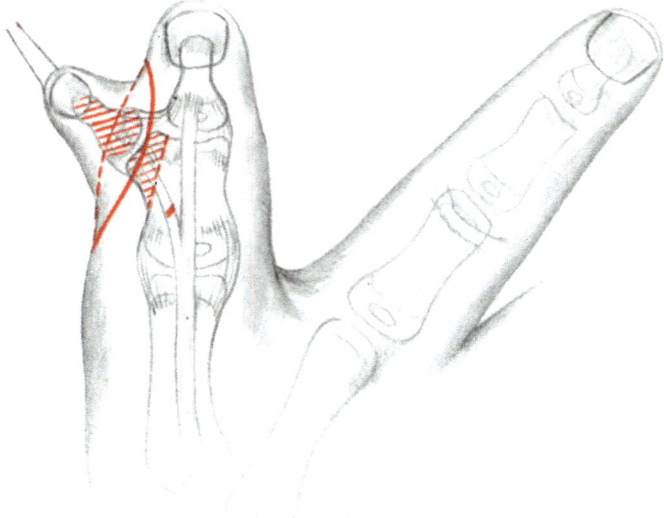

1

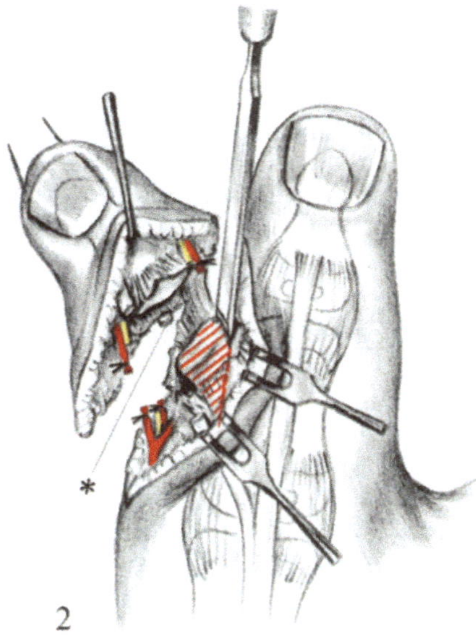

2

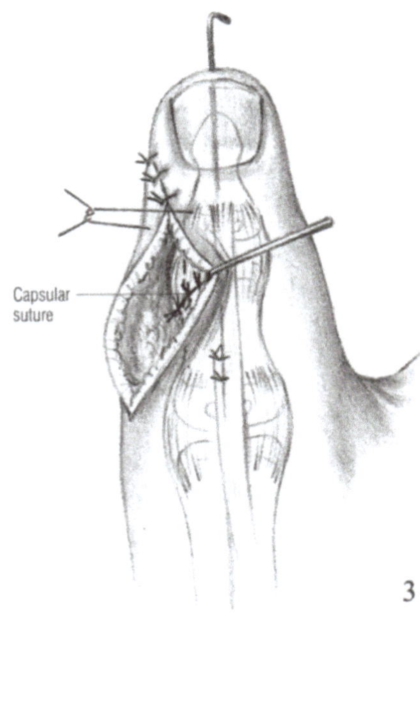

3

4.4.4 Thumb Duplication with Triphalangeal Radial Element

Goal of Surgery

Removal of the dysplastic element.

Fig. 1, 2 Preoperative appearance and incision, dorsal *(1)* and radial *(2)* aspects.
The extensor tendon of the thumb bifurcates in the area of the first metacarpal. *Hatched areas* of bone will be removed. Incision starts on the dorsal side. The position of the palmar incision depends on the size of the remaining skin defect after mobilization and resection of the dysplastic finger.

Fig. 3 Radiodorsal aspect.
The extensor tendon of the supernumerary thumb has been transected and mobilized distally. The palmar artery has been ligated and the nerve transected. The MP joint is opened after dissection of the insertions of the thenar musculature. The bases of both proximal phalanges are located in one common joint capsule.

Fig. 4 Radiopalmar aspect. The dysplastic thumb has been amputated, the excess portion of the first metacarpal is being removed.

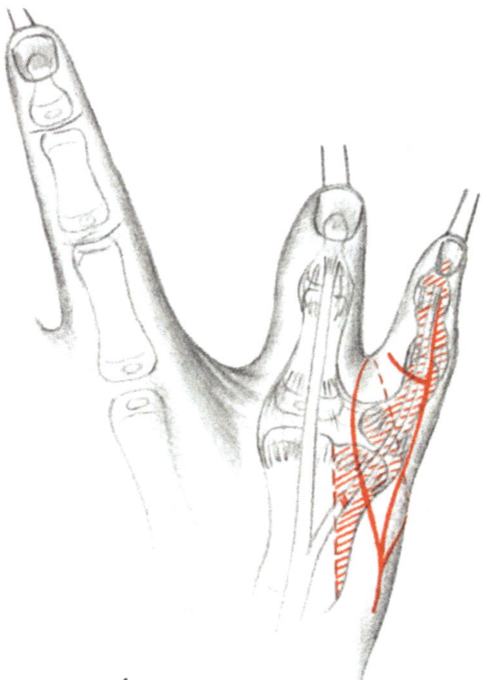
1

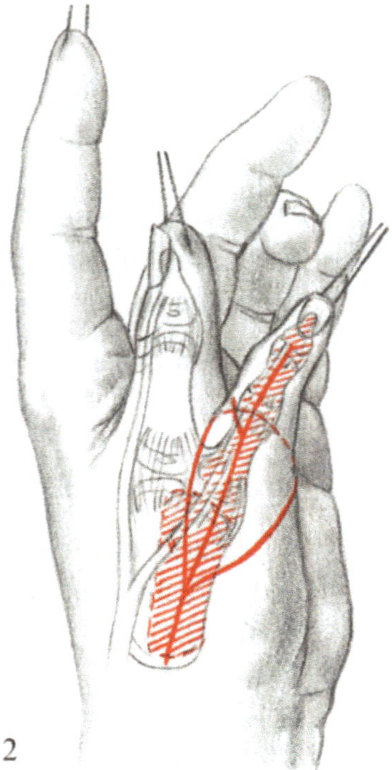
2

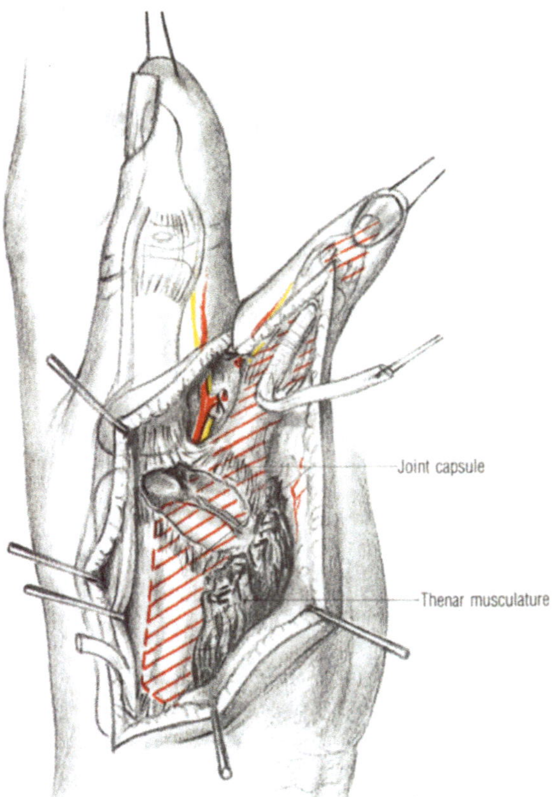

3

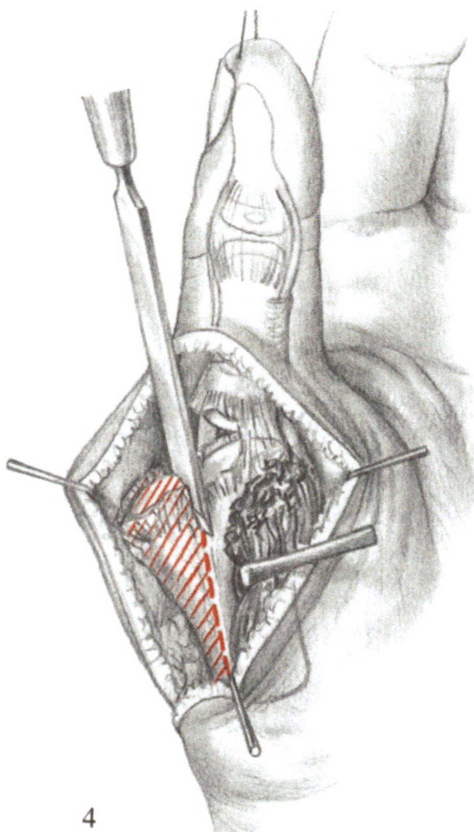
4

Fig. 5 The resection site of the first metacarpal is covered with the thenar musculature; the capsule of the MP joint has been closed (*). Fixation by transarticular Kirschner wire (not shown). Wound closure.

Fig. 6 Postoperative appearance.

Postoperative Care

As described in operative examples, Sect. 4.4.2 and 4.4.3. In this case deepening and widening of the thumb commissure will be carried out at a later date (see Sect. 4.2.1).

Errors and Their Consequences

E. The width of the metacarpal has not been reduced.
C. A cosmetically unsatisfactory bulge persists. It will become even more noticeable with further growth.

E. The epiphyseal plate of the first metacarpal has been damaged.
C. Growth deformities have to be expected, particularly if surgery is performed at an early age.

See also Sect. 4.4.2.

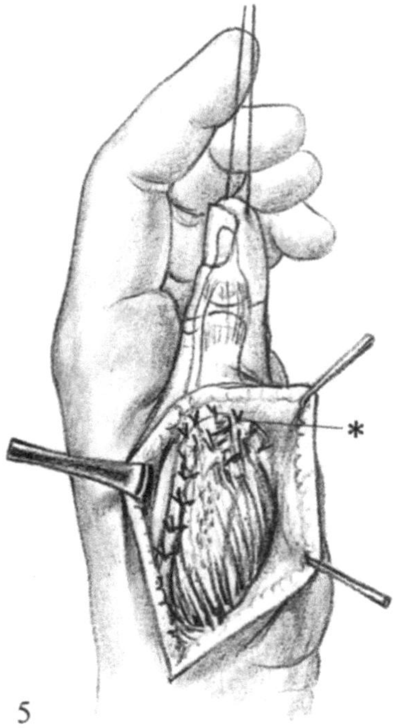

5

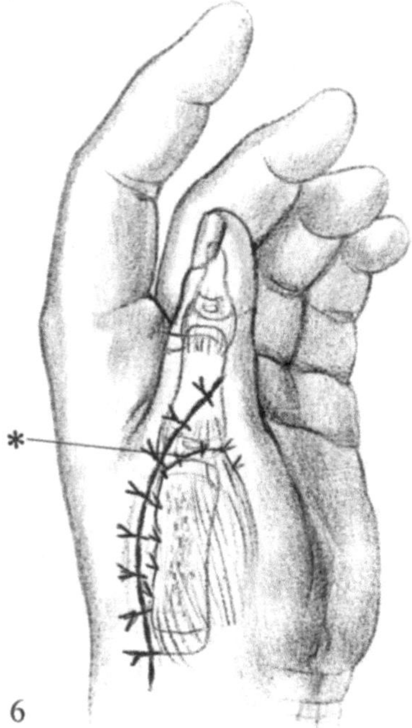

6

4.4.5 Thumb Duplication with an Ulnar Rudimentary Metacarpal

Goal of Surgery

Removal of the ulnar elements of the thumb duplication, construction of a well-functioning commissure.

Fig. 1 Preoperative appearance and incision, dorsal aspect.
The extensor tendon of the thumb is bifurcated. *Hatched* bony elements will be removed.

Fig. 2 Dorsal aspect after dissection of the dorsal skin flap.
Excision of the rudimentary metacarpal begins at its proximal end.

Fig. 3 The palmar flap has been dissected; nerves and the flexor tendon have been transected and the main artery has been ligated.

Fig. 4 Postoperative appearance.
The proximal end of the transected tendon has been sutured to the tendon of m. extensor poll. long. Temporary fixation with two crossed Kirschner wires.

Postoperative Care

Short-arm plaster cast. The Kirschner wires will be removed 2–3 weeks postoperatively. Night splint.

Errors and Their Consequences

E. Palmar vessel and nerves have been damaged.

E. The palmar triangular flap is too small or too short.
C. The skin suture line will be under tension. Necrosis of the flap may occur. Thick-split thickness skin transplants are required.

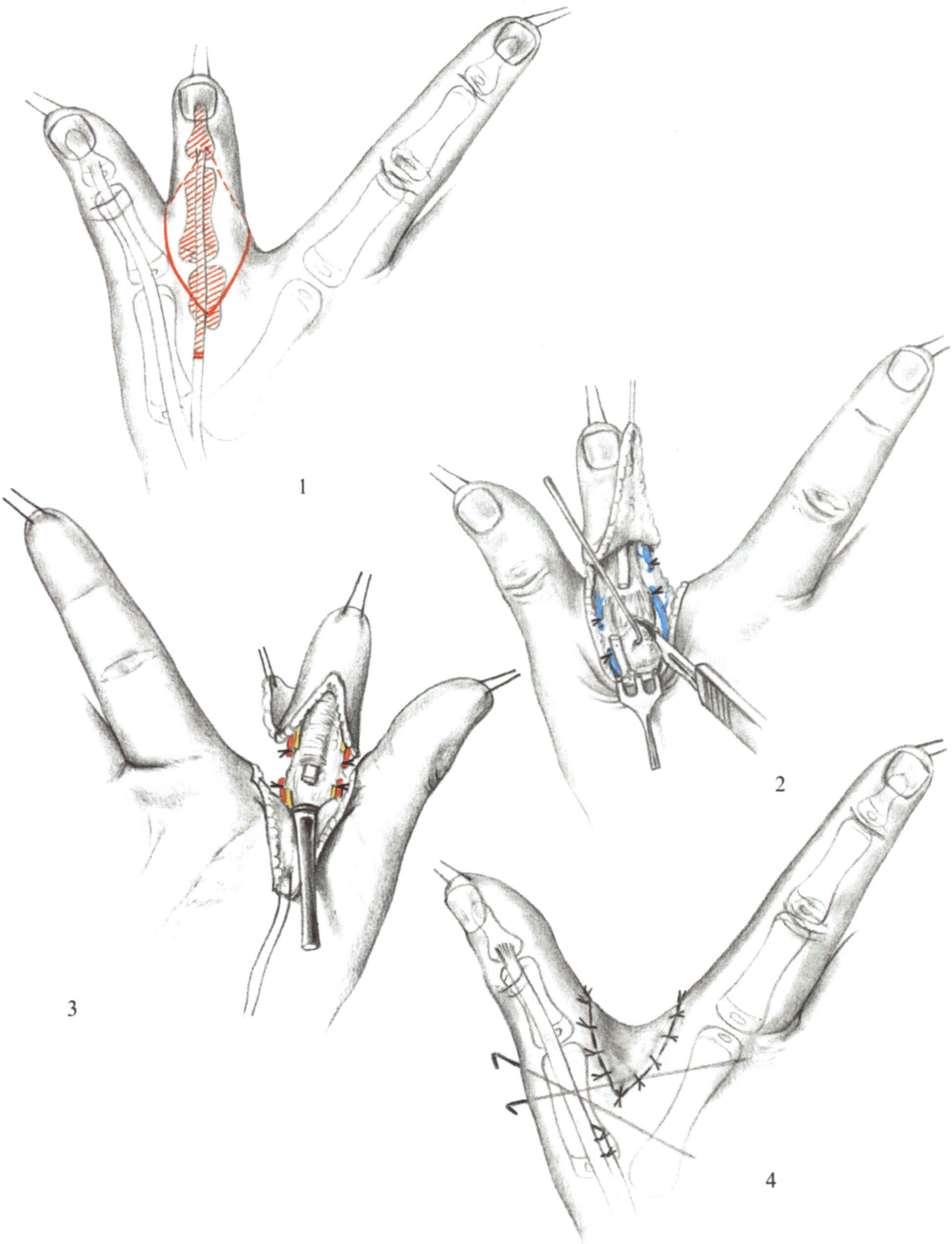
1
2
3
4

4.4.6 Thumb Duplication with Smaller Radial Element and Deformed Metacarpal

Goal of Surgery

Removal of the smaller thumb element. Correction of the longitudinal axis of the first metacarpal by wedge osteotomy (see also Sects. 4.4.3 and 4.4.4).

Fig. 1 Preoperative appearance and incision, dorsal aspect.
A thin extensor tendon inserts at the distal phalanx of the smaller thumb element ("bifurcation tendon"). The *hatched areas* of bone will be removed.

Fig. 2 Palmar aspect during removal of the smaller element.
The flexor tendons and nerves have been transected; the vessels have been ligated. The radial thenar musculature has been cut (not shown).
Resection of the metacarpal boss (*hatched area*) will follow.

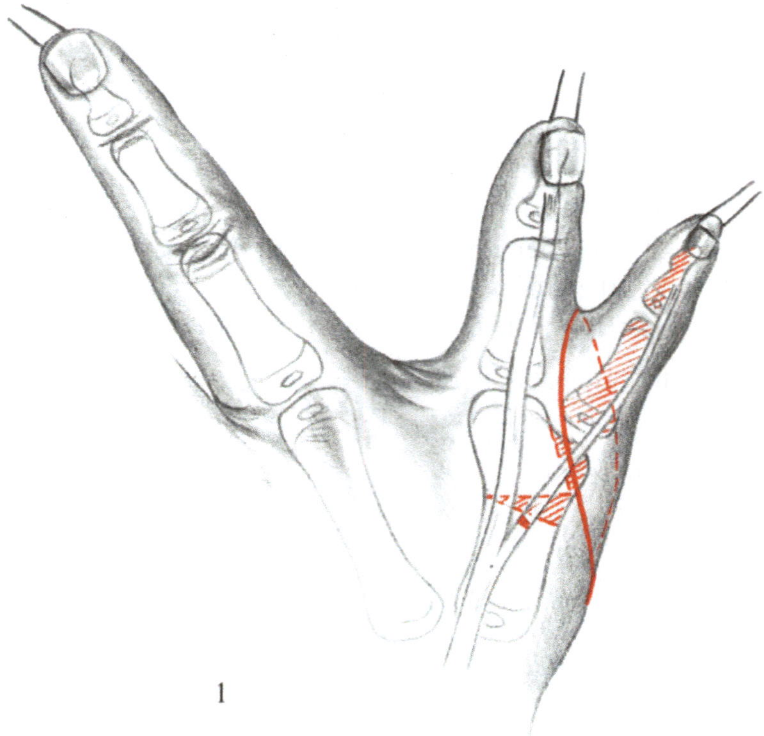

1

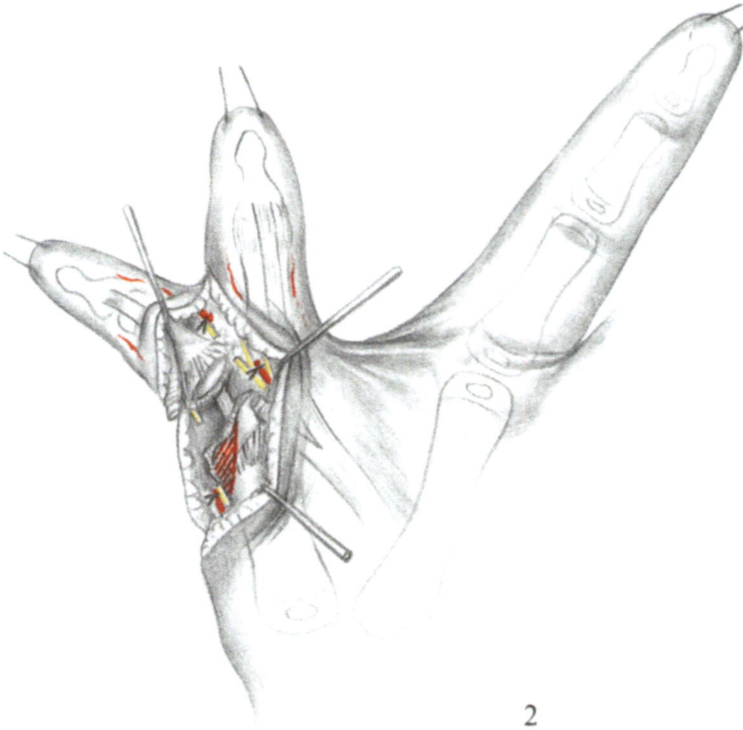

2

Fig. 3 Radially based wedge osteotomy of the first metacarpal. The size of the wedge had been determined preoperatively (x-ray tracing). The neurovascular bundles and other soft tissues are protected by retractors.
Rotation at the osteotomy site is possible if thumb opposition is inadequate.

Fig. 4 The fragments have been stabilized with crossed Kirschner wires. Wound closure in layers.

Fig. 5 Postoperative appearance.
The sites of the osteotomy and resection of the first metacarpal are *marked in red.*

Postoperative Care

Long-arm cast, removal of the Kirschner wires 4 weeks postoperatively. Night splint.
Physiotherapy.
An enlargement of the thumb commissure is planned for a later date (after good mobility in the MP joint has been achieved).

Errors and Their Consequences

E. Surgery is limited to removal of the smaller thumb element without correction of the longitudinal thumb axis and without resection of the bulging metacarpal boss.
C. An increase of the metacarpal boss has to be expected with further bone growth; cosmesis of the Ist ray remains unsatisfactory.

E. Palmar vessels and nerves of the remaining thumb have been damaged.

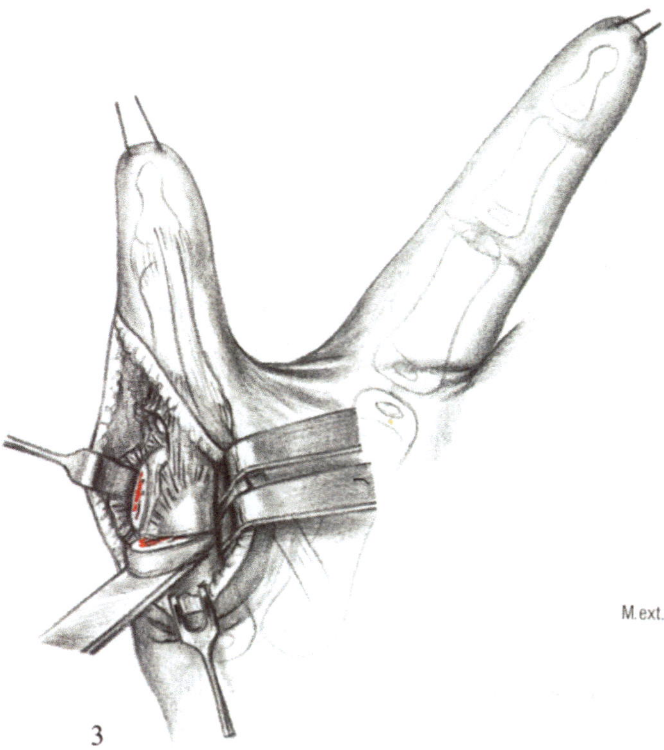

3

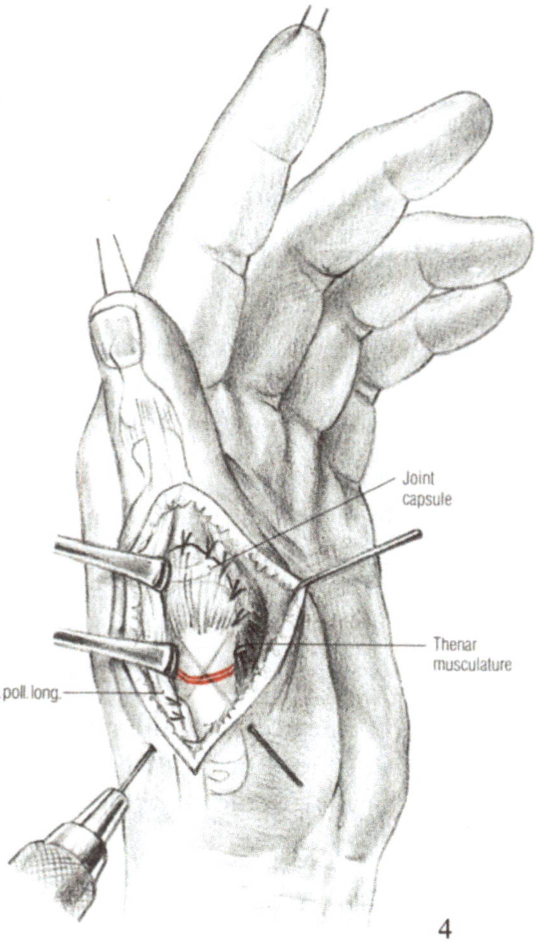

4

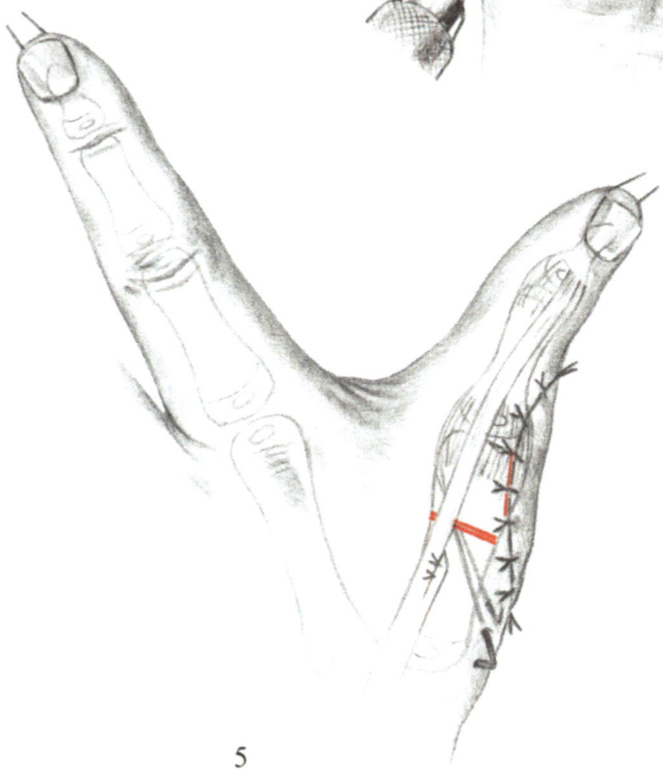

5

4.4.7 Thumb Duplication: Floating Thumb

Goal of Surgery

Removal of the (accessory) rudimentary thumb.

Fig. 1 Preoperative appearance and incision, dorsal aspect.
The basis of the thumb rudiment is small and stemlike. The rudiment contains two skeletal elements (*).

Fig. 2 Radial aspect.
Injury of the radiovolar vessel and nerve of the true thumb has to be avoided during amputation of the rudiment.

Errors and Their Consequences

E. The accessory thumb has been amputated by "strangulation."
C. A necrotic area located at the amputation site can increase the risk of infection; at a later date a wartlike excrescence develops.

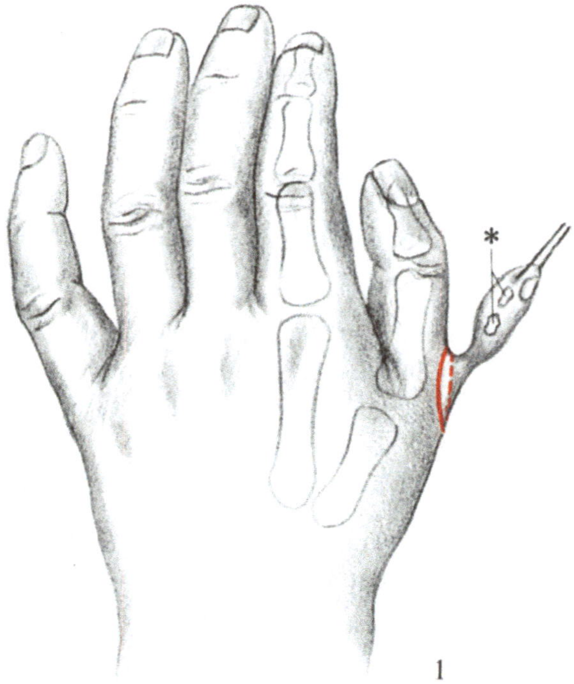

1

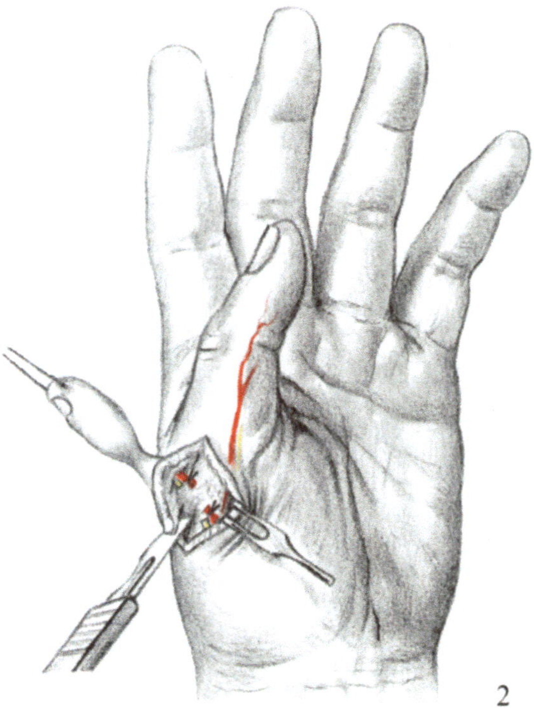

2

4.5 Other Finger Duplications

4.5.1 Duplication of the Little Finger

Goal of Surgery

Removal of the ulnar element.

Fig. 1 Preoperative appearance and incision, dorsal aspect.
The ulnar and radial elements have a common metacarpal. The *hatched bony areas* will be removed. The incision on the palmar side and the possible lengthening of the dorsal incision are indicated by the *broken lines*. The *dotted skin areas* may have to be resected during skin closure.

Fig. 2 Dorsal view after dissection of the skin flaps.
The palmar vessels and nerves have been ligated and transected respectively. The capsule of the common MP joint is being incised and the extensor tendon of the ulnar element will be cut as marked. (The extensor aponeurosis is not shown.) Next, exposure and transection of the m. abd. dig. quinti at the ulnar base of the proximal phalanx of the little finger. The flexor tendons will be cut at the level of the MP joint (not shown).

Fig. 3 Dorsal view after amputation of the ulnar duplication element.
The size of the common fifth metacarpal is being reduced (as shown in *Fig. 1*), followed by smoothing of the osteotomy site.

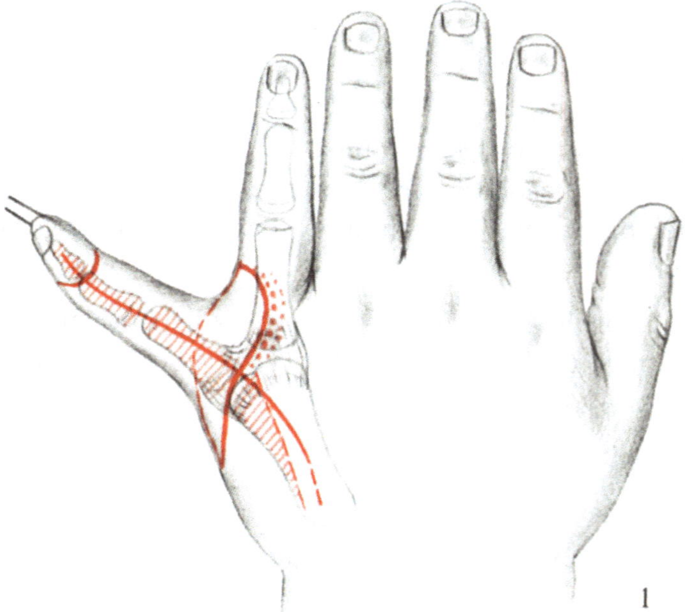

1

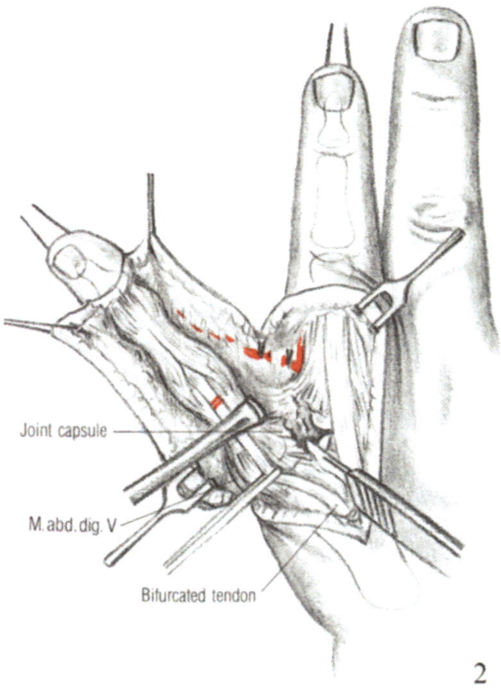

2

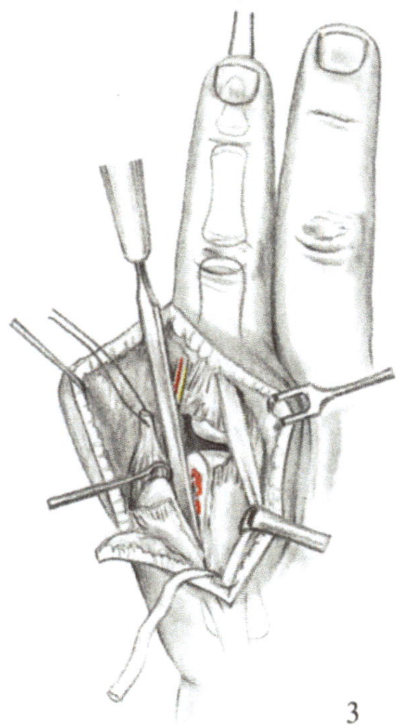

3

Fig. 4 The m. abd. dig. quinti has been sutured to the ulnar lateral expansion. The stump of the extensor tendon of the amputated finger is attached to the other little finger extensor tendon. The capsule of the MP joint has been closed with interrupted sutures.

Fig. 5 The resection area of the metacarpal is covered by hypothenar musculature. Skin closure with adaption of the skin flaps. The *black hatched areas* will be removed (see also *Fig. 1*).

Fig. 6 Postoperative appearance.

Postoperative Care

Short-arm cast for 3 weeks, followed by physiotherapy and night splint.

Errors and Their Consequences

See Sects. 4.4.3 and 4.4.4.

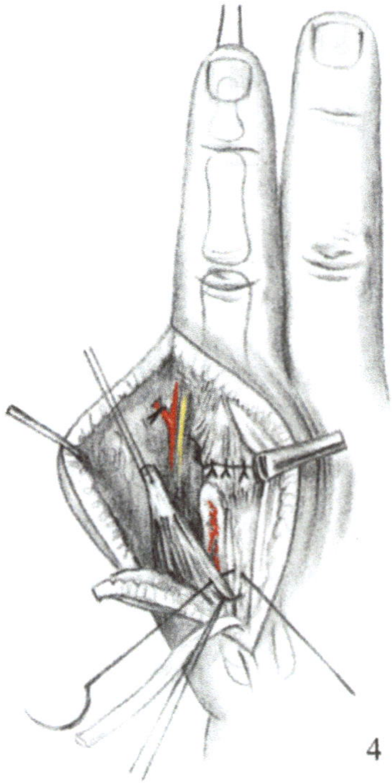

4

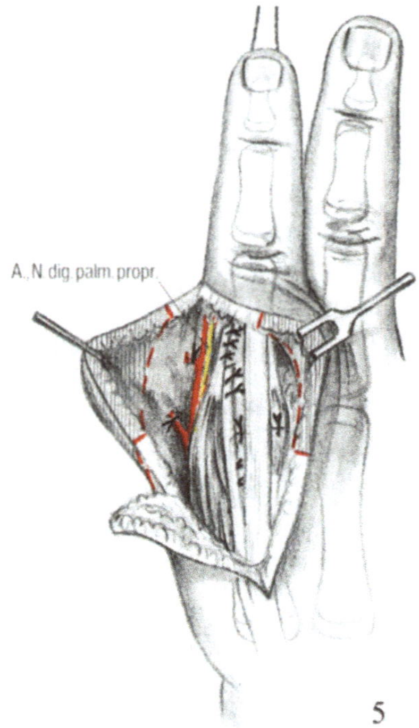

5

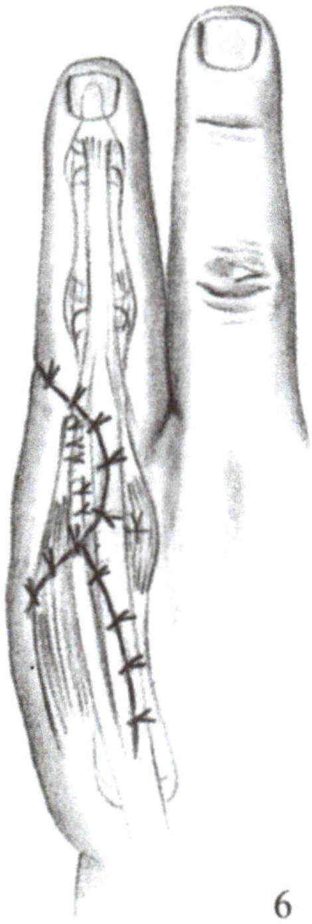

6

4.5.2 Little Finger Duplication with Metacarpal Bifurcation

Goal of Surgery

Resection of the supernumerary little finger and its metacarpal part.

Fig. 1 Preoperative appearance and incision. Dorsal aspect.
Hatched areas will be removed. The supernumerary finger has two phalanges.

Fig. 2 Palmar–ulnar aspect.
The palmar nerves and vessels of the supernumerary finger have been cut and ligated. The abnormal course of the palmar finger artery is visible (*). Subsequently, the flexor tendons will be severed as marked.

Fig. 3 Partial dorsal view.
The junctura tendinum as well as the extensor tendon will be severed just proximal to the bifurcation (as marked). The hypothenar muscles will be freed peripherally where they join the tendons.

Fig. 4 Appearance after amputation of the smaller element at the proximal joint.
The metacarpal boss will be resected (see *Fig. 1*); the resection site will be smoothed with a fine rasp.

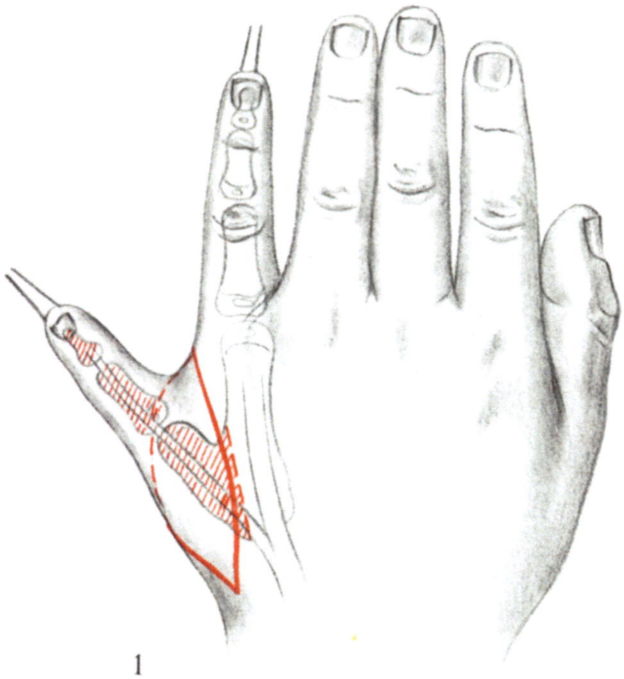

1

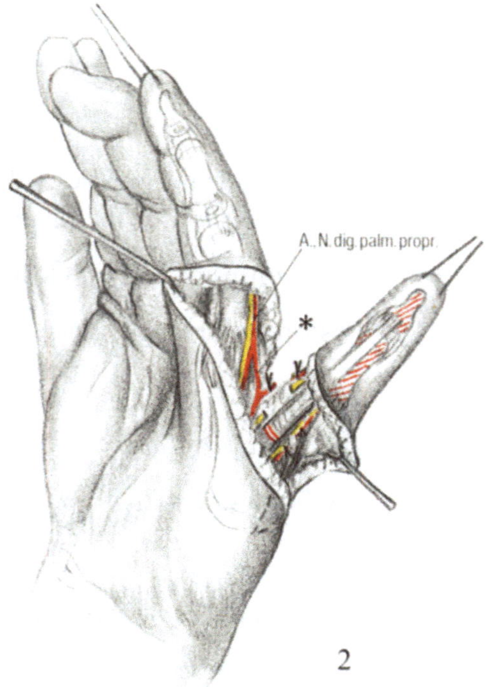
A., N. dig. palm. propr.
*

2

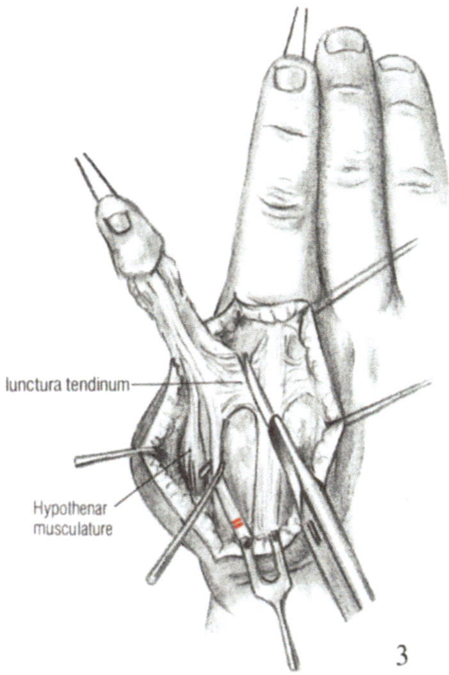
Iunctura tendinum
Hypothenar musculature

3

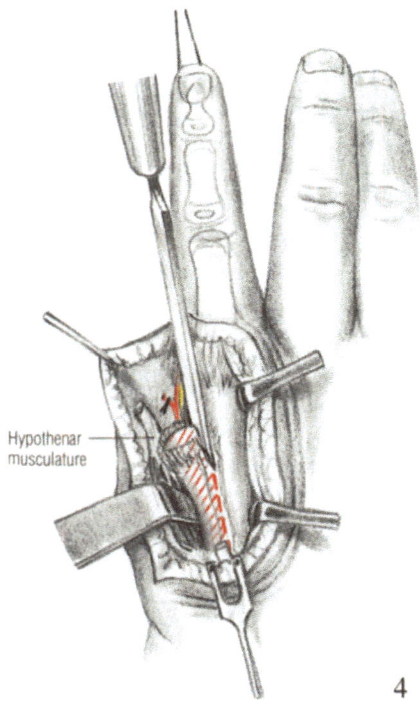
Hypothenar musculature

4

Fig. 5 The hypothenar muscles will be sutured to the resected bone surface and attached to the insertion of the ulnar lateral band.

Fig. 6 Situation prior to skin closure.

Fig. 7 Postoperative appearance.

Postoperative Care

See Sect. 4.5.1.

Errors and Their Consequences

Failure to resect metacarpal boss (see "Remarks," Sect. 4.4.3).

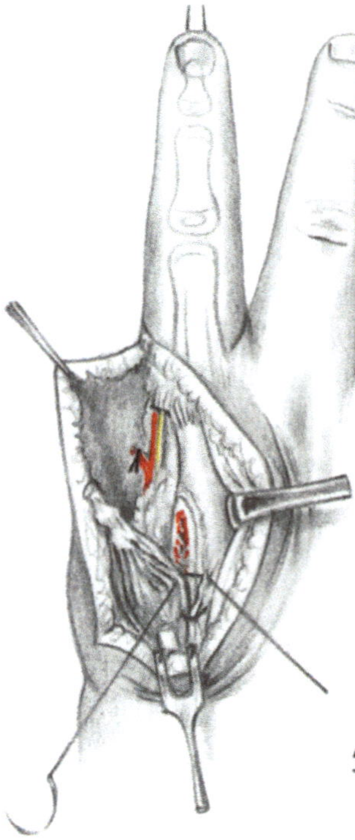

5

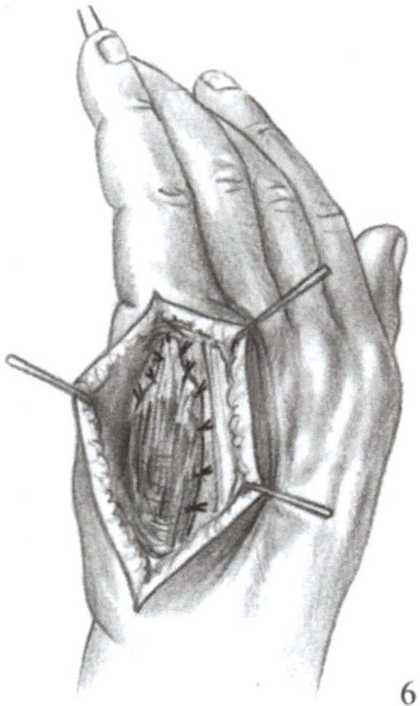

6

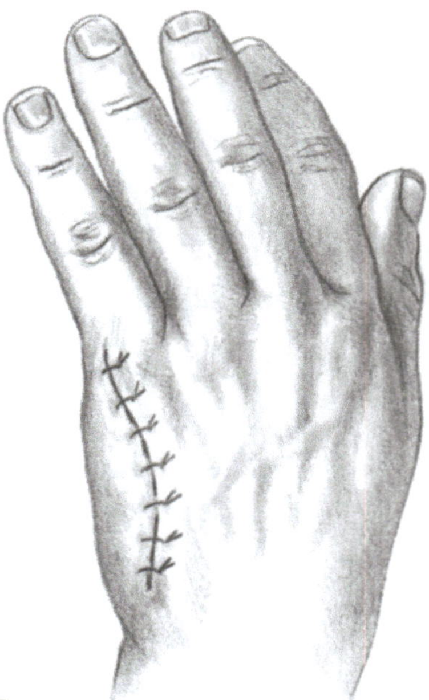

7

4.5.3 Duplication of the IVth Ray with Complete Syndactyly

Goal of Surgery

Removal of the supernumerary ray, separation of the soft tissue bridge between the middle and ring finger, and formation of a smooth commissure in its appropriate location.

Figs. 1, 2 Preoperative appearance and incision.
The commissure is constructed from two local triangular pedicle flaps. *Hatched bony areas* will be removed; *red dotted areas* of skin will be excised prior to closure. For further surgical procedure, see Sect. 4.5.6a.o.

Figs. 3, 4 Postoperative appearance.

Postoperative Care

Long-arm plaster cast, not including thumb, for 3–4 weeks, followed by physiotherapy.

Errors and Their Consequences

E. No tethering of third and fourth metacarpals (see Sects. 4.5.6 and 9.4).
C. Diminished gripping ability etc.
See also comments in Sects. 4.5.6 and 2.1.

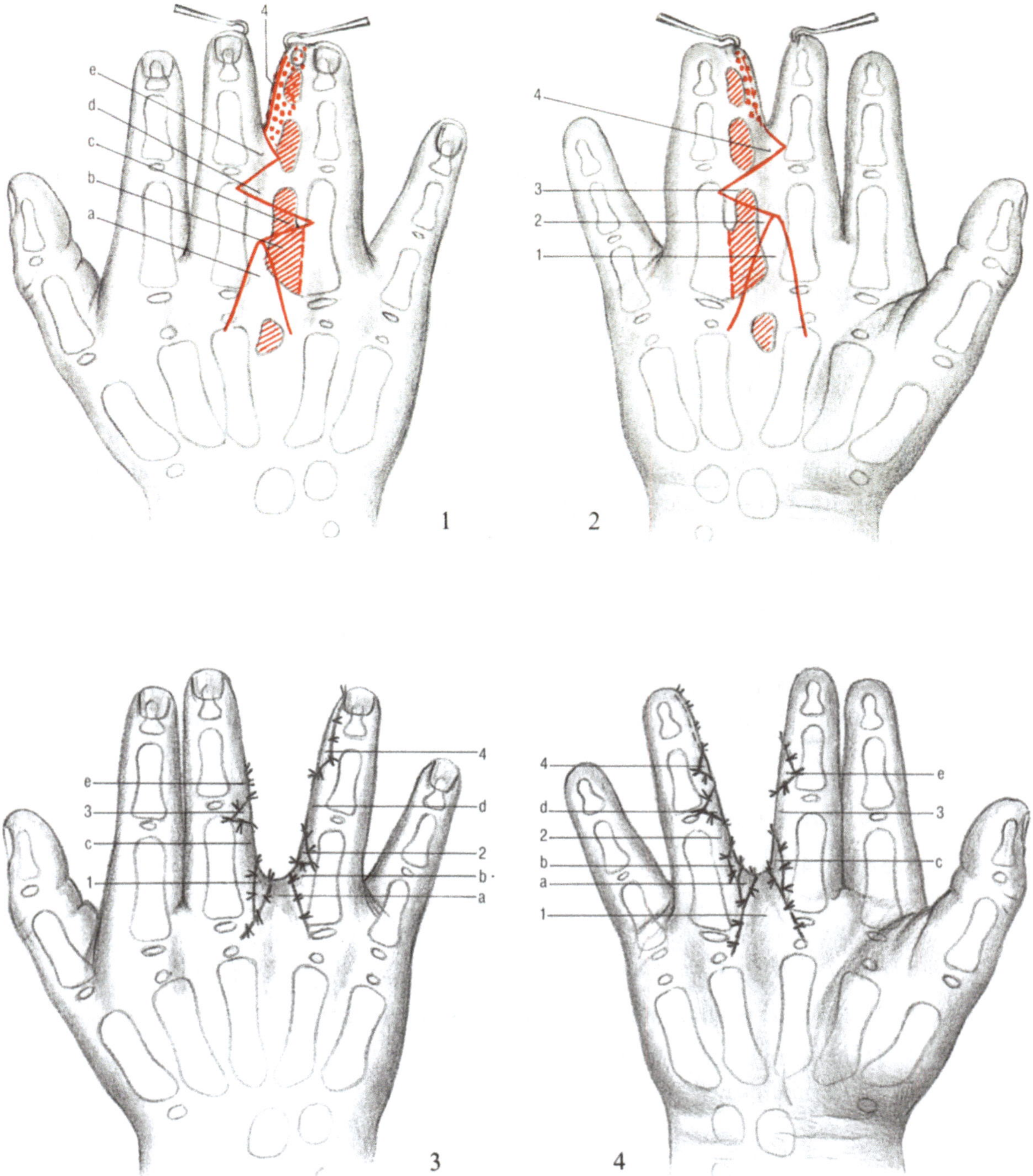

4
e
d
c
b
a
1
4
3
2
1
2
e
3
c
1
4
d
2
b
a
3
4
d
2
b
a
1
e
3
c
4

4.5.4 Ring Finger Duplication with Syndactyly, Deviation, and Bifurcation of the Proximal Phalanx

Goal of Surgery

Resection of the supernumerary digit, removal of the webbing between middle and ring finger, and correction of malalignment.

Figs. 1, 2 Preoperative appearance and incision.
Hatched areas of bone will be resected (wedge osteotomy of the proximal phalanx of the ring finger to correct axial deformity).
Essentially, the operation is performed as outlined in Sect. 4.5.6.

Fig. 3 Postoperative appearance, dorsal aspect.
Correcting the PIP joint of the ring finger necessitated a radial capsulotomy; the ligamentum collaterale was replaced by a tendon transplant (from the resected finger). The osteotomy is secured by two crossed Kirschner wires (or a plate from a self-compressing small fragment set). The proximal phalangeal joint has been temporarily immobilized by transarticular Kirschner wire fixation.
Skin flaps had to be shaped and trimmed for closure (*dotted areas, Figs. 1 and 2*).

Fig. 4 Postoperative appearance, palmar aspect.
Remaining open areas are covered by thick-split thickness skin transplants *(Tr)*.

Postoperative Care

See Sect. 4.5.6.

Errors and Their Consequences

E. Damage to palmar and dorsal main vessels and nerves.

E. Damage to epiphyseal plates.
C. Abnormal growth.

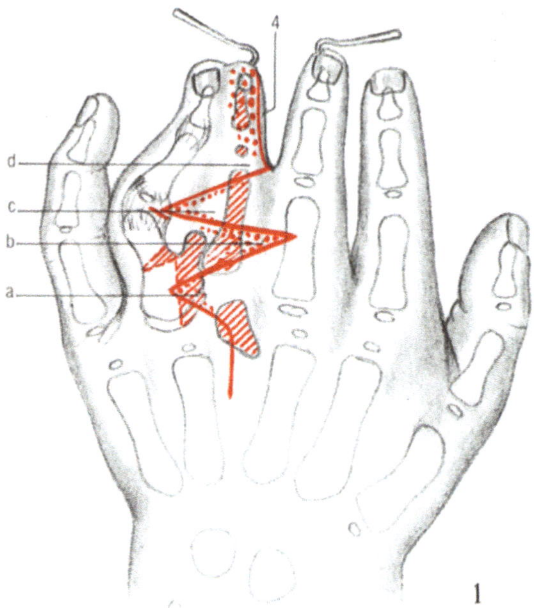

1

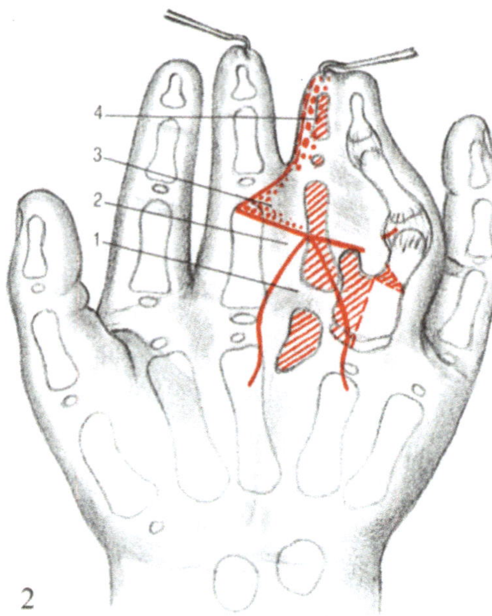

2

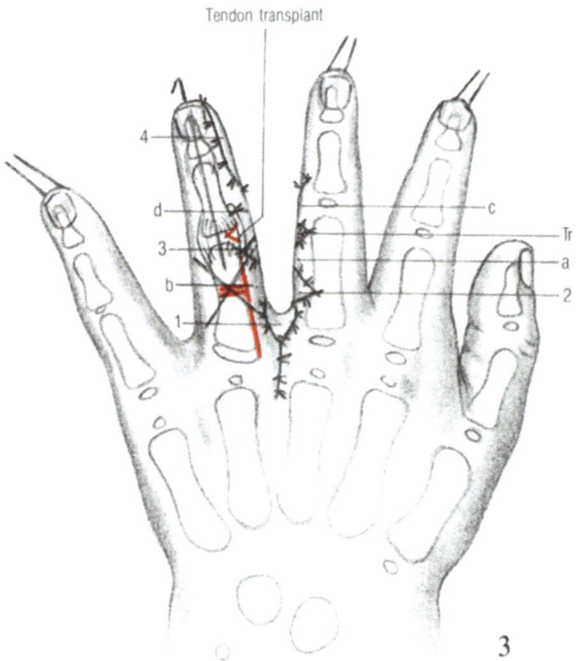

3

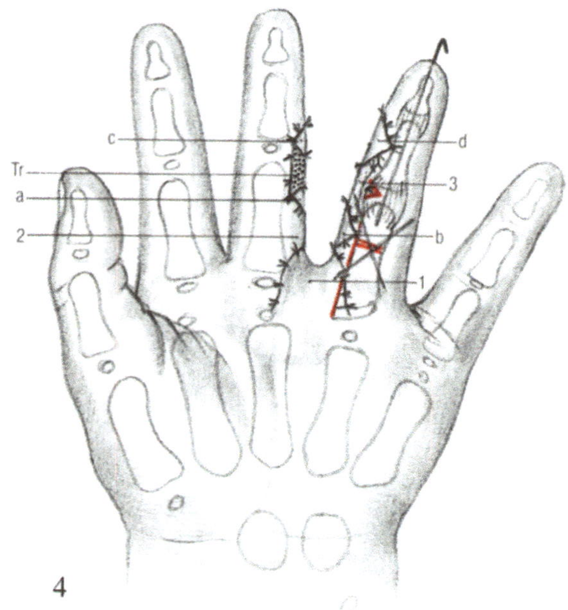

4

4.5.5 Ring Finger Duplication with Acrosynostosis and Total Syndactyly of the IIIrd/IVth Rays

Goal of Surgery

Separation of fingers and removal of the supernumerary ray.

Fig. 1 Preoperative appearance and incision; dorsal aspect.
Hatched bony areas will be resected.

Fig. 2 Preoperative appearance and incision; palmar aspect.
The commissure has been formed by two triangular, proximally based pedicle flaps. Closure of the skin flaps may require an additional horizontal incision *(thick broken line)*. Incision on opposite side is marked by *thin broken lines.*

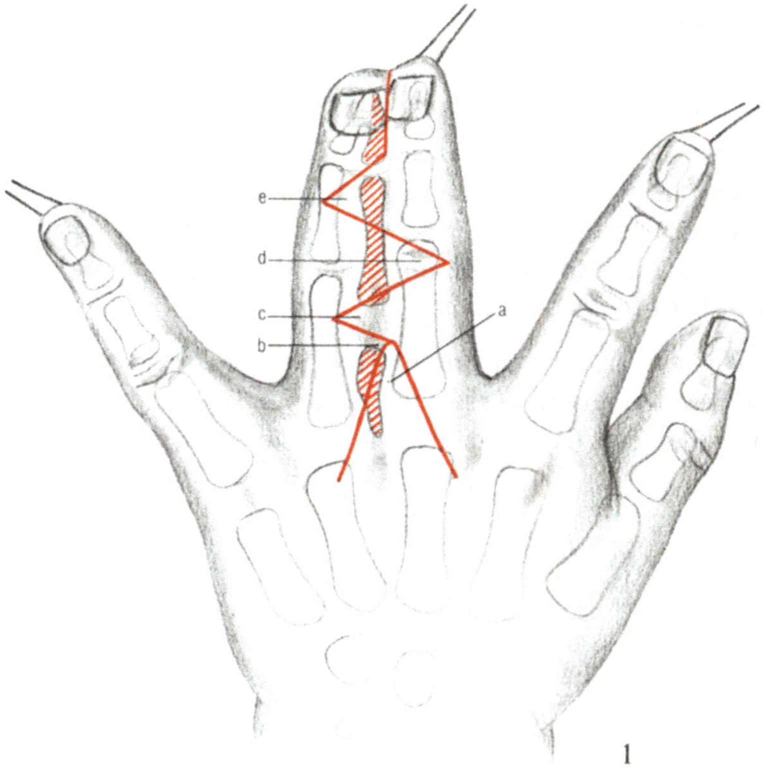

1

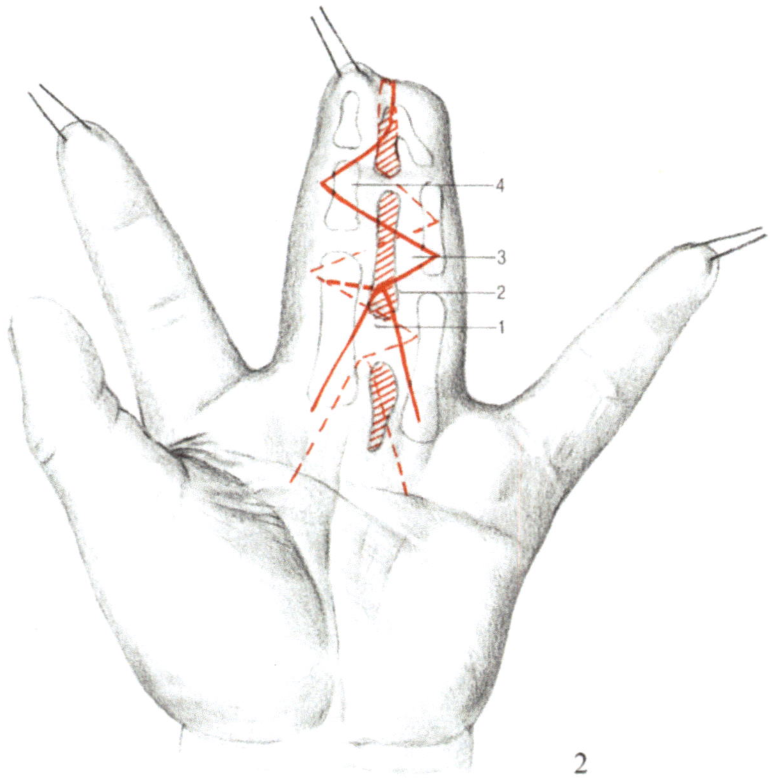

2

Fig. 3 Dorsal aspect after raising of dorsal (and palmar) skin flaps.
A thin extensor tendon reaches to the dysplastic digit. The bony bridge between the distal phalanges of the ring finger and the dysplastic supernumerary finger is severed with a narrow osteotome.

Fig. 4 The distal phalanx of the supernumerary digit has been removed.
Working from the extensor side, the remainder of the digit is removed from surrounding soft tissue. (Avoid damage to palmar neurovascular bundles.)

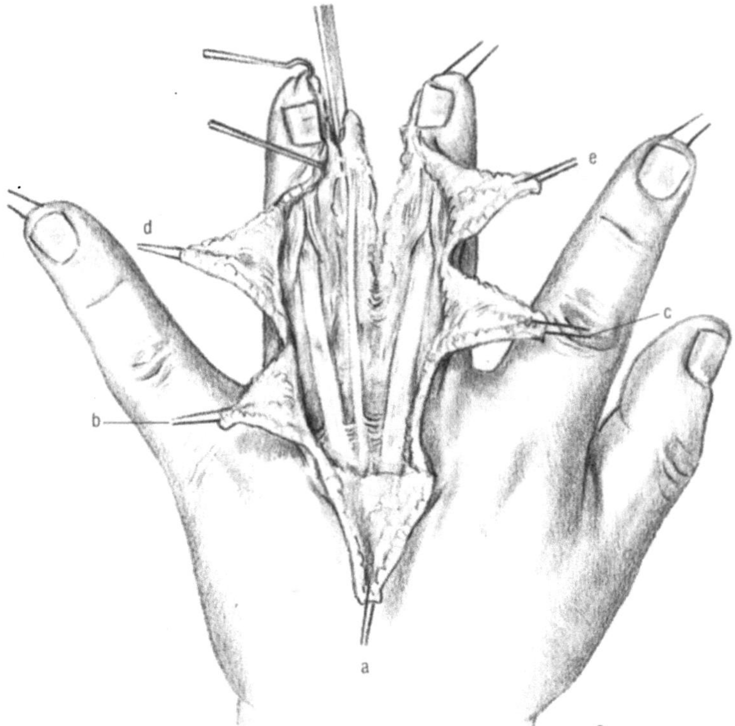

3

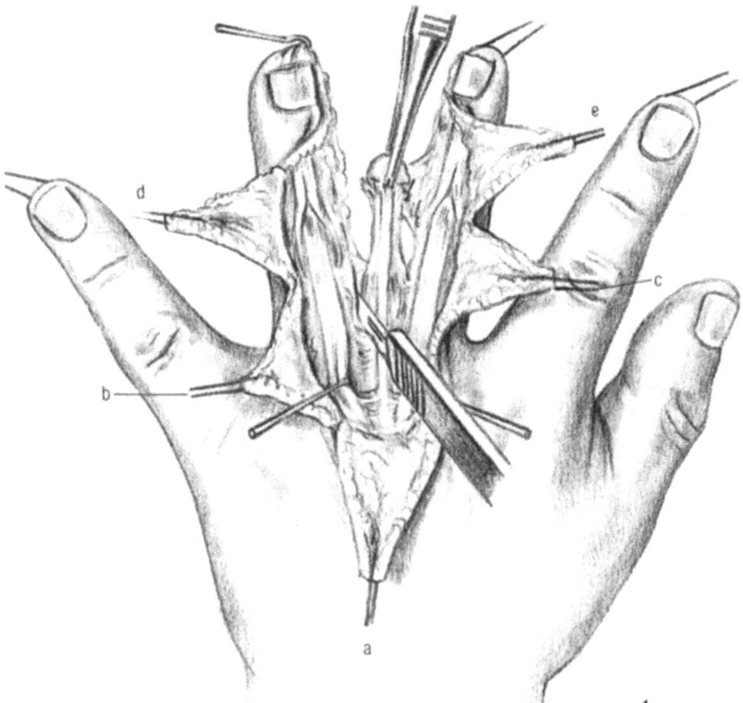

4

4.5.5 Ring Finger Duplication with Acrosynostosis and Total Syndactyly of the IIIrd/IVth Rays

Fig. 5 Palmar aspect.
Subsequent to removal of metacarpal rudiments, the severed juncturae tendinum are sutured. (To achieve better tethering, a tendon loop may be required; see Sect. 4.5.6.)

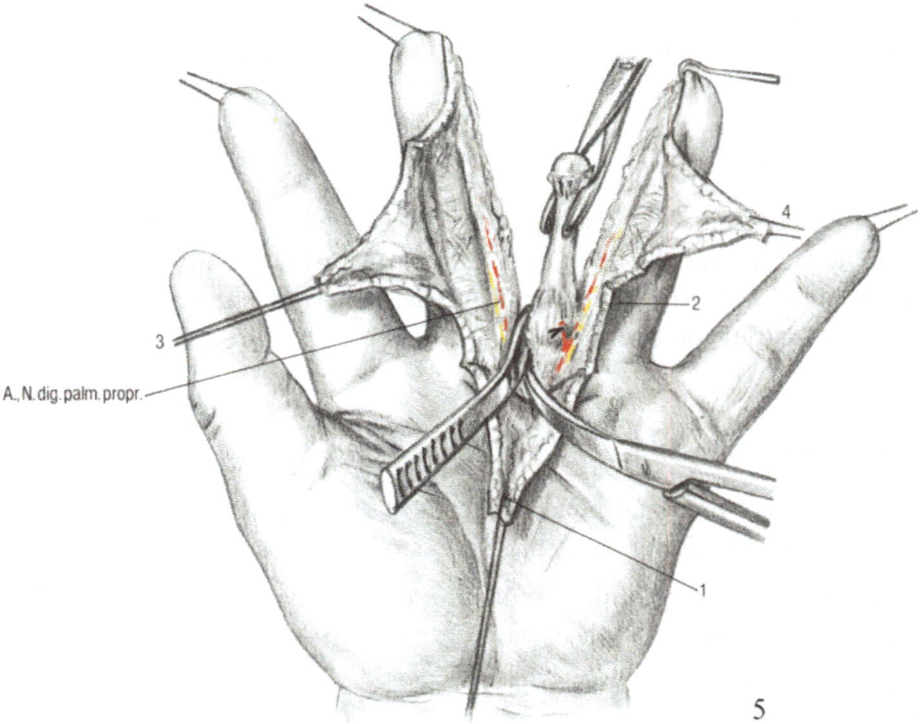

5

4.5.5 Ring Finger Duplication with Acrosynostosis and Total Syndactyly of the IIIrd/IVth Rays

Fig. 6,7 Postoperative appearance.
Open skin areas are covered by thick-split thickness skin transplants *(Tr)*.

Postoperative Care

The wound is covered with vaseline gauze. The light compression bandage is split approximately 2 h after the operation. Long-arm cast for 2–3 weeks (first dressing change after 8–10 days); then short-arm cast. Physiotherapy will begin approximately 4 weeks after the operation.

Errors and Their Consequences

E. Failure to resect proximal bone rudiment of supernumerary digit.
C. Insufficient width, depth, and smoothness of commissure.

E. Failure to resect matrix during reduction of fingernail.
C. Annoying, abnormal growth of nail.

E. Inadequate tethering of metacarpal heads.
C. Weak grip etc.

See also Sect. 2.1.

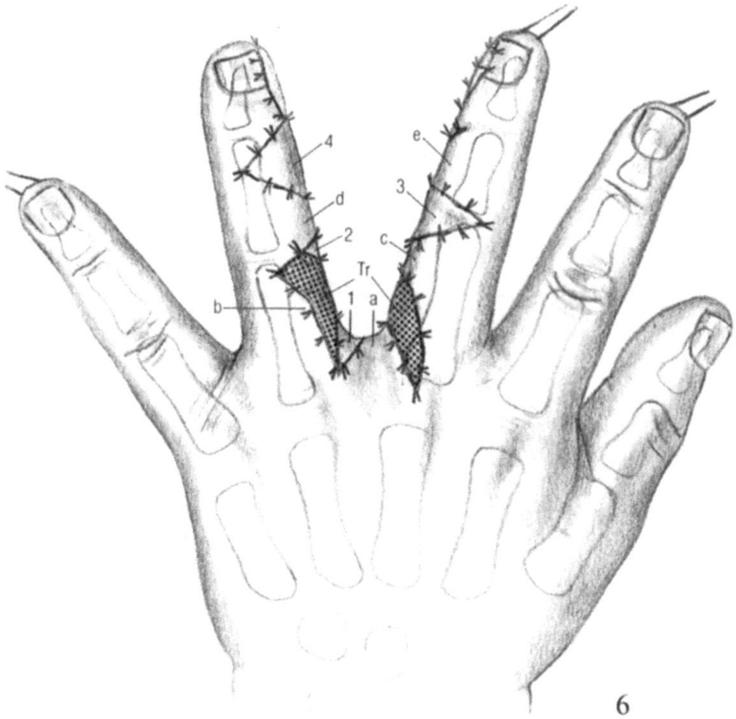

6

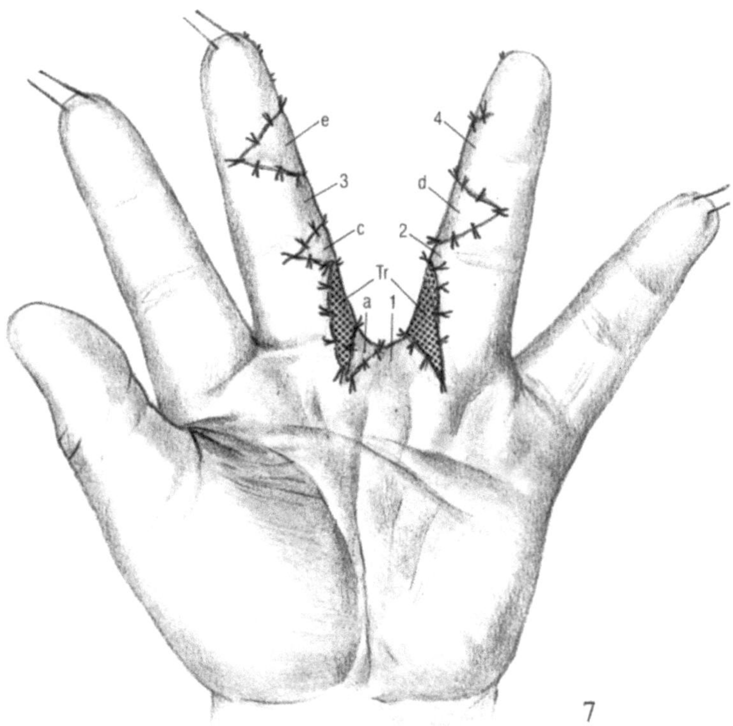

7

4.5.6 Index Finger Duplication

Goal of Surgery

Resection of the supernumerary dysplastic digit and its metacarpal part and tethering of the remaining index finger to the middle finger.

Fig. 1 Preoperative appearance and incision, dorsal aspect.
The extra digit appears to be shortened due to abnormal flexion of the MP joint. *Hatched areas* of bone will be excised.

Fig. 2 Dorsal aspect after exposure of extensor aponeurosis and transection of junctura tendinum.
Transection of extensor tendon as marked.

Fig. 3 The proximal joint has been opened, exposing the adjacent metacarpal. The dysplastic index finger will be amputated after its flexor tendons and palmar neurovascular bundle have been transected. (Ligate vessels!)
Raise the extensor tendon of the amputated finger as far distal as possible and protect it in moist sponges.

Fig. 4 Situation after amputation.
Palmar finger arteries have been ligated. The excessive metacarpal portion of the supernumerary index finger will now be osteotomized.

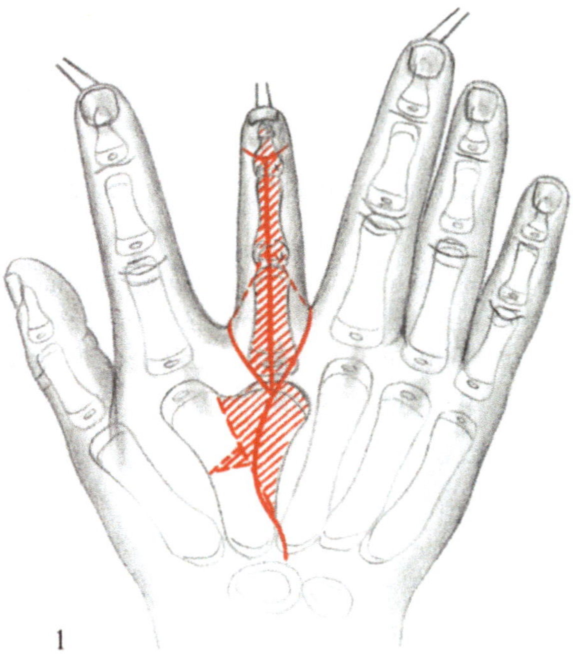

1

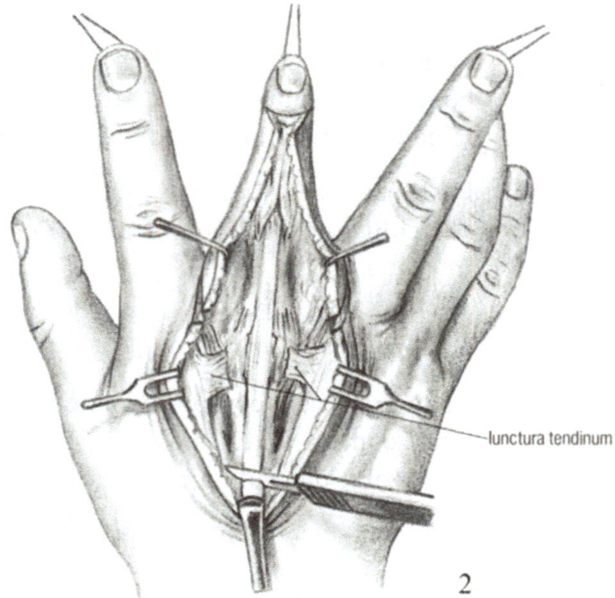
Iunctura tendinum

2

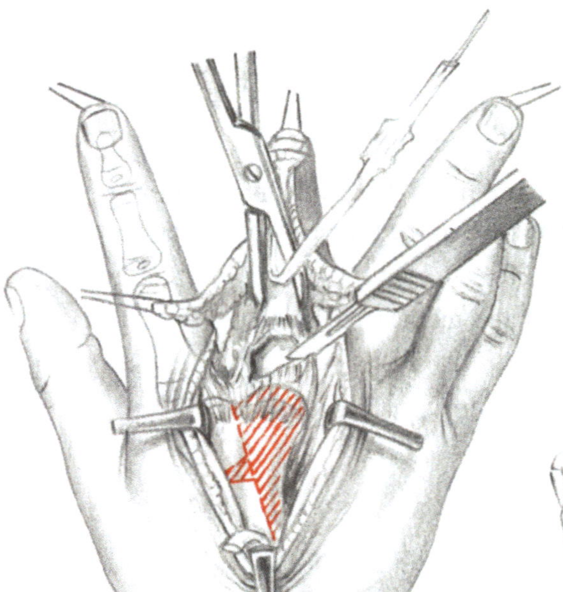

3

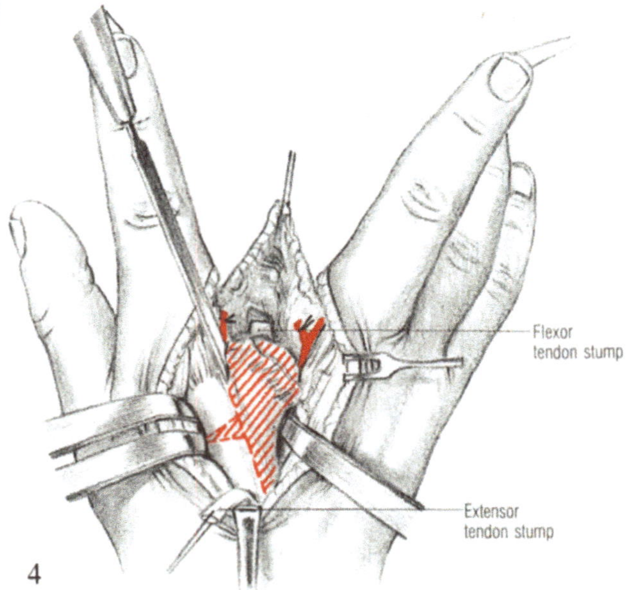
Flexor tendon stump
Extensor tendon stump

4

Fig. 5 To correct the longitudinal finger axis, a wedge is removed from the remaining part of the second metacarpal bone.

Figs. 6,7 The osteotomy site is held in position by two Kirschner wires (or a small fragment set plate). The transected tendon is wound around the second and third metacarpal bones as a subperiosteal "figure of eight," tightened and sutured to itself. The remains of juncturae tendinum of both extensor tendons are tied down.

Fig. 8 Postoperative appearance, partial dorsal aspect.
Sketchlike presentation of index finger tethering.

Postoperative Care

Long-arm cast for approximately 4 weeks, leaving thumb and fingers free. Then x-ray control and removal of Kirschner wires. Short-arm cast for an additional 2–4 weeks, depending on x-ray findings, to be followed by physiotherapy.

Errors and Their Consequences

E. Damage to palmar and dorsal main vessels and nerves.

E. The tethering effect of the tendon is inadequate. It has been passed over rather than under the extensor tendons of the IInd and IIIrd fingers around the metacarpal bones.

E. Osteotomy does not adequately correct the metacarpal bone.

E. Insufficient osteosynthesis.
C. The healing process is delayed and malposition may occur later.

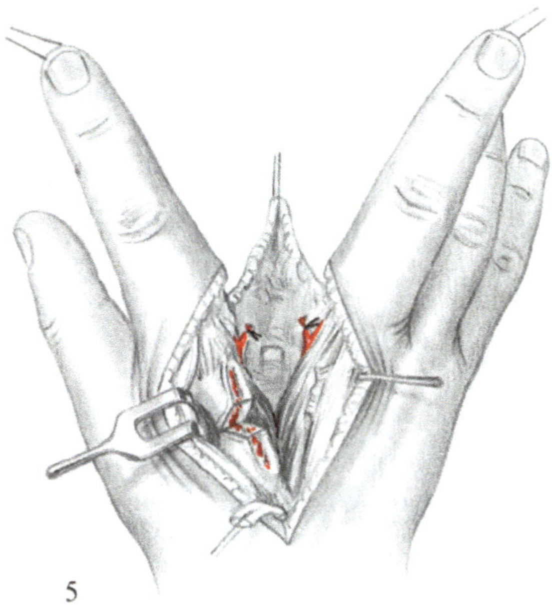

5

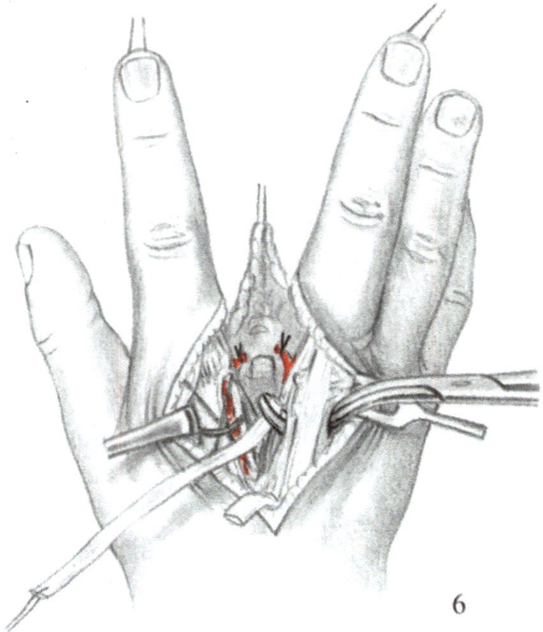

6

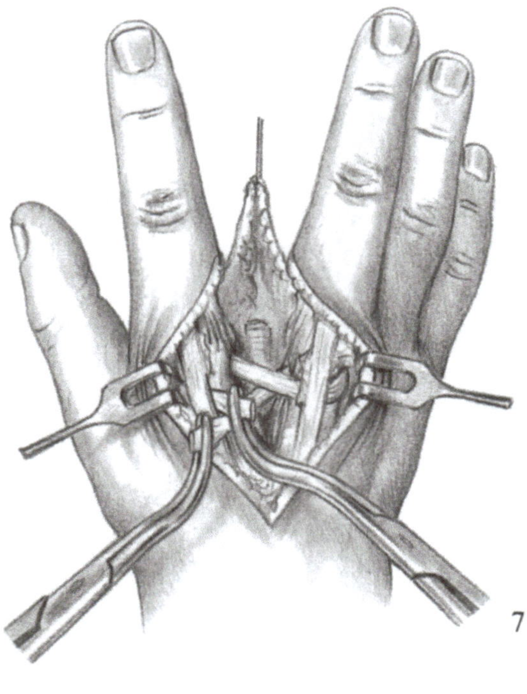

7

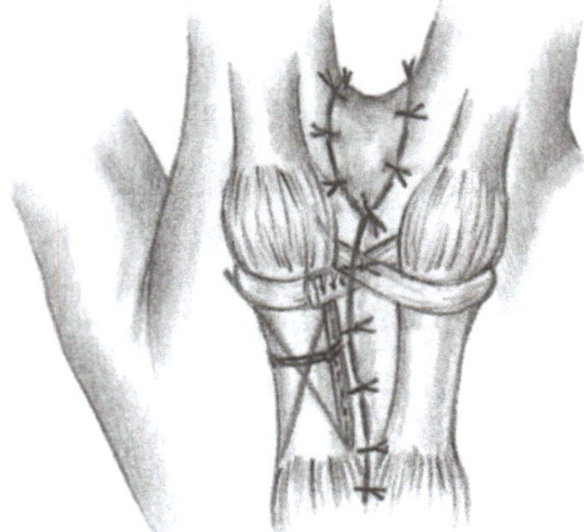

8

4.5.7 Hexadactyly (Six Triphalangeal Fingers)

Goal of Surgery

Formation of a functional thumb by amputation of the outermost radial ray and pollicization of the IInd digit.
For details of the technique, see also Sect. 4.2.4.

Figs. 1,2 Preoperative appearance and incision.
Both hands have six complete three-phalangeal finger rays (as well as bilateral partial aplasia of the tibia and polydactyly of the feet). These conditions defy classification into any of the more common groups of anomalies. During the operation, the muscles of the radial border ray showed certain thenar characteristics, and a lumbricalis muscle was found at its *ulnar* side.
Incisions on the opposite side are marked by *broken lines*. Large parts of flaps *(2)* and *(3)* (*dotted areas*) will be eliminated during closure. The edge of flap *(3)* should be identical with the thenar fold of the new thumb. The skin incision on the extensor side of the IInd finger has to be extended to the level of the PIP joint.

The palmar triangular flap *(1)* may also be raised somewhat longer and more radial. This procedure permits one to use merely one flap for coverage of the defect between the index finger flaps on the radial side (not as shown in *Fig. 11.*)

Fig. 3 Partial palmar aspect.
Skin flaps have been developed, flexor tendons, vessels, and nerves are exposed. Use surgical telescopes! Stay close to the palmar aponeurosis while developing flaps *(1)* and *(3)* (not shown).

Only when palmar vessels and nerves are clearly in sight may the aponeurosis be excised to the level of the third metacarpal bone. It will then be easier to raise the palmar skin. Main arteries of the supernumerary finger will be ligated; tendons and nerves will be transected, as will the lig. capit. transversum between the Ist and IInd ray.

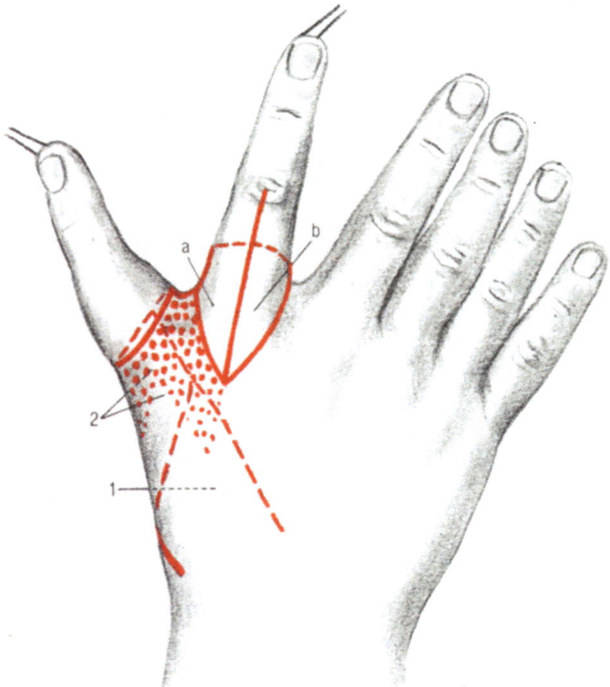

a
b
2
1

1

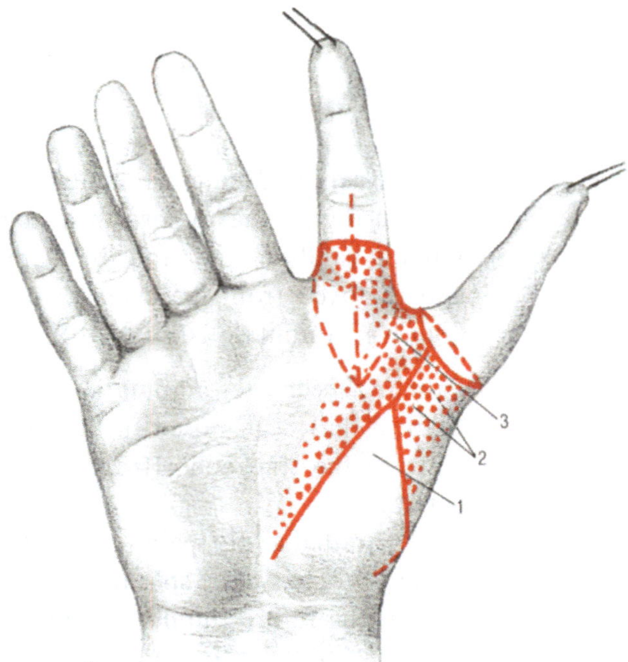

3
2
1

2

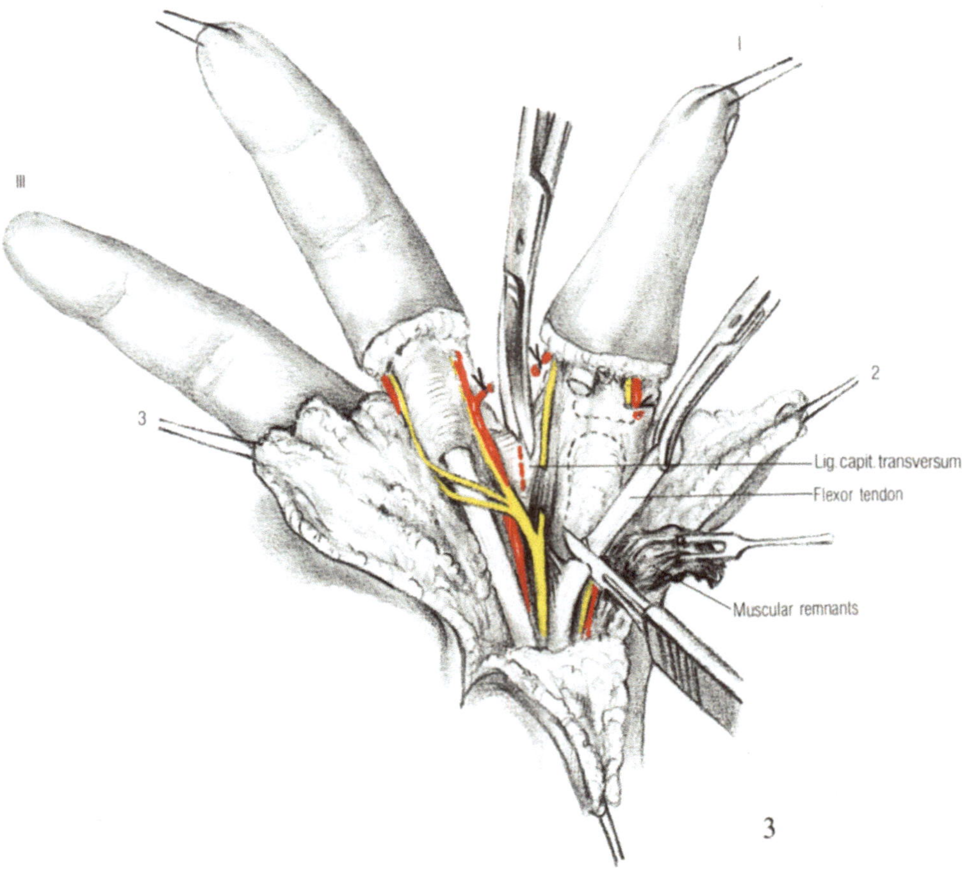

II
I
III
2
3
Lig. capit. transversum
Flexor tendon
Muscular remnants

3

Fig. 4 Dorsal aspect during amputation of supernumerary finger. Preserve main veins of IInd digit! Anastomoses near a main trunk are to be ligated, not coagulated! Lateral bands of the IInd digit are transected at their junction with the muscles and removed from the extensor aponeurosis to the level of the PIP joint of the digit (*). Amputate Ist digit at the carpometacarpal joint.

Fig. 5 Palmar aspect after amputation of Ist digit.
Flap *(3)* has been raised further ulnar; the palmar aponeurosis has been resected between the IInd and IIIrd digit after exposure of the bifurcation of vessels and nerves.

The radial a. dig. palm. propr. to the future index finger is ligated. The common nerve trunk has to be split interfascicularly so far proximally as to permit transposition of the future thumb without tension (*broken line*) (*). In this case we found the ulnar a. dig. palm. propr. to be encircled by a nerve (see figure).

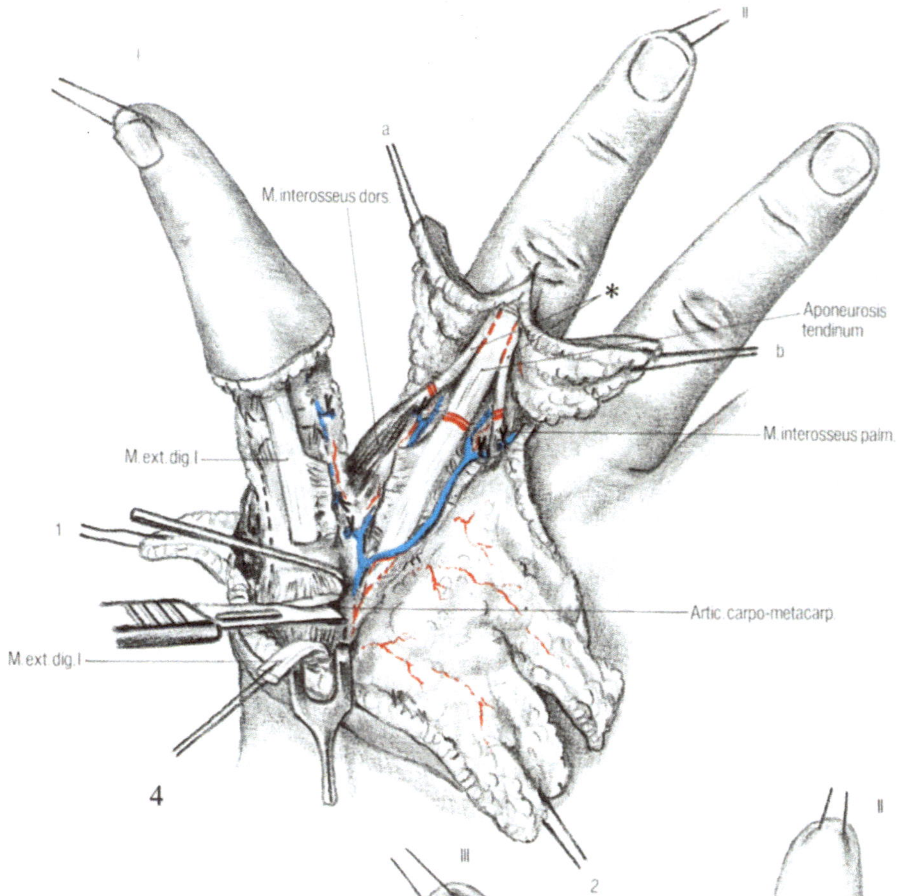
I
II
III
a
M. interosseus dors.
*
Aponeurosis tendinum
b
M. interosseus palm.
M. ext. dig. I
1
Artic. carpo-metacarp.
M. ext. dig. I
2

4

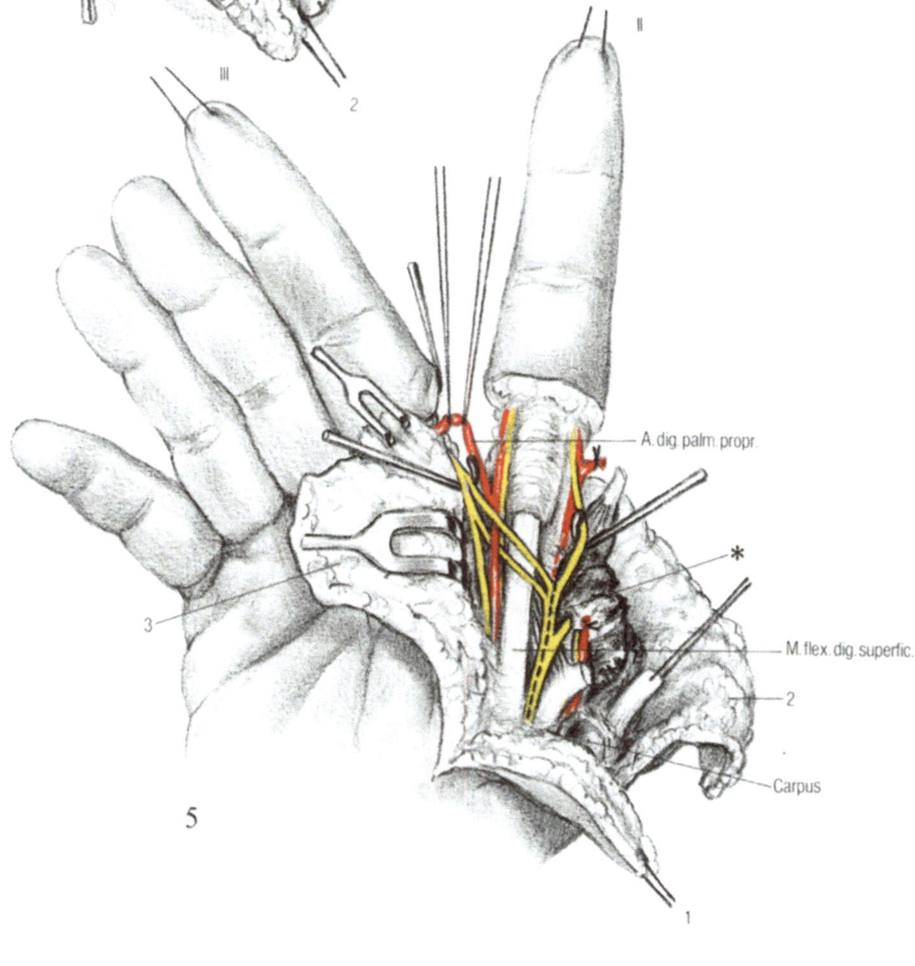
II
III
A. dig. palm. propr.
*
3
M. flex. dig. superfic.
2
Carpus
1

5

Fig. 6 Radial aspect.
Subperiosteal exposure and resection of the metacarpal bone of the future thumb without removing its head. The length of the finger has to be reduced to the normal length of a thumb. Excise the metacarpal with care: proximally the a. rad. may run close to the bone.

Fig. 7 Radial aspect after resection of the second metacarpal bone.
Resect the epiphyseal plate from remaining head of metacarpal bone. To prevent a hyperextension deformity, the resected surface is pulled dorsally with hooks and the metacarpal head is fixed in this position with a transarticular Kirschner wire (see insert).
Essentially, the finger is now merely suspended by the neurovascular bundle. It is then turned 130–150°, abducted approximately 30°, and fixed to the decorticated carpal bone (Kirschner wire).

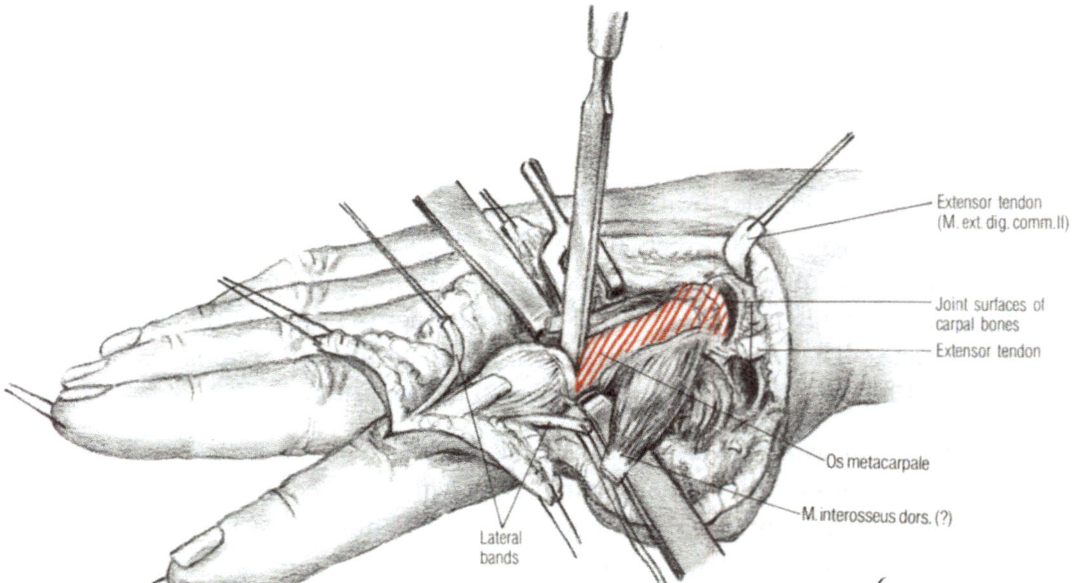
Extensor tendon
(M. ext. dig. comm. II)
Joint surfaces of
carpal bones
Extensor tendon
Os metacarpale
M. interosseus dors. (?)
Lateral
bands

6

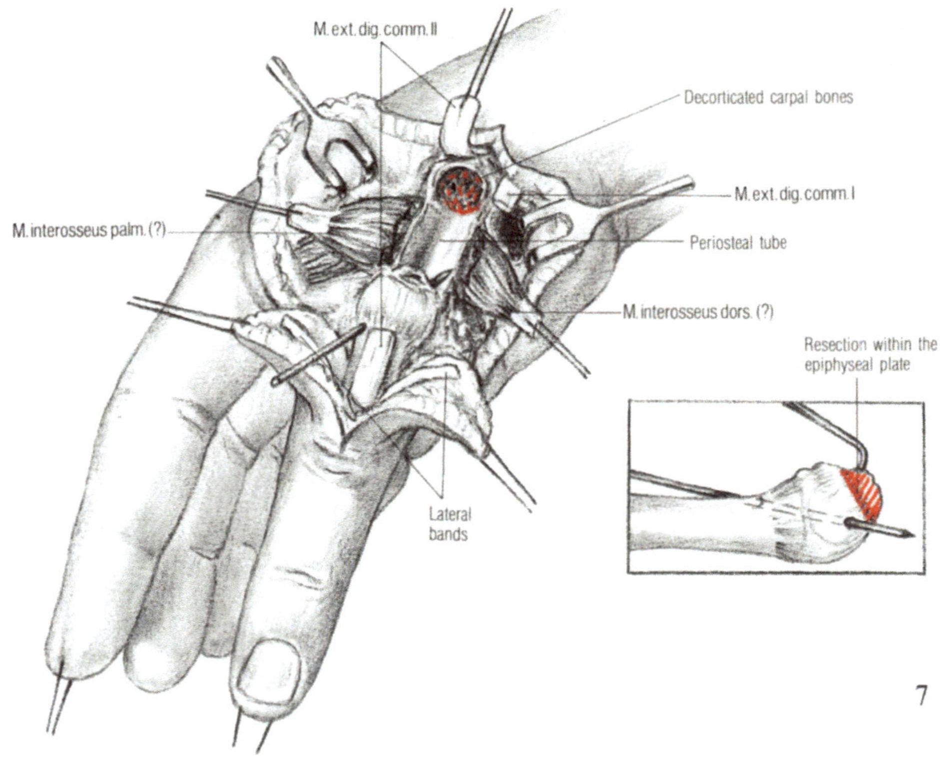
M. ext. dig. comm. II
Decorticated carpal bones
M. ext. dig. comm. I
M. interosseus palm. (?)
Periosteal tube
M. interosseus dors. (?)
Resection within the
epiphyseal plate
Lateral
bands

7

Fig. 8 Dorsoradial aspect after transposition of finger.
A second Kirschner wire is used (not shown), after adjustments have been made, to fix the head of the thumb in its ideal position opposite the head of the ring finger. Bone chips must be inserted in cases where large gaps remain toward the carpal bones. The ulnar lateral band will be woven into the palmar m. interosseus, the radial into the dorsal m. interosseus (Buck-Gramcko 1966).

Fig. 9 Radial–palmar aspect: anastomosis of the tendons.
For the sake of clarity, the new thumb is shown abducted and extended.
The stumps of the former IInd finger extensor tendons have been overlapped and sutured. The extensor tendon of the amputated Ist digit has been anchored to the radial basis of the new first metacarpal bone (formerly the second proximal phalanx).
The former Ist digit's extensor tendon now serves as an abductor. The dorsal mm. interossei of the Ist and IInd digits serve as opponens, and the palmar m. interosseus of the IInd digit serves as the abductor. Upon completion of suturing the tendons, the tourniquet is removed and all bleeding is stopped (microcoagulation!).

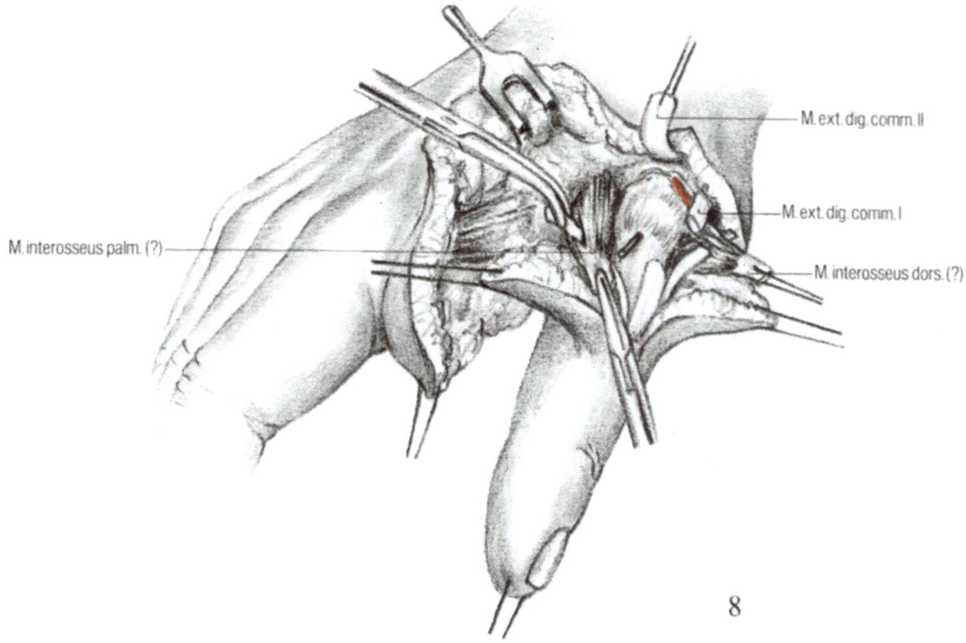
M. ext. dig. comm. II
M. ext. dig. comm. I
M. interosseus palm. (?)
M. interosseus dors. (?)

8

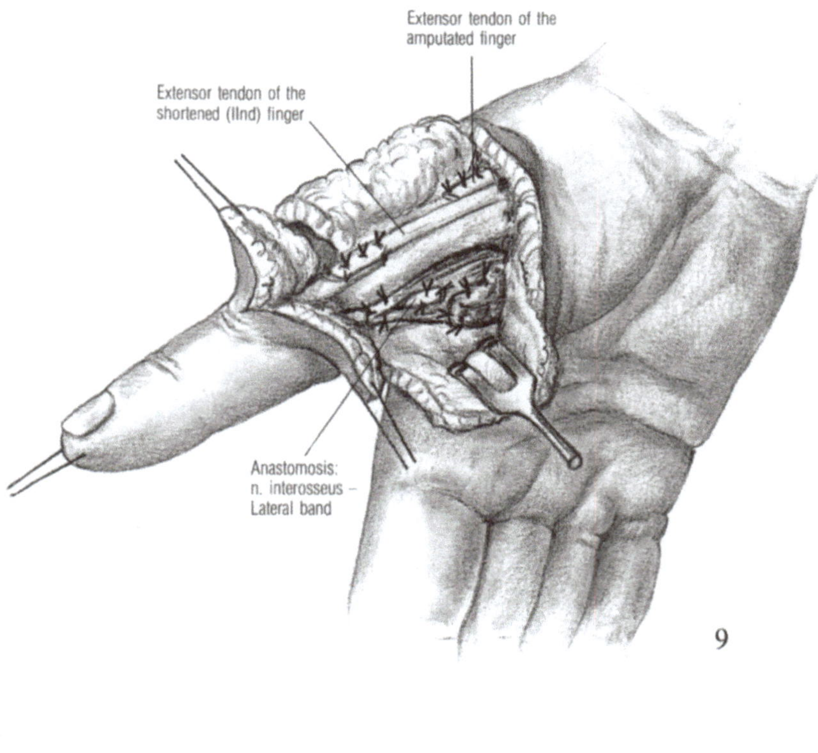
Extensor tendon of the amputated finger
Extensor tendon of the shortened (IInd) finger
Anastomosis: n. interosseus - Lateral band

9

Figs. 10,11 Postoperative appearance, radial and palmar aspects.
Tension-free skin closure. Several skin flaps, especially *(2)* and *(3)*, had to be trimmed and shaped considerably.

Postoperative Care

See Sect. 4.2.4.

Errors and Their Consequences

E. Instead of resecting excess thenar muscles, they have been inserted into extensors.
C. Muscular imbalance and impaired circulation of the skin (tension!)

See also Sect. 4.2.4.

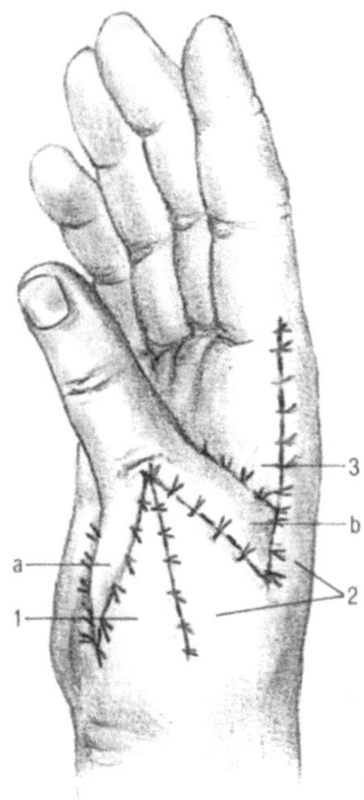

10

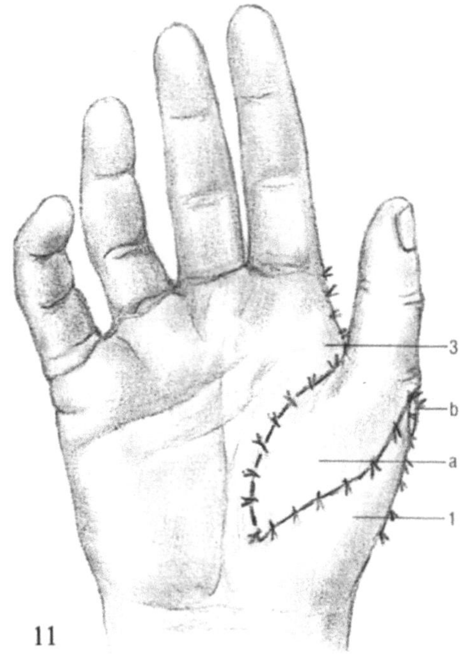

11

5 Metrical Variations

5.1 Introduction

5.1.1 General Remarks

The terms "metrical variations" (W. MÜLLER 1937) refers to congenital malformations of the hand characterized by *variations in the length of some fingers or phalanges* (W. MÜLLER: "Disorders in Differentiation of Length").

Generally speaking, variations of the triphalangeal thumb are referred to as "plus forms," whereas "minus variants" are the relatively common brachydactylies.

5.1.1.1 Triphalangy of the Thumb

A triphalangeal thumb features an additional middle phalanx, either rudimentary or complete.

Of the many theories regarding the origin of the triphalangeal thumb the most widely accepted today is Gegenbaur-Pfitzner's hypothesis of assimilation (PFITZNER 1898). It attributes the usual lack of a middle phalanx in the thumb to "assimilation" into the distal phalanx; accordingly, a triphalangeal thumb is considered a phylogenic atavism (see POL 1921, 1937; WERTHEMANN 1952; ROCHLIN and ZEITLER 1968; etc.).

However, it is difficult to reconcile this idea with the early phylogenic development of the biphalangeal system: almost without exception the Ist rays of mammals, reptiles, and amphibians have only two phalanges (NAUCK 1938). Completely unfounded is JOACHIMSTHAL's theory (1900), later taken up by HOPF (1959) and others, that a triphalangeal thumb represents *duplication of the index finger combined with an aplastic thumb.* There are no morphological findings to support this theory, nor do minor abnormalities indicate the existence of a teratologic progression (SCHNEIDER-SICKERT and HIPPE 1975).

However, plus forms do show *teratologic progression* (W. MÜLLER 1937; POL 1937). Their most important stages are as follows:

- Small wedge-shaped skeletal segments between proximal and distal phalanges (*Schaltstück* or connecting link);
- Rudimentary middle phalanges of varying lengths whose epiphysis has *no* nucleus of its own;
- More or less fully developed middle phalanges whose epiphysis *does have* a separate nucleus.

As a rule the latter are described as *"dolichophalangy,"* as opposed to other forms of triphalangeal thumbs which are collectively referred to as *"brachymesophalangeal forms."*

The above-mentioned skeletal conditions are merely one aspect of these abnormalities: the Ist ray loses its characteristics as a thumb and comes to resemble a long finger *(Dolichophalangy)* as the development of the middle phalanx progresses. The radial border digit resembles other long fingers both in form and function. The first metacarpal is tethered proximally and distally by the tight metacarpal ligaments. The carpometacarpal joint lacks normal freedom of movement and all (?) or most of the thenar muscles (personal observations); opposition of the thumb is lacking, resulting in or deriving from loss of rotation of the entire ray in regard to the long fingers. The skeletal diameter adapts to that of the nearest finger. Of the frequently observed two epiphyses of the first metacarpal, the proximal one is sometimes only a pseudoepiphysis. Aberrant nerves and vessels similar to those seen in hypoplastic thumbs have been observed (see Sect. 4.1.1.2). If accompanied by camptodactyly, additional abnormalities of the muscles and tendons have to be expected (see Chap. 12).

Hypoplastic middle phalanges present a different clinical picture. The thumb's important function of opposition is retained; it decreases, however, as development of a middle phalanx increases. From the point of view of their function KELIKIAN (1974) describes this "opposional three-phalangeal thumb" as the counterpart of the nonopposional thumb. As a rule the thenar eminence is atrophied. Despite the additional middle phalanx, such a thumb may be shorter and thinner than a normal one; the commissure may be narrower. Quite frequently it is in a less rotated position.

These conditions are therefore comparable to thumb hypoplasias of the first and second degree as described in Chap. 4. In many cases, the distal joint of the short middle phalanx deviates laterally, almost always in an ulnar direction. Its shape is wedgelike or trapeziform ["delta phalanx," (JONES 1964)]. If still less developed (connecting link, see Sects. 5.3, 9.3), the only clinical finding is a slanted distal phalanx.

All known forms of familiar triphalangism have proven to be *autosomal dominant*. It is interesting to note that this condition is on occasion coupled with a duplication of the thumb (MÜLLER 1937; a.o.). The so-called dysmelia syndrome often includes triphalangeal as well as hypoplastic and aplastic thumbs.

5.1.1.2 Brachydactyly

Its basis is a selective hypoplasia of a single ray element involving one or more fingers.

Important questions regarding the teratology of brachydactylies remain to be answered. There are many indications that they originate from disturbances of the enchondral ossification process.

The correlation between the disposition to hypoplasia of the phalanges and their respective diaphyseal ossification in the embryo is of interest: the earlier their ossification normally begins, the more frequent is the involvement of that particular part of the skeleton (FÜRST 1900; POL 1937). Hence the frequency of affected middle phalanges which ossify first.

Depending on the exact location of the shortening, we distinguish *brachytele-, brachymeso-, and brachybasophalangy* as well as brachymetacarpy. As a rule, the width of the reduced finger is normal [exception: butt thumb, (brachytelephalangy I)]. Genetically, certain combinations of brachydactyly are *autosomal dominant* with differing variance (see classifications by Pol 1937; Schinz 1943; Bell 1951). Brachydactyly occurs in isolation as well as an obligatory or facultative symptom of numerous syndromes (see Kelikian 1974; McKusick 1975; etc.). We emphasize its combination with soft tissue defects in *symbrachydactyly* (see Chap. 8).

The *tetratological staging* of the affected middle and proximal phalanges corresponds to that of the middle phalanx of the thumb (see above).

The great majority of brachydactylies do not impede the function of the finger to any substantial degree and are therefore in many cases diagnosed by sheer coincidence. Few of them require an operation. Exceptions are the brachydactylies that are accompanied by lateral deviations of the fingers *(clinodactyly)*. They occur mostly in so-called anepiphyseal middle phalanges, usually in the little finger but also in the IInd and IVth digits. The deviation points almost without exception toward the middle finger and disappears upon flexion. Major deviations, especially of the index finger, are also seen in brachybasophalangies.

Based on appearance and teratogenetic differences, we distinguish the following *irregularities in the transversal segmentation* of individual rays:

Assimilation hypophalangy (biphalangy), which results in finger shortening due to lack of segmentation between middle and distal phalanges or (rarely) between middle and proximal phalanges. As a rule there is only one common diaphyseal nucleus (see schema by Schinz 1943; Cocchi 1965; Witt et al. 1966).

Brachyhyperphalangy (Schinz) (or pseudohyperphalangy) shows an additional segmentation of the proximal phalanx, which in most cases is not much shorter than the normal one. This form occurs in the IInd and IIIrd digits, always in connection with brachymesophalangy (so-called Vidal type). The proximal part of the proximal phalanx is quite frequently trapeze shaped, and the index finger deviates in an ulnar direction. There is a functionless joint between the two parts of the proximal phalanx (amphiarthrosis). Later on these parts can fuse, just as the proximal phalanx may fuse with the brachymesophalangeal middle phalanx.

Postnatal phalangeal fusions are related to *joint hypoplasias* (Chap. 6). Their pathomechanics are presumed to be closely related to brachydactyly.

Unusual types of brachydactyly can show strange variations of epiphyseal plate configuration, i.e., a dome-shaped plate coursing from the proximal to the distal end of the shortened phalanx instead of in its usual parallel direction: so-called *Bogenepiphyse* (Schneider-Sickert 1975). This is generally accompanied by a dysplasia of the distal phalanx and deviation of the distal section of the ray.

5.1.2 Indications for Surgery

Only a small percentage of brachydactylies require an operation, e.g., if major functions are impaired or appearance is cosmetically unacceptable.

Essentially they are either cases of metrical variations with *axis deviations* of the thumb or cases with pronounced involvement of the other fingers (especially IInd and Vth or *dolichophalangy* and more extreme grades of *brachymesophalangeal* thumbs. A few attempts have been made to lengthen metacarpals (KELIKIAN 1974; VERDAN 1975; v. ANDRIAN-WERBURG 1975). Personally, however, we have not yet seen a patient where a lengthening attempt justified the risk of impairing function.

An operation may also be indicated in the presence of *concomitant malformations*, especially in cases of phalangeal aplasia or dysplasia, duplication of the thumb, and camptodactyly (see also Chap. 8: Symbrachydactyly).

5.1.3 Timing of Surgery

Where *pollicization* of a triphalangeal thumb is indicated, we refer to our recommendations outlined in Sect. 4.1.2.

Other operations, too, should be performed in time to complete the entire program, including postoperative physiotherapy, before the patient enters school. Exceptions are some corrective osteotomies for *clinodactyly* with trapeze-shaped middle phalanges of the thumb or long fingers. Such operations can be performed more accurately and the risk of stunting growth by damaging the epiphyses is lessened if they are delayed as long as functional impediments permit. Similar considerations are valid for axis deviations in brachyphalangy with abnormal epiphyseal plates (Sect. 5.4).

In regard to *concomitant malformations*, we refer to the corresponding chapters (particularly 6, 8, and 12).

5.1.4 General Surgical Directives

The preferred operation for correction of *dolichophalangy* is a subtotal metacarpectomy and transposition of the finger on its neurovascular pedicle *(pollicization)*. Recommended procedures are the same as for other pollicizations (see Sects. 4.1 and 4.2.4–4.2.6). Amputation and pollicization by transposition of the IInd finger may be indicated in some cases where triphalangy is combined with major hypoplasia of the entire ray (see Sect. 4.2.4).

Functional disturbances of the *brachymesophalangeal thumb* may be caused by clinodactyly, narrow thumb commissure, limitation or total lack of opposition, decreased rotation as well as instability of the MP joint. These disturbances necessitate a series of operations, a fact to consider in determining the initiation of treatment. If practicable, correction of the axis should be combined with deepening and widening of the commissure (Z-plasty or dorsoradial swivel flaps; see Sect. 2.2.3 etc.) (BLAUTH 1975) and/or a rotation osteotomy of the first metacarpal. In another operation, an opponens plasty might be combined with stabilization of the first

MP joint. These are measures described in Sect. 4.2 (examples 4.2.1–4.2.3), aimed at correcting first- and second-degree thumb hypoplasia. In cases of brachydactyly, *extensor rigidity* is rarely a cause for performing a flexion osteotomy.

5.1.5 Postoperative Care

See individual examples.

Goal of Surgery

Improvement of function and appearance of the hand by shortening the Ist ray and rotating the triphalangeal thumb on its neurovascular pedicle.

Figs. 1, 2 Preoperative appearance and incision.
Diaphysis and metaphysis of the first metacarpal (*hatched areas*) will be resected. In hypoplastic triphalangeal thumbs it may be more expedient to retain a proximal portion of the metacarpal in order to assure a thumb of adequate length. The *dotted skin areas* will be resected as needed during closure.
To assure tension-free rotation, the incision along flap *(1)* may have to be extended proximally.
Lately we have placed the semicircular palmar incision at the finger even farther distal, approximately midway between the flexor creases of the MP and PIP joints (not shown, see Sect. 4.5.7). Initially the tip of flap *(1)* extends farther distal. It can be trimmed later if necessary. From a cosmetic point of view, even better results are achieved in this manner.

Specific Surgical Directives
In general, one should follow operative guidelines and suggestions described in Sects. 4.2.4–4.2.6.
Any vestiges of thenar muscles may be utilized once the dolichophalangeal thumb has been transposed. (This also applies to advanced cases of brachymesophalangeal thumbs for which operations outlined in Sects. 4.2.1–4.2.3 may be inadequate and for which a transposition with a neurovascular pedicle may be indicated.) However, these muscles should not be permitted to interfere with skin closure; if this occurs they have to be resected.

Figs. 3, 4 Postoperative appearance, radial *(3)* and palmar *(4)* aspects.
The thumb is now in opposition and has been turned ca. 140°. Fixation in position of function with two Kirschner wires (metacarpal head flexed dorsally! See Sect. 4.5.7 a.o.). The tip of the thumb is near the PIP joint of the adjacent finger.
For the sake of clarity, Fig. 4 shows only part of the desired fixation in functional position prior to postoperative physiotherapy.

Postoperative Care and Errors and Their Consequences

See Sect. 4.2.4 a.o.

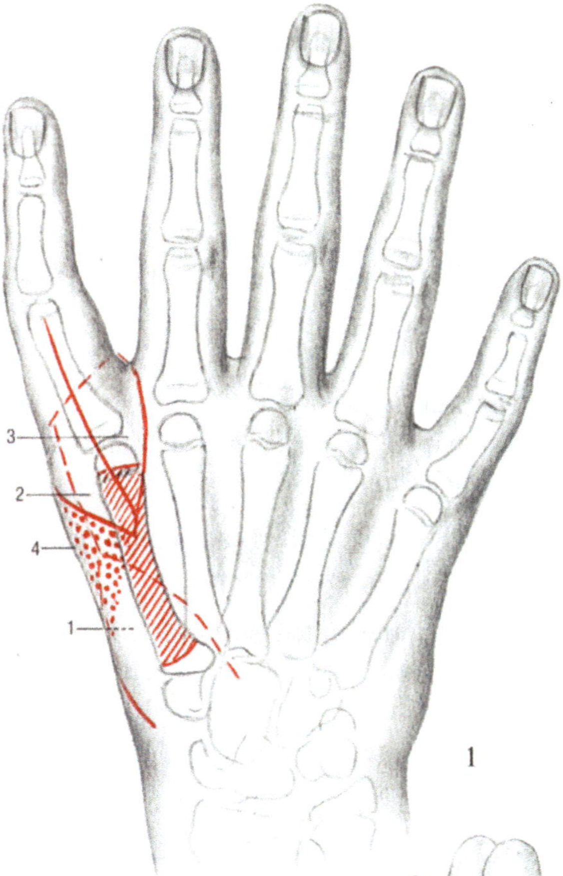

1

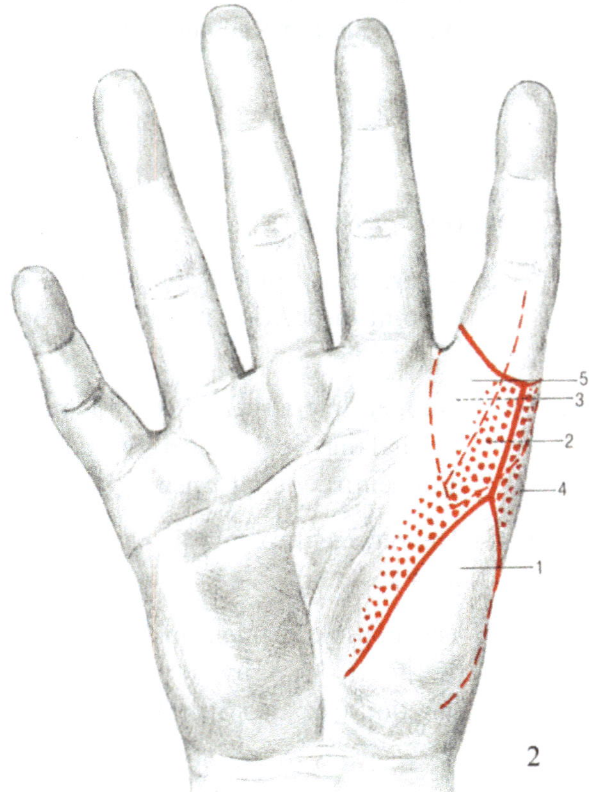

2

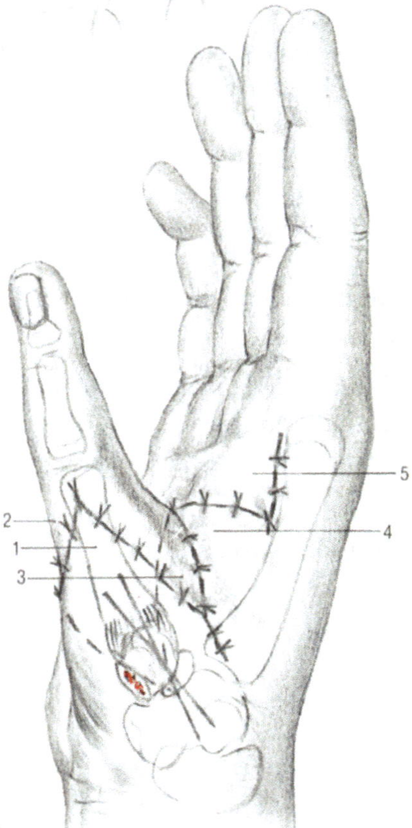

3

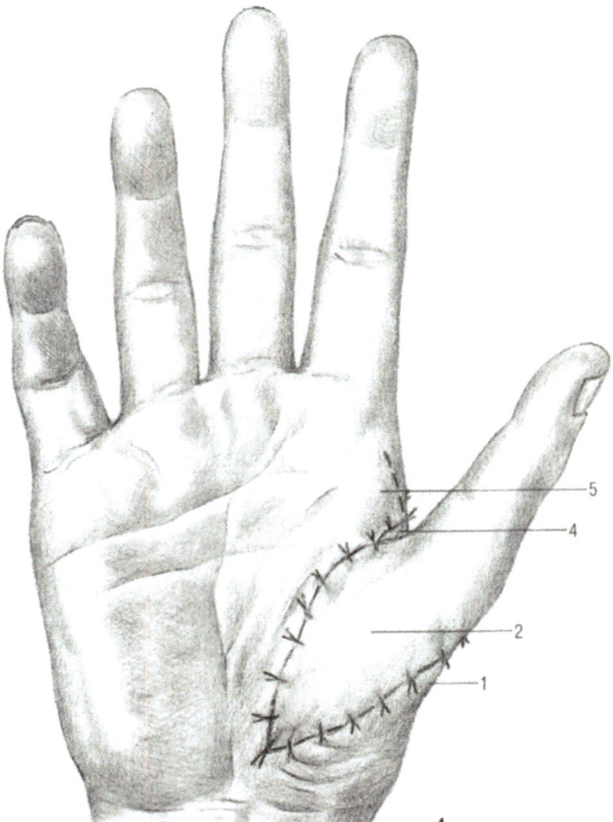

4

5.3 Brachymesophalangeal Thumb: Ulnar Clinodactyly with Wedge-Shaped Rudimentary Phalanx

Goal of Surgery

Straightening of the longitudinal thumb axis and creating fibrous rigidity of the IP joint in position of function.

Fig. 1 Preoperative appearance and incision, dorsal aspect.
Triphalangy is limited to a rudimentary, wedge-shaped phalanx which is removed in its entirety after opening of the capsule (*hatched area*).

Fig. 2 The rudimentary middle phalanx has been completely divested of its capsuloligamentous structures.

Fig. 3 The capsuloligamentous structures are closed with interrupted sutures. Fixation of the IP joint by a transosseous, transarticular Kirschner wire in position of function (see also Sect. 9.3).

Postoperative Care

Short (or long)-arm cast for approximately 4 weeks. Removal of the Kirschner wire at that time, splint application (day and night) for an additional 4 weeks. A night splint will be worn for another 6 months.

Errors and Their Consequences

E. Recurrence is possible despite removal of the cuneiform rudiment.
C. Follow-up examinations are required.

E. This method is used to remove a larger phalangeal rudiment when a *wedge osteotomy* as described in Sect. 5.5.1 is actually indicated.
C. The soft tissues may not shrink sufficiently postoperatively to attain fibrous rigidity.

E. The period of postoperative immobilization is too short.
C. The joint will remain unstable.

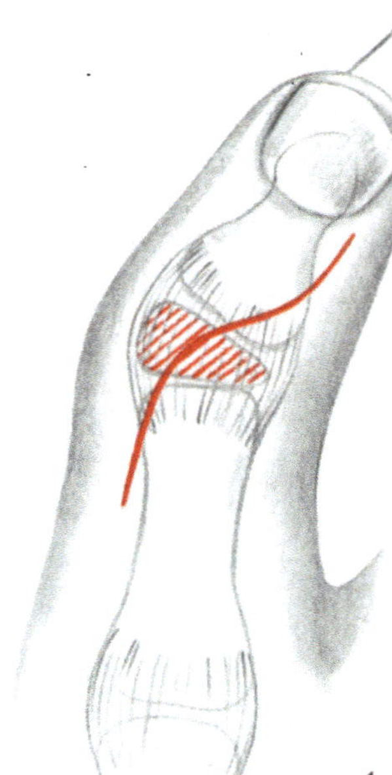

1

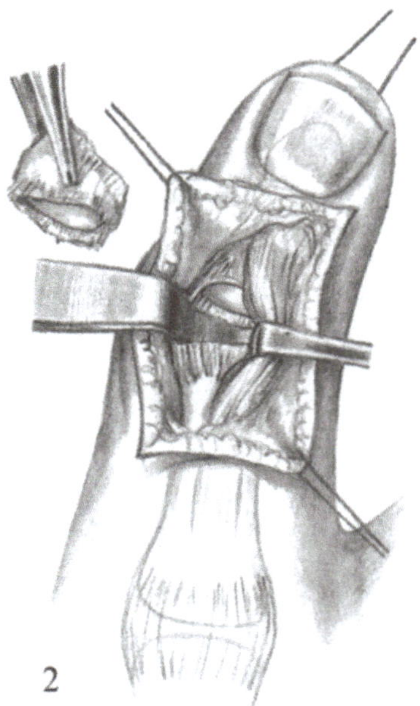

2

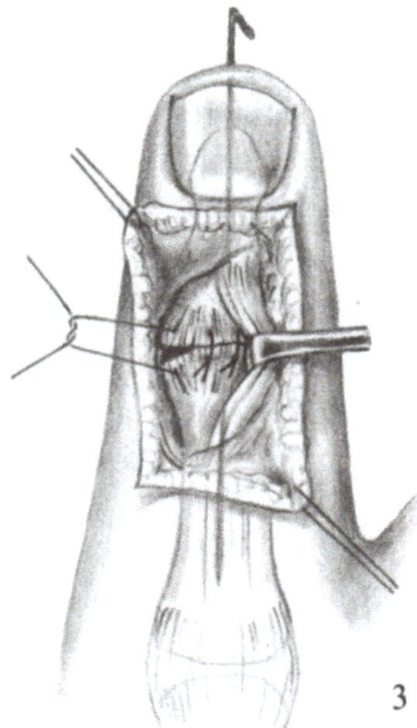

3

Goal of Surgery

Improving grip by correcting the thumb's malposition and deepening of the commissure between the Ist and IInd finger.

Fig. 1 Preoperative appearance and incision, dorsal aspect.
Familial brachydactyly: brachybasophalangy of the thumb, with trapeze-shaped epiphysis ("delta phalanx"). The first commissure is narrow, the thumb is in marked radial abduction. A Z-plasty (as shown in Sect. 2.2.5) would not provide sufficient depth and width. Therefore, an additional dorsoradial swivel flap *(a)* is required. The malposition of the thumb is corrected by a cuneiform osteotomy of the proximal phalanx with an ulnar base *(red hatched area)*. Remaining excess skin on the extensor side of the thumb is resected during wound closure *(black hatched area)*.

Fig. 2 Dorsal aspect.
The thumb's longitudinal axis has been corrected; the dorsoradial swivel flap forms the center of a deep and wide commissure. One or two transosseous–transarticular Kirschner wires keep the fragments of the thumb's proximal phalanx in place (a slight additional rotation of the thumb at the base of the osteotomy may improve opposition). Functional position of the thumb is secured by a transosseous Kirschner wire through the first metacarpal. A thick-split thickness skin graft *(Tr)* covers the area from which the flap *(a)* was taken.

Fig. 3 Postoperative appearance, palmar aspect.
Kirschner wire fixation is not shown; opposition of the thumb omitted to show commissure in detail.

Postoperative Care

Long-arm cast for approximately 4 weeks with subsequent removal of Kirschner wires. First dressing change after 8–10 days. Upon removal of the cast a night splint is prepared to keep the Ist ray in a position of maximum abduction and medium opposition.

Comment

Recurrence of abnormal growth is possible at the osteotomized hypoplastic proximal phalanx of the thumb (e.g., by partial damage of the epiphyseal plate during osteotomy). This may require correction by further osteotomies or, in the presence of dysplastic MP or IP joints, by soft tissue operations (or "chondrodesis," see Chap. 7).

Errors and Their Consequences. See Sects. 2.2.5 and 2.2.3.

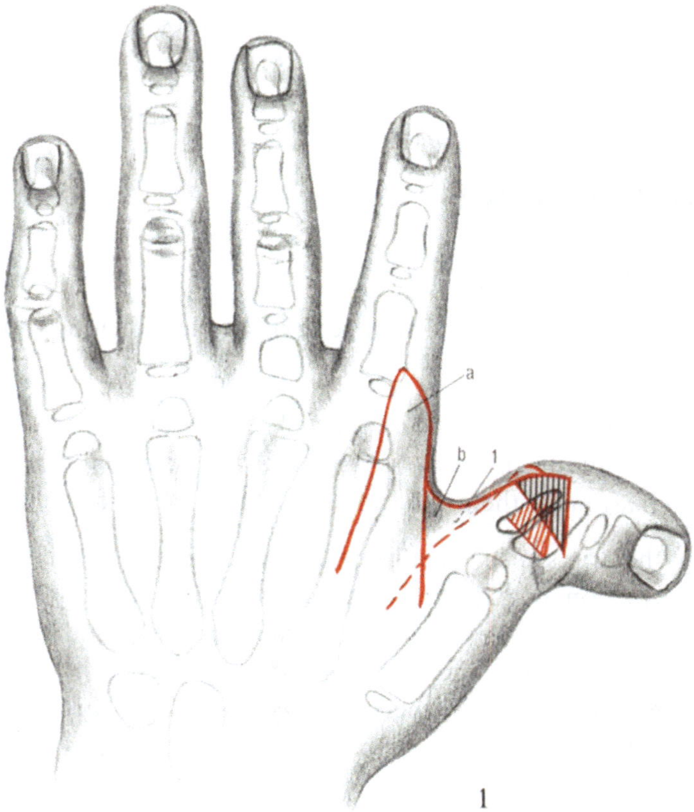

1

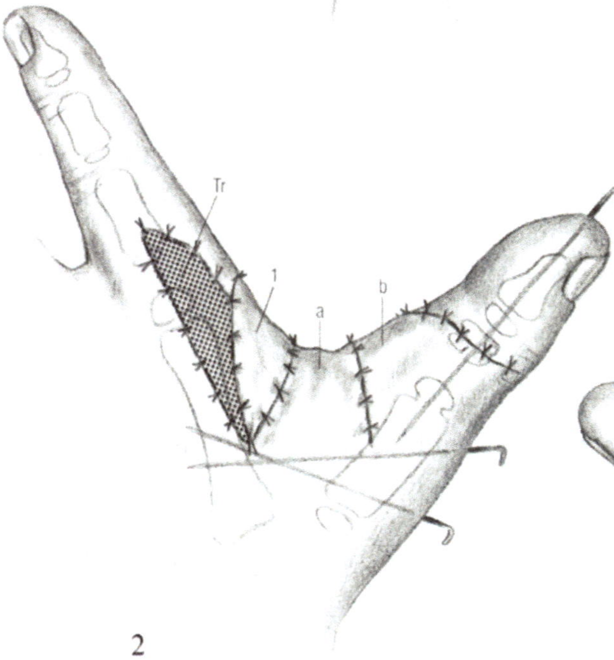

2

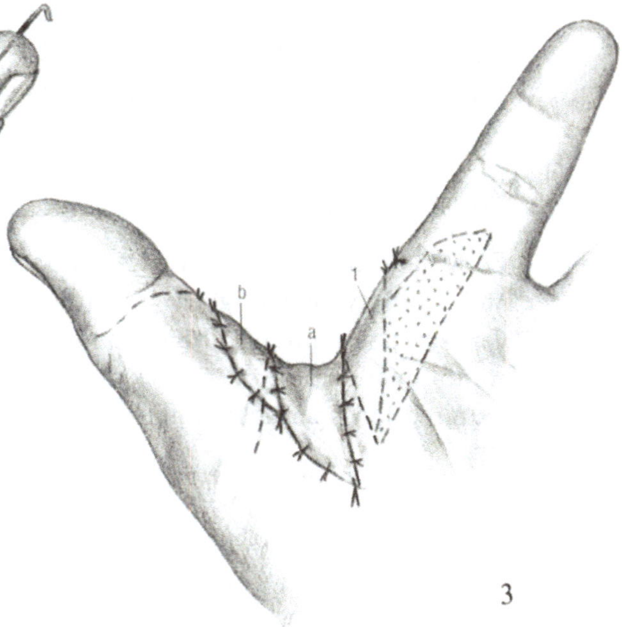

3

5.5 Brachymesophalangeal Long Finger

5.5.1 Radial Clinodactyly of the Index Finger

Goal of Surgery

Straightening of the longitudinal finger axis and lengthening of the middle phalanx.

Fig. 1 Preoperative appearance, dorsal aspect.
Access to the middle phalanx is gained by a longitudinal dorsoradial incision. The *broken lines* mark the osteotomy site. It is exposed by a circular periosteotomy.

Fig. 2 Following the transverse osteotomy and the filling of the defect resulting from the axis correction with pieces of autologous spongiosa, the fragments are fixed by crossed Kirschner wires with the middle phalanx in medium position of flexion. The radial Kirschner wire should be cut subcutaneously. Instead of the transarticular vertical wire, a second Kirschner wire may be driven through the middle phalanx (distal radial to proximal ulnar).

Postoperative Care

(Long-) or short-arm cast, including index and middle fingers, in position of function. The transarticular Kirschner wire will be removed after 4 weeks and a finger splint will be applied. The second Kirschner wire will be removed 2 weeks later, and gradual, careful physiotherapy will be instituted.

Errors and Their Consequences

E. An additional cuneiform resection has been omitted despite soft tissue tension and inability to straighten the finger fully even after a circular periosteotomy.
C. A certain amount of malposition remains.
Joint function may decrease even with consistent physiotherapy because of the required long period of immobilization.

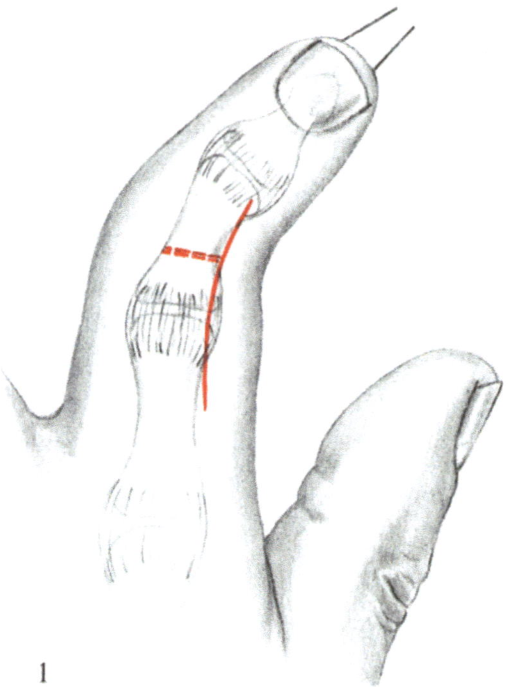

1

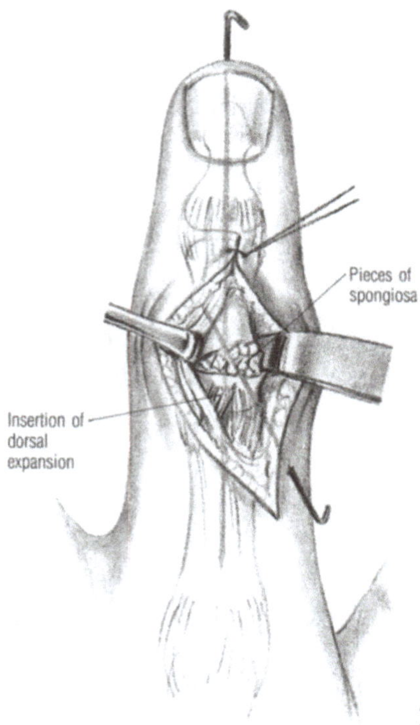

2

5.5.2 Radial Clinodactyly of the Index Finger (Alternative Method)

Goal of Surgery

Straightening of the longitudinal axis of the finger.

Fig. 1 Preoperative appearance, dorsal aspect.
The middle phalanx is exposed by a curvilinear skin incision or by a dorsoulnar approach *(broken line)*. Removal of excessive skin prior to wound closure is facilitated by the curvilinear incision *(dotted area)*.

Fig. 2 Postoperative appearance.
An ulnar-based wedge has been removed from the middle phalanx. The osteotomy is stabilized by two crossed Kirschner wires. The radial wire should be cut off subcutaneously. The PIP joint is in medium flexion.

Postoperative Care and Errors and Their Consequences

See Sect. 5.5.1.

Remarks

We recommend this method if the middle phalanx is relatively long. Its advantage is a shorter period of immobilization and a lesser risk of partial joint stiffness.

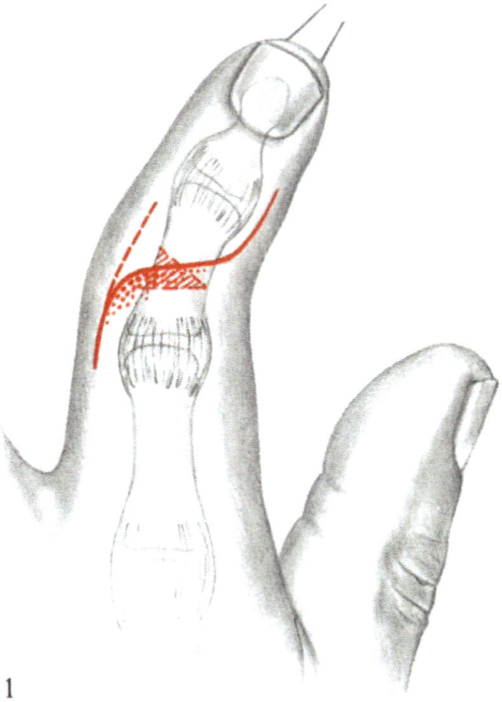

1

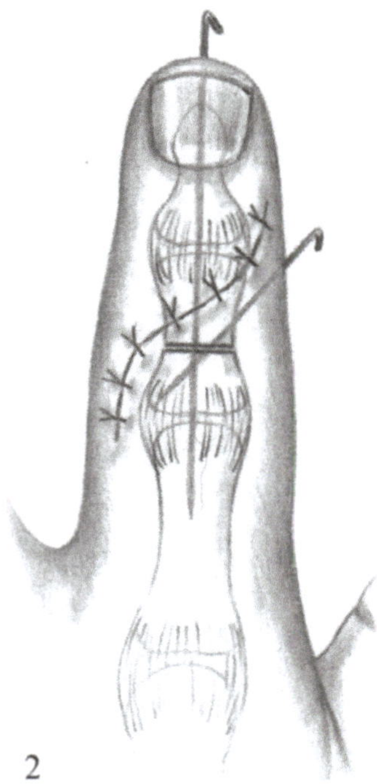

2

6 Hypoplasias and Aplasias of Finger Joints

6.1 Introduction

6.1.1 General Remarks

Joint hypoplasias and aplasias are characterized by *congenital extension rigidity* (Pol 1921, 1937). They may occur in *isolation* as well as in combination with other defects. They are always part of *Apert syndrome* (see Chap. 2.2) and are also seen in more severe malformations of the extremities such as *ectromelia, partial giantism,* and *symbrachydactylies*. Occasionally, rigidity occurs in individual fingers in connection with other abnormalities, e.g., syndactyly, polydactyly, and cleft hands (for review, see Kelikian 1974; Pol 1937). The Anglo-American term commonly applied to these malformations is "symphalangism" (Cushing 1916).

Isolated forms occur sporadically as well as repeatedly within families; autosomal dominance is irregular and clearly subject to variation in its manifestations; alternating incidence combined with perodactylous shortening of the distal phalanges has been described (Weyers 1968). It is assumed that there is a close pathogenetic *correlation between this and other anomalies involving segmentation* (Duken 1921; Pol 1921; Werthemann 1952; Drinkwater 1917), since brachymesophalangism, brachytelephalangism, double epiphyses, and assimilation hypophalangism (on various rays) are frequently seen in the same patient or in patients' relatives (see also Chap. 5).

Symphalangism – which is often bilaterally symmetrical – affects almost exclusively the IP joints of the *long fingers*. The *PIP joints* (one or all) are predominantly involved, the DIP joints more rarely. Only in exceptional cases are both IP joints or MP joints affected.

The little finger is most frequently and most severely affected whenever more than one finger is involved. Cases of hypoplasia and aplasia of the thumb's carpometacarpal, metacarpal, and interphalangeal joints have been reported sporadically (see Pol 1937, etc.).

Clinically, all cases of hypoplasia and aplasia of the finger joints are characterized by rigidity in complete or near-complete extension (as opposed to acquired ankyloses). *Palmar and dorsal skin folds* in the area of the expected joint are conspicuously absent in assimilation hypophalangy and severe brachymesophalangy. Shortening of the finger or its segments may develop during extrauterine growth; however, it is usually minimal, in contrast to biphalangy.

Clinical appearance and, above all, x-ray and histologic findings are best understood by considering *pathogenesis:* under normal circumstances the phalanges begin to develop during the precartilaginous stage between two precartilaginous nuclei in the so-called *intermediary zone* of the primitive skeleton (see Duken 1921; Pol 1937, etc.).

Hypoplastic and aplastic phalanges also have two separate precartilaginous nuclei which later change into cartilage and bone, each with an epiphyseal plate (x-ray). However, *development of the joints* in the intermediary zone is *terminated prematurely*.

Without development of a mesenchymal space, a single, longer phalanx develops instead of two; it has *one* diaphyseal ossification zone and *one* nucleated epiphysis. If it affects the distal joint, this *joint agenesis* is referred to as *assimilation hypophalangy* (PFITZNER 1898) or, more generally, as *biphalangy* (see Chap. 5). For details see DUKEN (1921), POL (1921, 1937) a.o.; additional remarks in BARSKY (1958).

Of interest is Blechschmidt's theory on formal genesis: he reasons that there exists a disturbance of the so-called (muscular) *articulation slings* which, together with the *pressure of the growing cartilage (Stemmkörperwachstum)*, ordinarily produces formation of the joints (for details see BLECHSCHMIDT and PETERSEN 1967).

MESTERN's recommendation (1934) to categorize joint hypoplasia according to histomorphological criteria seems questionable from a formal genetic point of view, and meaningless from a clinical one.

In cases of *minimal inhibition anomally* a joint line is still present *(joint hypoplasia)* although its surfaces are nearly flat *(amphiarthrosis)*. Where growth has been inhibited more severely, development is limited to a *synarthrosis* either in the form of syndesmosis or synchondrosis. In the vast majority of cases, the latter forms a synostosis during early childhood. The springlike elasticity of the hyaline cartilage in synchondrosis can clinically simulate the presence of a joint. In contrast to joint agenesis, the x-ray will almost always reveal in such cases the area where development of the joint stopped (even after completion of ossification) by a more or less pronounced irregularity of the outer bone contour. Since osseous union of the hypoplastic joints occurs prior to the closing of the epiphyseal plate, radiographs may be misinterpreted: a persistent epiphyseal plate may be erroneously diagnosed as a joint.

6.1.2 Indications for Surgery

In a large percentage of cases the unpropitious extensor rigidity of the affected fingers diminishes the hand's usefulness only slightly. Therefore, isolated rigid fingers rarely require an operation. Occasionally, however, a flexion osteotomy may be indicated, especially where other malformations exist simultaneously.

6.1.3 Timing of Surgery and General Surgical Directives

Upon completion of bone growth a *cuneiform osteotomy* at the level of the hypoplastic joint may be considered, possibly combined with the removal of a persistent syndesmosis or synchondrosis (palmar wedge, fixation with Kirschner wires or small fragment screw).

Prior to completion of growth, further reduction of length can only be avoided by a *diaphyseal osteotomy* unless one wants to attempt a *"chondrodesis"*, i.e., removal of a cuneiform slice of cartilage directly from the joint surface. The cartilaginous areas of resection are fixed temporarily (4–6 weeks) by fine Kirschner wires. The result is a rigid joint in an improved position. Optimum functional position of the distal joint is an angle of 10–20°, and that of the proximal joint is 30–50° (with increasing flexion toward the little finger).

With the possible exception of the MP joint, *arthroplasty* should be performed sparingly. Insertion anomalies of finger tendons are to be expected; FISCHEL (1909) described a case of an aplastic PIP joint where the mm. flexores superficiales inserted at the proximal phalanx (in relation to this, see BLECHSCHMIDT's theory).

Details of operative techniques are outlined in Chap. 5 and Sect. 2.2.1 in connection with other malformations.

7 Joint Dysplasias

7.1 Introduction

7.1.1 General Remarks

The term "joint dysplasia" covers *anomalies of cartilaginous and bony parts of the joints* as well as *ligamentous–capsular* ones. Their etiology and pathology is unclear. The appearance and location of these malformations is quite *inconsistent;* they may be isolated incidents or part of a generalized connective tissue weakness (e.g., Marfan syndrome, Ehlers-Danlos syndrome); they may accompany endochondral dysostoses or, occasionally, complex malformations of the hand such as cleft hands, symbrachydactyly, oligodactyly, or polydactyly.

Their *principal clinical symptom* is inadequate stability or total absence of stability of the affected joint: excessive hyperextension, lateral instability, lax joints that can be easily subluxated or dislocated.

Joint dysplasias may be *caused* by interference of primary cartilage and bone formation and/or by inadequate firmness of ligamentous–capsular elements caused either by anomalies of the ligaments or by a generalized weakness of connective tissues.

Function of the fingers may be severely limited or even totally lost.

From a morphological and functional point of view, dysplasias of the *thumb ray* belong to a separate group: according to personal observations and to the few existing references in medical literature, they are extremely rare, but cause much greater problems than dysplasias of individual long fingers. Subluxation and dislocation of the thumb's carpometacarpal and MP joints reduces pinching strength, results in insecurity of grasp, and may lead to loss of typical forms of grip such as the key grip.

These *dislocations of the first carpometacarpal joint* are thought to be cause or symptom of the so-called *flat hand,* first mentioned by GOLDTHWAIT (1914). Primary malformations, especially of the os trapezium, are considered to be its leading cause (GOLDTHWAIT 1914; G. HOHMANN 1949); in some cases this has been verified (KELIKIAN 1974). Connections between these dislocations and dysostoses are under discussion, and patients showing unmistakable signs of Ehlers-Danlos syndrome are known.

Dysplasias and subluxations of the first MP joint, on the other hand, are most frequently seen in first- or second-degree hypoplasias of the thumb and in diastrophic dwarfism ("hitchhiker's thumb": hypoplasia of the first metacarpal). The thumb is usually in a position of radial abduction, and due to inadequate ligamentous protection it veers farther radial or hyperextends during pinching activities (BLAUTH 1967).

7.1.2 Indications for and Timing of Surgery

Dysplastic joints may be treated either by conservative means, such as splints, or by stabilizing operations. The age of the patient and the degrees of malfunction and cosmetic impairment determine the treatment and its timing.

7.1.3 General Surgical Directives

The simplest and most effective way to stabilize affected joints in a functionally favorable position is by *arthrodesis* (see Chap. 6). This should be done after closure of the epiphyseal plate to prevent excessive loss of longitudinal growth.

A few accounts of attempts to stabilize thumbs with subluxations of the carpometacarpal or MP joint by means of *extra-articular tendomyoplasty* have been reported. However, no information is available regarding long-term results. *Hohmann* reports on successful treatment by conservative means as well as by simple tightening of the capsule. Others report on reinforcement of the ligamentous–capsular structures by various methods of a free tendon transplant (EDGERTON et al. 1965; WITT 1957; WITT et al. 1966; BUNNELL 1959; BLAUTH 1972). To repair subluxations of the thumb's MP joint, WITT (1957) shortened the flexor side of the capsule in combination with transplantation of distal parts of the m. opponens or the m. abd. poll. brev. and m. flex. poll. brev. palmar to the basis of the proximal phalanx. He considers this method reliable and recommends early arthrodeses only in the most severe cases of uncontrollable dislocation during adolescence. WECKESSER (1954, 1955) recommends arthrodesis of the thumb or external stabilization with a splint combined with muscle-strengthening exercises. He claims to have achieved good results in several cases by fixation of the extended thumb in a cast, starting during the 1st–3rd month of life for periods totaling at least 1–7 months.

We, ourselves, have tightened capsules in combination with collateral ligament plasties (transosseous tendon loop) in patients with dysplasia and subluxation of the first MP joint (BLAUTH 1972). Occasionally, we have performed a so-called *chondrodesis* on children: we merely resected a narrow disk of cartilage from each side of the joint and placed the resected surfaces in a position of function. The position was secured with Kirschner wires and plaster casts for 4–6 weeks and with splints for an additional 6–8 weeks. This method should prevent growth problems and assure adequate stabilization of the joint.

However, we do not have any long-term results relating to this procedure, nor to a soft tissue operation necessitated by congenital dislocation of the first carpometacarpal joint.

8 Symbrachydactylies

8.1 Introduction

8.1.1 General Remarks

The manifold variations of symbrachydactyly are easily classified within a *teratologic order* with four degrees of severity (BLAUTH and GEKELER 1971):

Group I ("short-finger type"), consists of shortening (or aplasia) of some or all middle phalanges *(brachymesophalangy→biphalangy)* combined with more or less extensive interdigital skin bridges (syndactyly). These symptoms led to the term "symbrachydactyly" (POL 1921). Most frequently affected are the center rays. The thumb usually retains its shape and size, but it may be located at the level of the metacarpus and may have lost its oppositional and rotational abilities at the carpometacarpal joint (joint dysplasia). In such cases the thumb commissure is narrow and is displaced distally.

Group II ("cleft-hand type") includes more severe hypoplasias of one or more center rays, increasingly affecting the ulnar part of the hand (in contrast to *cleft hand,* in which the radial side is more affected!). Such an involution may extend proximally to the metacarpus ["atypical cleft hand" (M. LANGE 1936; BARSKY 1964, a.o.)]. There always remain budlike excrescences of the affected fingers, sometimes containing cartilage or bone rudiments, and in all cases at least single finger rudiments show (small) nails (in contrast to peripheral hypoplasia). Adjoining fingers will show an increased incidence of clinodactyly, biphalangy, joint aplasia, dislocations, and subluxations of the MP, PIP, and DIP joints.

Group III ("monodactylous type") comprises hands in which every three-phalangeal finger has been reduced to mere budlike rudiments with nails. The thumb ray retains its shape, but is short and of limited mobility.

In *group IV ("peromelus type")* all that is left of the fingers are humplike protuberances.

In all cases *anomalies of the blood vessels, nerves, and tendons* have to be expected. However, even the most severely deformed rays have rudimentary tendons.

Symbrachydactylies are relatively *rare.* As a rule, they occur *unilaterally* and, on occasion, combined with a thoracic wall defect *(Poland syndrome).* If *bilateral,* they are usually accompanied by peromelia and micrognathia *(Hanhart syndrome).*

8.1.2 Indications for Surgery

Almost all types of symbrachydactyly cause *malfunctions* of the hand which, as a rule, can only be remedied successfully by surgery. Hence, operations are almost always indicated.

For groups II–IV the main goal, essentially, is improved *grasp and pinch.*

Attempts to *separate syndactylous digits* are justified only if they are of reasonable size and able to function. Correction of syndactyly makes the fingers appear longer, therefore the operation also improves the appearance of the hand.

Construction of a *natural post* in a *monodactylous* hand hinges upon preoperative development of the thumb's strength and mobility through physio- and occupational therapy, as well as the simultaneous use of a temporary artificial gripping abutment device (see Fig. 42, Blauth and Gekeler 1973).

8.1.3 Timing of Surgery

The most effective time for surgery of groups I and II is the preschool years. Third-degree symbrachydactyly should be corrected earlier, i.e., during the 2nd or 3rd year of life, in order to attain natural pincer action as soon as possible. Arthrodeses are not performed until the epiphyseal plates are closed.

8.1.4 General Surgical Directives

Operative procedures in cases of *interdigital skin coalescences* (Sects. 8.2, 8.5) are similar to those for simple cutaneous syndactyly (Sect. 2.1).

Special problems arise when the *commissure of the thumb is very narrow or entirely missing:* its enlargement by means of two local triangular pedicle flaps similar to a Z-plasty is rarely satisfactory. What is needed is an additional swivel flap from the dorsal side of the thumb or index finger (see Sects. 4.2.1, 3.4). If the thumb is in very close apposition to the index finger, a tubed pedicle flap serves best to cover the skin defect caused by the separation of the thumb ray (Sect. 4.2.2).

Along with *lengthening osteotomies* of the Ist and/or Vth rays, consideration should be given to potentially helpful measures such as *corrective osteotomies* of border metacarpals (Sect. 8.3), *extension* of the commissures *into the metacarpus* (Sect. 8.5), *resections* of nonfunctioning hypoplastic rays (Sect. 8.4), and *operations at the first carpometacarpal joint* (Sect. 8.3).

Monodactylous hands can be reconstructed to permit *natural grasp* (Sect. 8.7) (Blauth 1972); the position of the opposing structure depends on the range of motion and alignment of the thumb ray. Since the implanted bone will not grow, it may have to be *lengthened* at a later date. The rigid "finger" usually is sufficiently sensitive for its own protection. In some cases a lengthening osteotomy may be a suitable alternative to a bony supplementary operation.

8.1.5 Postoperative Care

For *syndactyly* and other *soft tissue* operations, see Sect. 2.1.

For *bony supplementary operations:* long-arm cast that includes the pincer structures. The limb has to be elevated until the wound is healed! Cast change after

2 weeks. Total duration of fixation is ca. 6–8 weeks, then x-ray control. Kirschner wires will be removed after the bone transplant has been incorporated; at that time one may have to diminish the diameter of the tubed pedicle flap. As a rule, physio- and occupational therapy may be started about 12 weeks after the operation. To protect the hands of very active children one should provide them with a forearm orthosis, applied to the ulnar side.

Conventional *arthrodeses* (Kirschner wire fixation, bone pegging) call for approximately 8 weeks of immobilization. Where phalanges are long enough to permit stabilization of the rigid osteosynthesis by a small lag screw, external fixation of the finger may be omitted.

8.2 First-Degree Symbrachydactyly Combined with Total Syndactyly of Two Long Digits and Partial Syndactyly Between Thumb and Index Finger

Goal of Surgery

Deepening and widening of the thumb commissure; separation of the IVth and Vth digits.

Figs. 1, 2 Preoperative appearance and incision.
The long digits will be separated by dorsal and palmar zig-zag incisions; the web space between them is to be constructed from a palmar leaf-flap with a proximal pedicle *(flap 1)*. For details of technique, see Sect. 2.1.2.
The thumb commissure will be constructed from two local triangular flaps *(5, e)* and a dorsoulnar swivel flap from the Ist ray *(f)*. After the skin incision, flap *(f)* should be raised directly from the thumb extensor aponeurosis. Avoid damaging proximally inserting vessels (see *Fig. 3*)!

Fig. 3 Radial–dorsal aspect of the deepened and widened commissure.
Fasciae and m. add. poll. are sufficiently indented to effect maximal abduction of the Ist ray. Temporary Kirschner wire fixation of the metacarpal in a position of maximal abduction and medium opposition. Skin closure. The remaining skin defects at the thumb will be covered with thick-split thickness skin transplants.

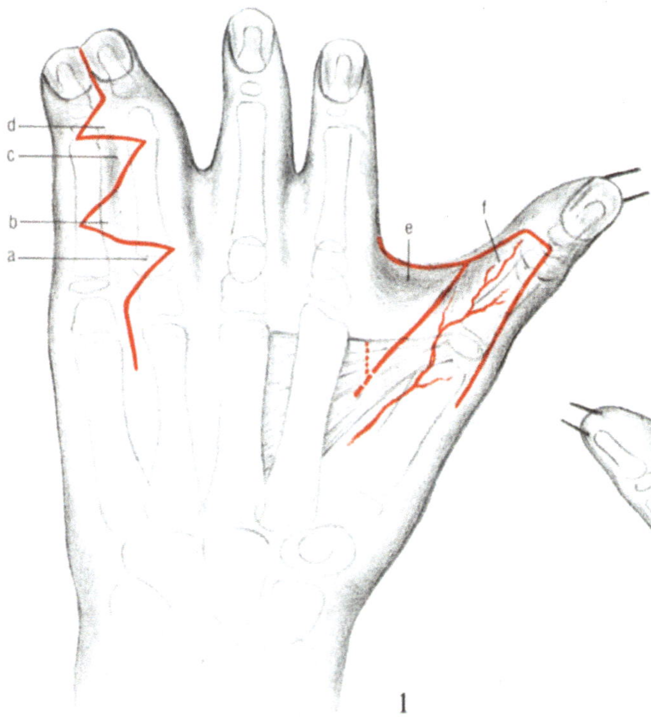
d
c
b
a
e
f
1

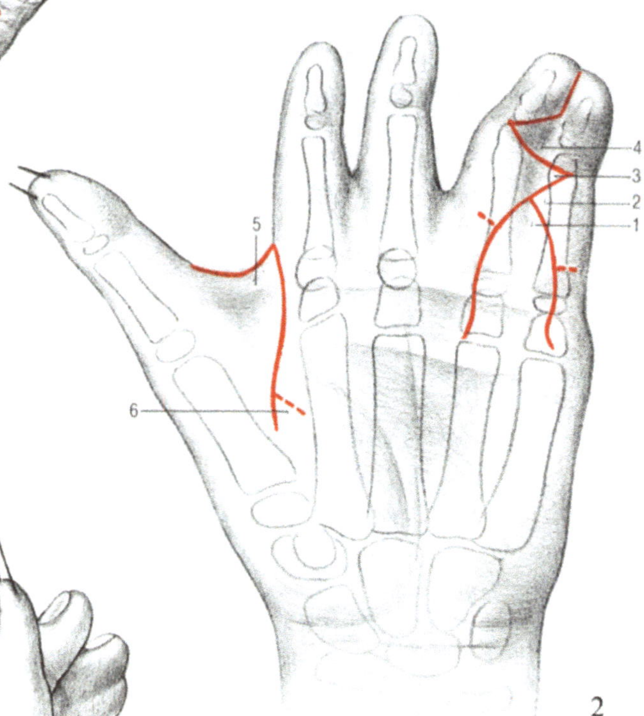
5
6
4
3
2
1
2

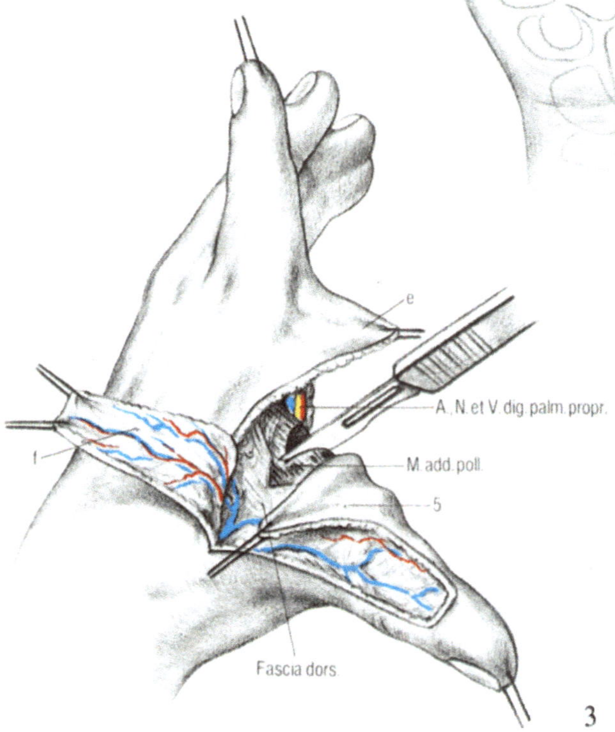
e
A. N. et V. dig. palm. propr.
f
M. add. poll.
5
Fascia dors.
3

Fig. 4 Postoperative appearance of the thumb commissure, dorsal aspect.
For clarity, the thumb is shown in abduction only (disregarding its opposition).

Fig. 5 Postoperative appearance of the thumb commissure, palmar aspect.
Flap *(6)* has been formed during wound closure to eliminate tension at the tips of flaps *(f)* and *(e)* (see incision, *Fig. 1*).

Figs. 6,7 Postoperative appearance after separation of digits IV and V.
To prevent longitudinal scars and to reduce tension, small triangular skin areas (see *Fig. 2*) have been excised on the palmar side of the fingers. The defects have been covered with thick-split thickness skin transplants *(Tr)*.

Postoperative Care

Sutures will be covered with vaseline gauze; the commissures are filled with loosely packed fluffs and gently compressed with a narrow elastic bandage. Long-arm cast. Kirschner wires will be removed after $2^1/_2$–3 weeks. Active physiotherapy is begun approximately 3 weeks after operation. As a rule, night splints are not required.

Supplementary Operations

The procedure for deepening the web space between digits II and III as well as between III and IV is described in detail in Chap. 2: either a dorsal commissure flap or two triangular flaps of dorsal and palmar origin can be used.

Errors and Their Consequences

E. Underestimating the extent of the skin defect after separation of syndactylous digits I and II *and* transposition of thumb. Some commissures remain too narrow if a tubed pedicle flap is not employed (Sect. 4.2.2).
See also remarks in Sect. 2.1.2.

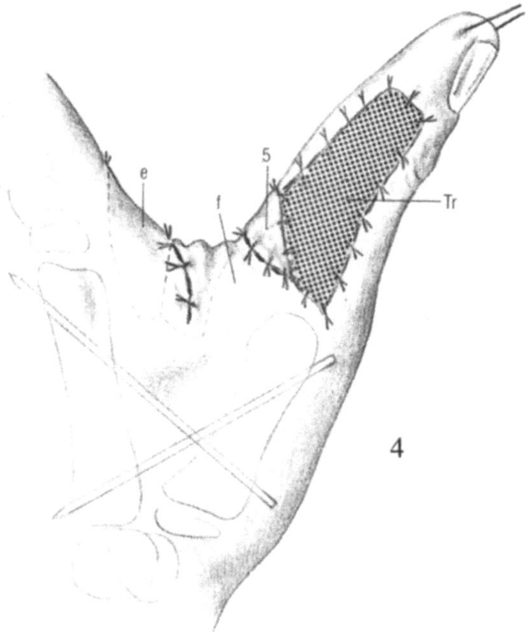

4

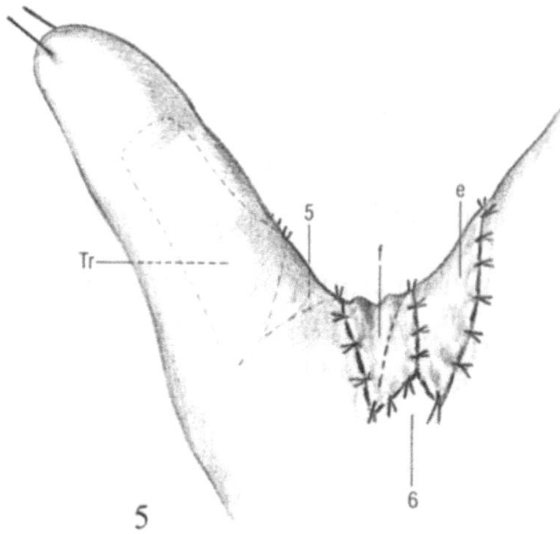

5

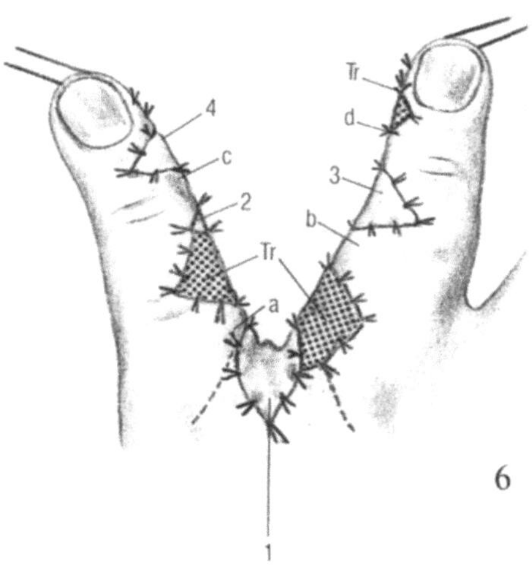

6

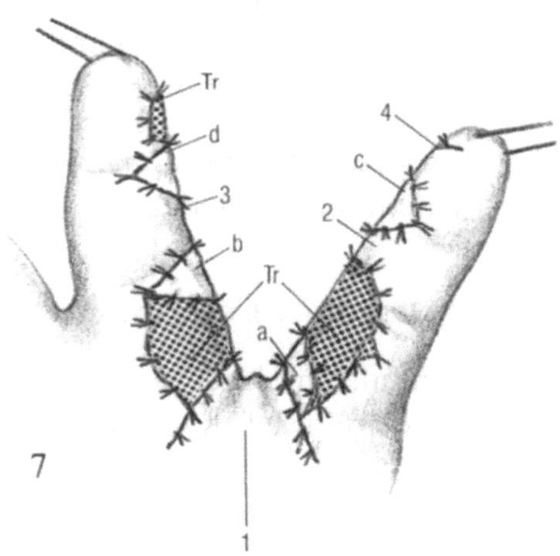

7

Goal of Surgery

Creating pinch between thumb and the tip of the index finger by transposing the Ist and Vth rays in combination with an opponens plasty.

Fig. 1 Preoperative appearance and incision, palmar aspect.
The operation is completed in three steps:
First step: Resection of the os trapezium (in case of rigidity of the first carpometacarpal joint) and interposition plasty according to BUCK-GRAMCKO: the Ist ray is placed in a position of function (mitigated opposition); the space created by resecting the os trapezium is filled by one half of the longitudinally split m. flexor carpi radialis tendon (with distal pedicle) as an interpositum. Two crossed Kirschner wires are drilled through the base of the first ray and the os scaphoideum to keep the bones separated.

Fig. 2 Resection of the os trapezium and the interposition plasty has been completed.
Second step: Opponens plasty. The entire length of the m. palmaris longus tendon is removed and connected by braiding it to the distally severed tendon of the m. flexor carpi ulnaris. It is then pulled through a loop formed by a piece of split-off tendon (hypomochlion) and passed subcutaneously to the MP joint of the thumb. There it is fixed to the proximal phalanx on its ulnar side with minimal tension. (The thumb is kept in functional position.) The tendon of m. abd. poll. long. is severed at its point of insertion and reinserted closer toward the extensor side.
Third step: Rotation osteotomy of the Vth metacarpal.

Fig. 3 Postoperative appearance.
Thumb and biphalangeal little finger are facing each other in opposition.

Postoperative Care

Carefully molded cast. Removal of Kirschner wires not before the 4th or 5th week, followed by intensive physiotherapy. Night splint.

Errors and Their Consequences

E. The magnitude of the operation has been underestimated. Formation of an ample commissure, surgical release of the first carpometacarpal joint, and/or the use of corrective plaster casts should precede the operation.

E. The course of sensory branches of n. radialis and of larger vessels has not been considered during skin incision and dissection.

E. The transplanted palmaris longus tendon has been fixed to the proximal phalanx of the thumb either with too much or without tension.

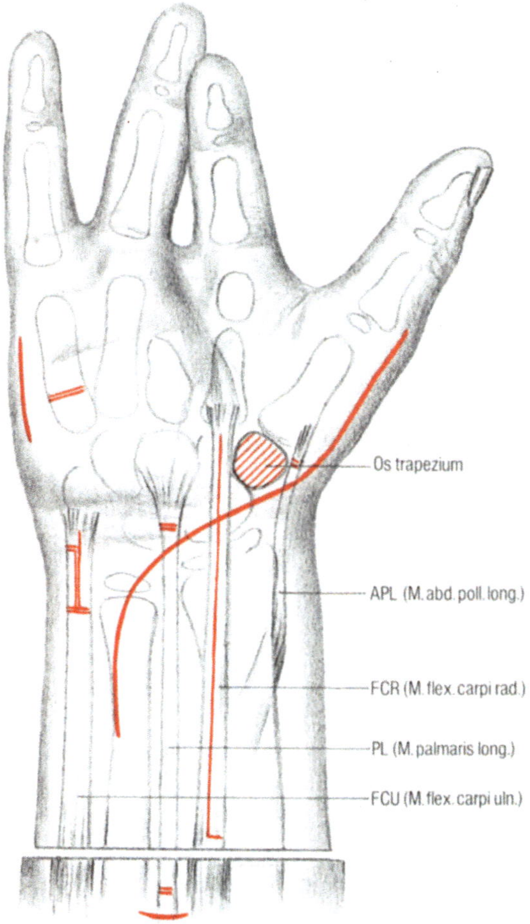
Os trapezium
APL (M. abd. poll. long.)
FCR (M. flex. carpi rad.)
PL (M. palmaris long.)
FCU (M. flex. carpi uln.)

1

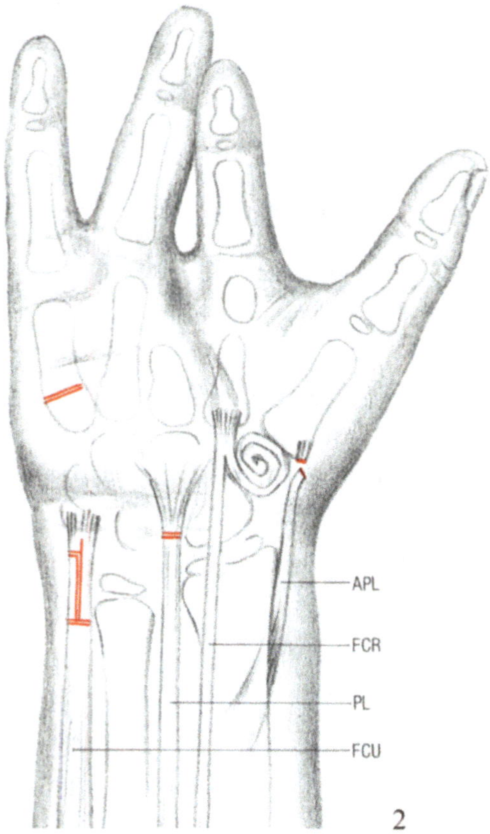
APL
FCR
PL
FCU

2

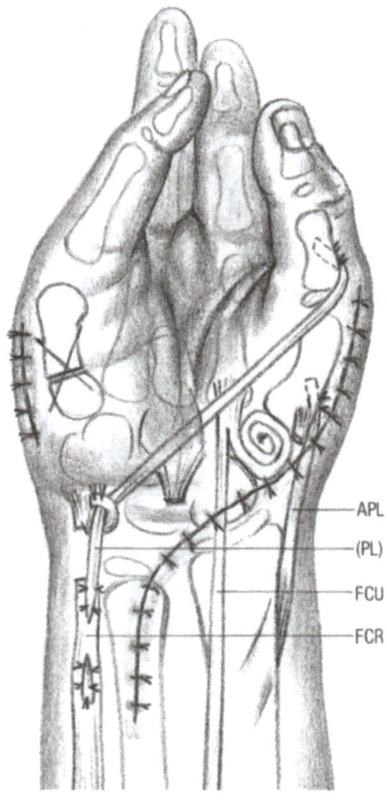
APL
(PL)
FCU
FCR

3

Goal of Surgery

Resection of the nonfunctional stumps to improve cosmetic appearance of the hand.

Fig. 1 Preoperative appearance, dorsal aspect.
Thumb and tip of the little finger permit good pinch and passable grasp. The finger rudiments will be slightly distracted and oval incisions made at their bases. Vessels are coagulated after release of the tourniquet.

Fig. 2 Postoperative appearance.

Postoperative Care

The incisions are covered with vaseline gauze. The interdigital space is loosely filled with fluffs. Light compression dressing. No special physiotherapy is required.

Errors and Their Consequences

E. Failure to stop bleeding after release of tourniquet.

E. Overly generous oval circumcision of finger rudiments; superfluous fatty tissue has been left behind.
C. Tension of skin sutures.

E. Omission of additional Z-plasty of the skin edges to counteract any tension on the commissure when thumb and little finger are abducted.

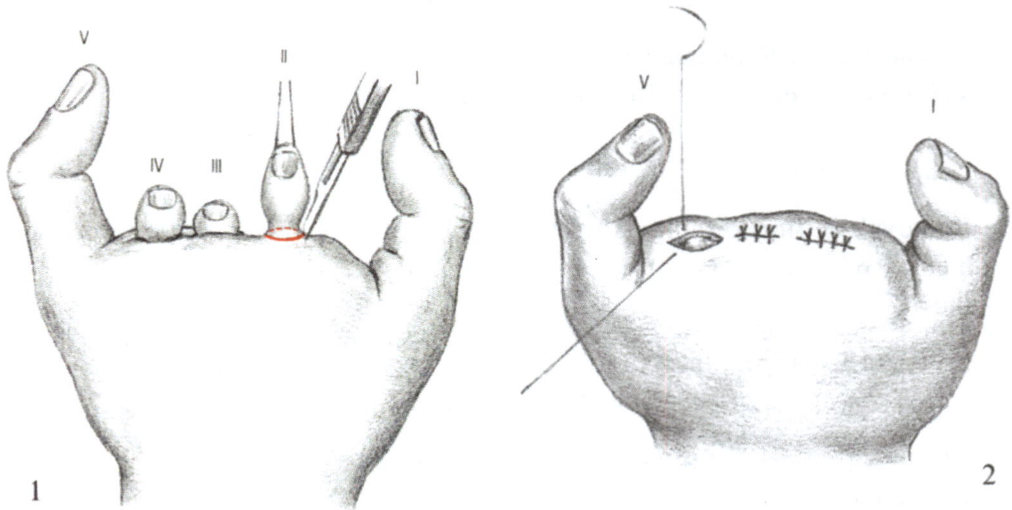
V
IV
III
II
I
1
V
I
2

8.5 Second-Degree Symbrachydactyly with Metacarpal and Syndactylous Finger Rudiments

8.5.1 Second-Degree Symbranchydactyly with Metacarpal and Syndactylous Finger Rudiments (Relatively Wide Commissure)

Goal of Surgery

Removal of finger rudiments, freeing of the little finger, and deepening of the metacarpal area.

Figs. 1, 2 Preoperative appearance and incision.
Hatched sections of bone and finger rudiments will be removed.

Fig. 3 Apical aspect after raising of individual skin flaps.
The *hatched skin areas* will be removed, the protruding sections of the second to fourth metacarpal bones will be trimmed with a Luer rongeur. Resected surface areas will be smoothed. The *black arrows* mark the points where the tips of skin flaps will be placed. The tourniquet will be released and bleeding totally stopped prior to suturing skin flaps.

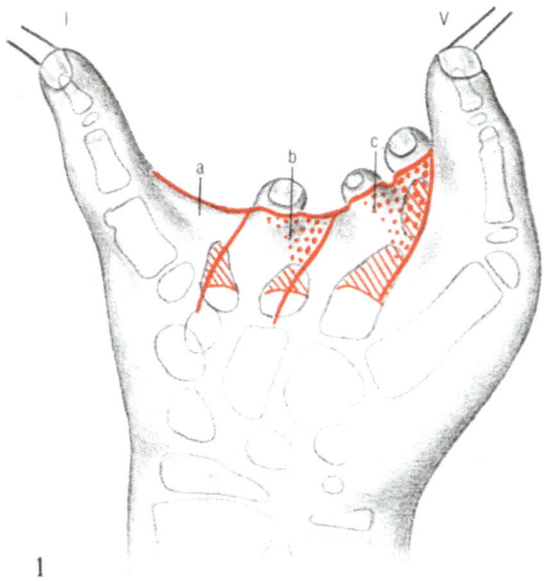
I
V
a
b
c

1

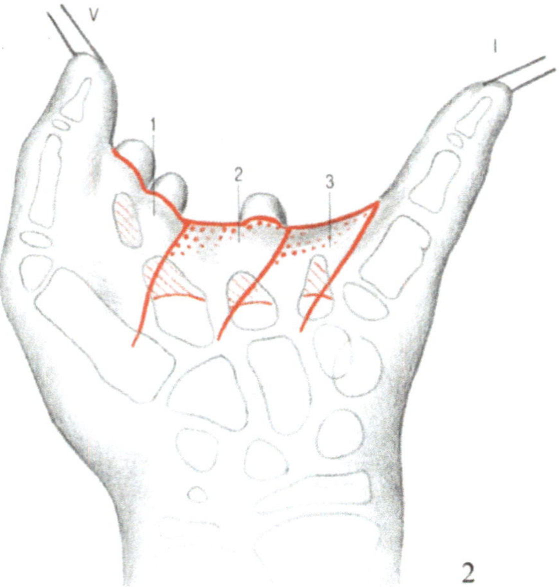
V
I
1
2
3

2

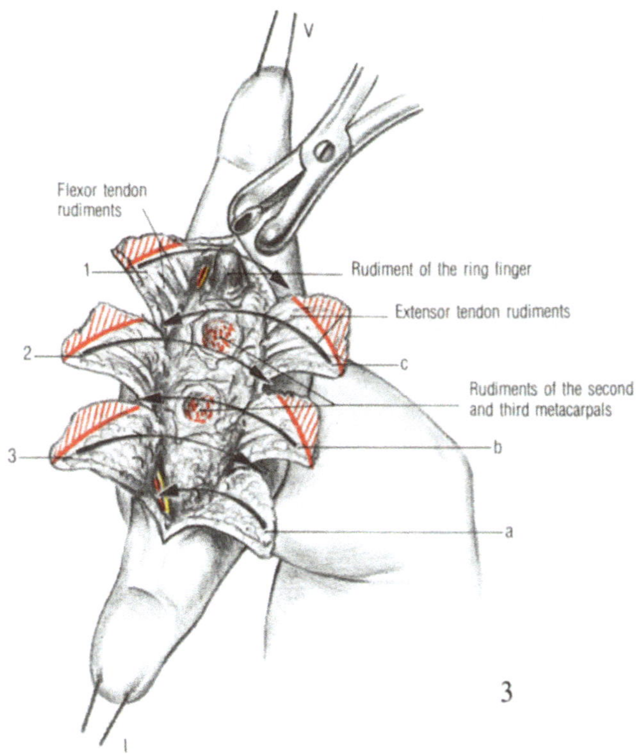
V
Flexor tendon rudiments
1
Rudiment of the ring finger
Extensor tendon rudiments
2
c
Rudiments of the second and third metacarpals
3
b
a
I

3

Figs. 4, 5 Postoperative appearance, dorsal and palmar aspects.

Supplementary Operations

In the case of insufficient or absent active abduction of the little finger, a transplantation of the tendon of the m. ext. dig. min. to the ulnar side of the basis of the proximal phalanx can be made; the proximal phalanx is then immobilized temporarily (ca. 3 weeks) by means of Kirschner wires.

Inadequate "commissure": see alternative operating technique described in Sect. 8.5.2.

Postoperative Care

See Sect. 8.2.

Physiotherapy will be instituted 2–3 weeks after surgery. Night splint for ca. 3 months.

Errors and Their Consequences

E. Damaging vessels and nerves of radial digits during dissection.

E. Neglecting to trim pointed or protruding metacarpal bones.

C. Skin suture under tension.

E. Inadequate control of bleeding; omission of suction drainage.

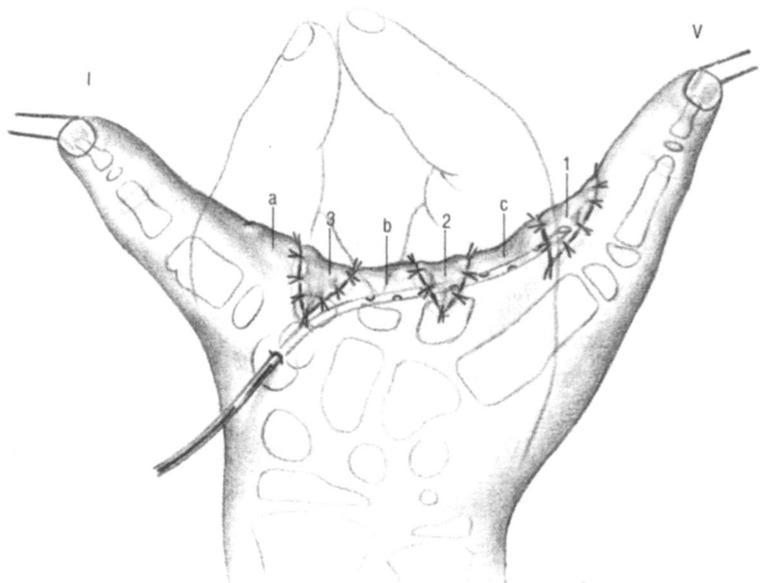

4

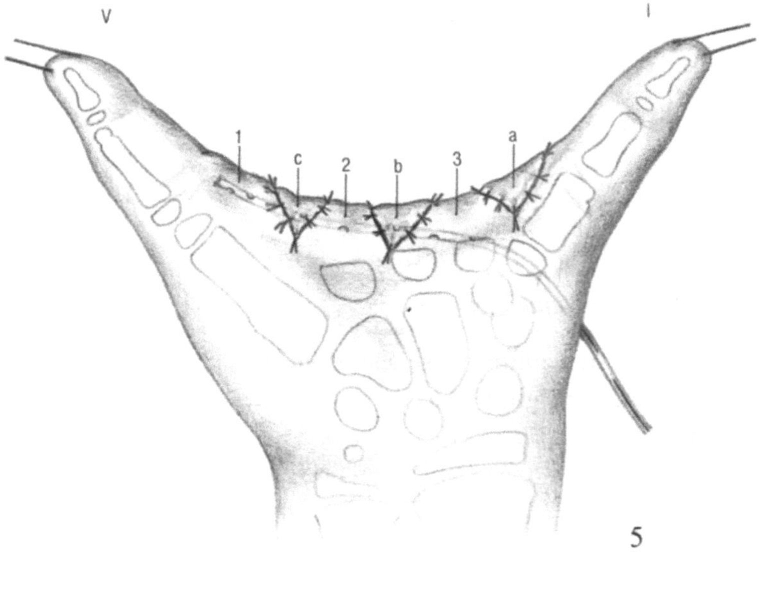

5

8.5.2 Second-Degree Symbrachydactyly with Metacarpal and Syndactylous Finger Rudiments (Narrow Commissure)

Goal of Surgery

Freeing the little finger ray by removing finger rudiments and metacarpolysis (improvement of function and appearance).

Figs. 1, 2 Preoperative appearance and incision.
The web space between thumb and little finger is considerably narrower and tighter than in the previous example (Sect. 8.5.1).
Hatched skeletal parts (IVth ray) and finger stumps will be removed. Local skin areas are adequate for closing the incisions after the axis of the little finger has been straightened.

Fig. 3 Skin flaps have been raised, the dysplastic IVth ray has been exposed. The little finger axis has been corrected.
Fixation by thin transarticular Kirschner wires is recommended (not shown). Palmar vessels and nerves of the border digits are visible. Parts of flap *(1)* will be trimmed, the ring finger rudiments dissected (*hatched areas*).

Figs. 4, 5 Postoperative appearance, dorsal and palmar aspects.

Postoperative Care

See Sect. 8.5.1.

Errors and Their Consequences

E. Damage to palmar main vessels and nerves during removal of the IVth ray and deepening of interdigital space.
See also Sect. 8.5.1.

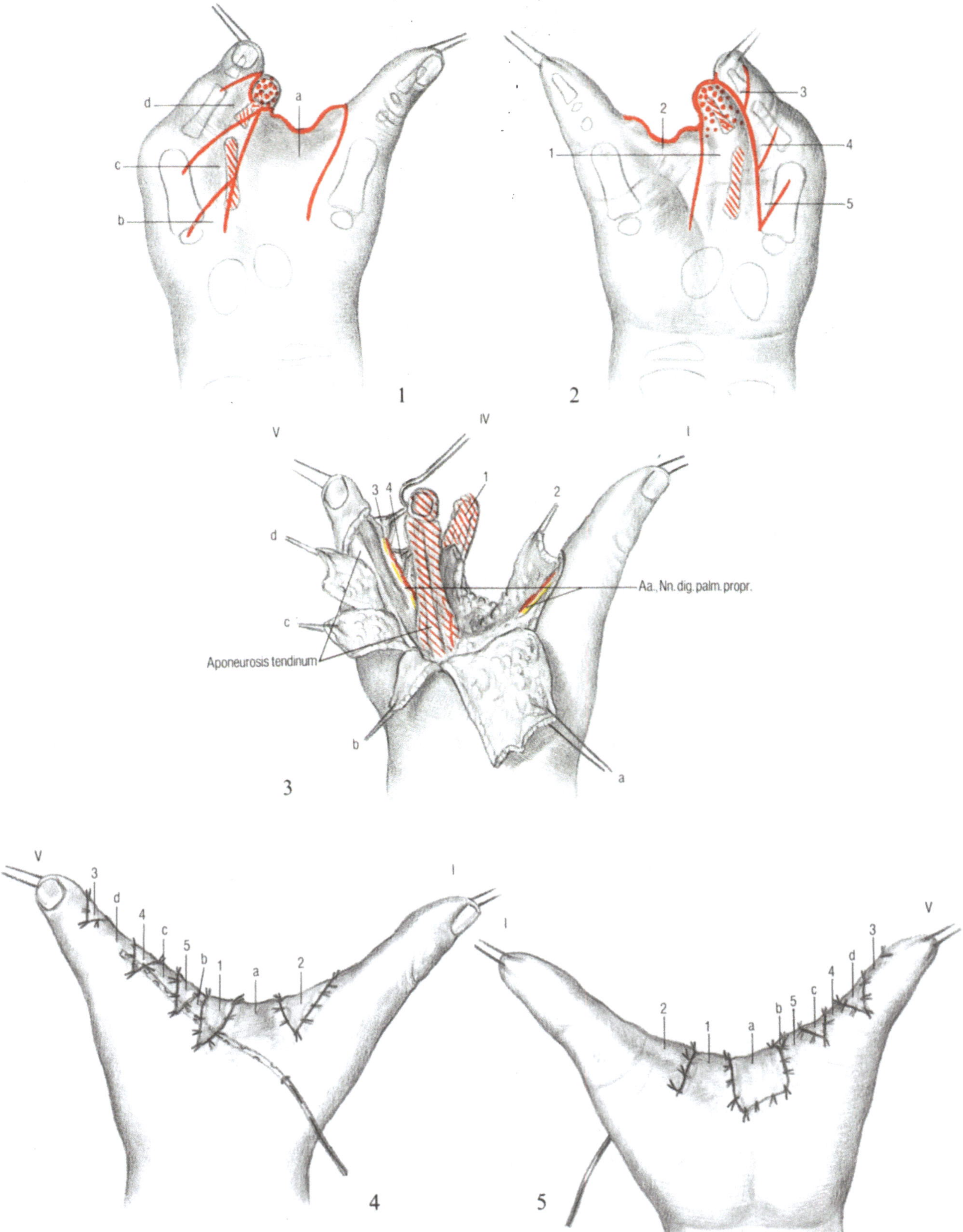
d
a
c
b
1
2
3
4
5
V
IV
I
Aa., Nn. dig. palm. propr.
Aponeurosis tendinum

8.6 Second-Degree Symbrachydactyly with Clinodactyly

Goal of Surgery

Correction of the malposition of the two long fingers and fusion of dysplastic finger joints.

Fig. 1 Preoperative appearance and incision, dorsal aspect. Rudiments of the IIIrd and IVth rays carrying fingernails have been removed previously (for technique see Sect. 8.4). The dysplastic IP joints of the two long fingers permit only minimal motion. The middle phalanx of the little finger is reduced to a wedge-shaped skeletal rudiment.
Hatched areas of bone will be resected. Correction of the little finger clinodactyly requires a Z-plasty. The palmar incision is outlined by the *broken line*.

Fig. 2 Dorsal and radial aspects of the index finger upon completion of arthrodesis and skin closure.
To provide satisfactory pinch of the two-phalangeal index finger, it has to be flexed at a 20–30° angle. Upon correction of the clinodactyly, excess medial skin is removed prior to wound closure (see *Fig. 1*).

Fig. 3, 4 Postoperative appearance; palmar, dorsal, and radial aspects of little finger following arthrodesis and wound closure. Lag screw arthrodesis is a good alternative to Kirschner wire fixation, if the finger is of adequate size. Flexion of 30–40°. Z-plasty on medial side, resection of superfluous skin from lateral areas.

Postoperative Care

See Sects. 5.3 and 5.4.
No cast is required if osteosynthesis is stable.

Errors and Their Consequences

E. Z-plasties and skin transplants have been omitted.
C. Axial correction of a more severely deflected finger will require a greater amount of skeletal shortening.

Where possible, arthrodesis should be performed after growth is completed to avoid further shortening of the finger. (Some operations are feasible prior to the completion of growth (see Sects. 5.3.1, 5.4.1, and 5.4.2), but success, i.e., permanent axis correction and stabilization, is doubtful.)

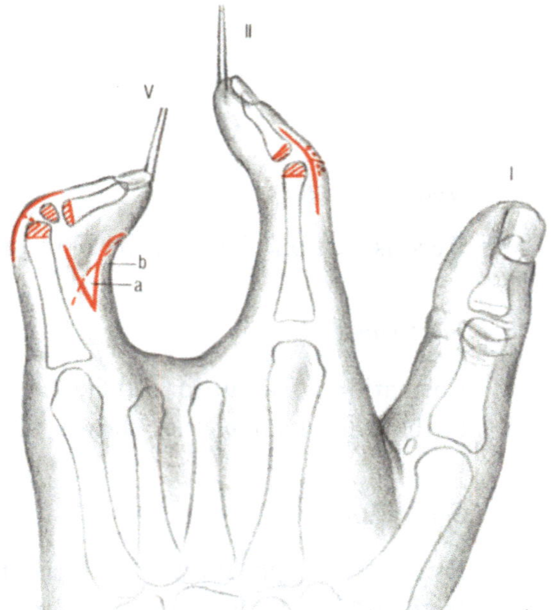

1

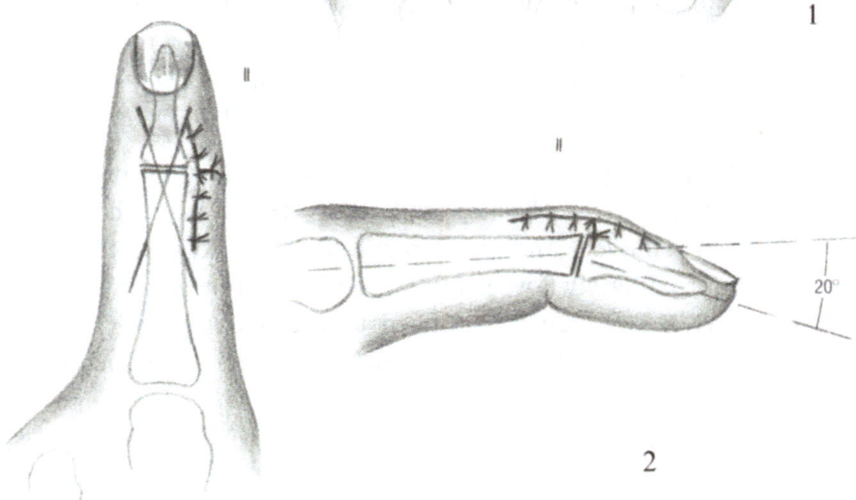

2

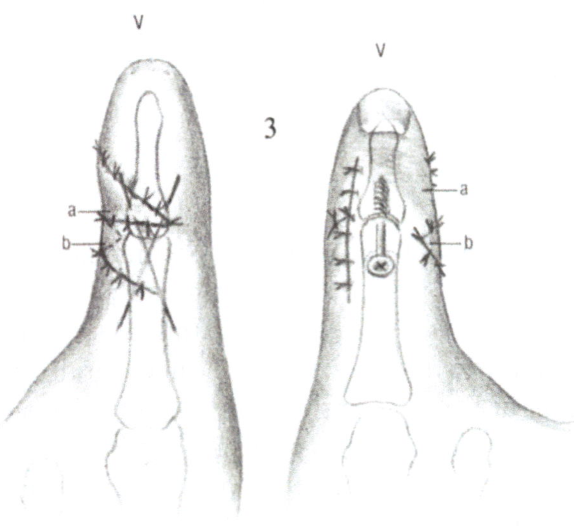

3

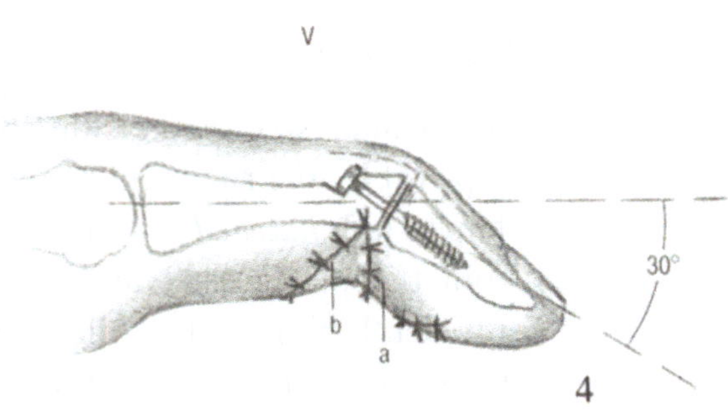

4

Goal of Surgery

Reconstruction plasty of the IVth ray as a natural post (four stages).

First stage

Formation of a tubed pedicle flap from abdominal skin of the ipsilateral side in the usual manner (not shown; see Sect. 4.2.2). Upon healing:

Second stage

Fig. 1 Preoperative appearance and incision, dorsal aspect.
Instead of the long fingers there are only four soft tissue rudiments with fingernails and short metacarpals.
The rudiments will be resected (*black hatched areas*). The incision has to correspond to the size of the tubed pedicle flap (see *Fig. 2*). *Broken red line:* palmar incisions.

Fig. 2. The tubed pedicle stem has been severed at its proximal end and the abdominal skin wound has been closed. Fatty tissue from the properly shaped flap end has been removed, and the flap end has been sutured to the metacarpal defect.
Approximately 3 weeks later, methodical development of circulation: Several times daily a *soft* clamp is applied to the distal pedicle stem; at first, circulation will be interrupted for a few minutes at a time, later for increasingly longer periods.

Third Stage

Transection and shortening of the distal pedicle stem. The stem should only be severed after optimal circulation from its proximal end has been established.

Upon wound healing and establishment of good circulation of the transplant (venous-filling time, see "Remarks" in Sect. 4.2.2):

Fourth stage

Fig. 3 The palmar side of the skin/soft tissue tube should be opened as parsimoniously as possible; the rudiment of the fourth metacarpal *(Fig. 1)* is exposed and properly shaped (see *hatched area* in *Fig. 1*). A bone graft of correct configuration is taken from the pelvic crest and fatty and connective tissue within the tubed graft is sufficiently removed to allow implantation of the bone graft. Since the bone transplant will not grow, operations done in infancy should provide a strong post with a graft length of approximately 3–5 cm. As the patient grows, the graft may have to be extended or a second bony supplementary operation may be required. (The insert shows two different osteosyntheses between graft and metacarpal.)

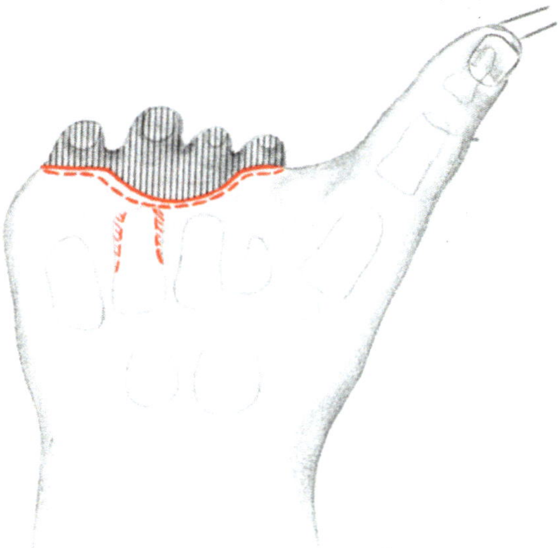

1

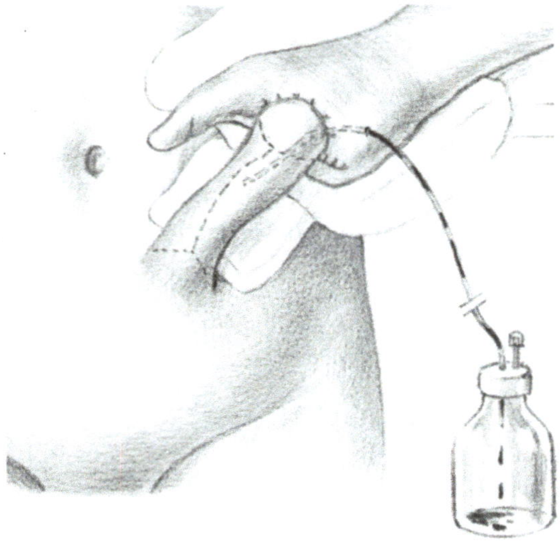

2

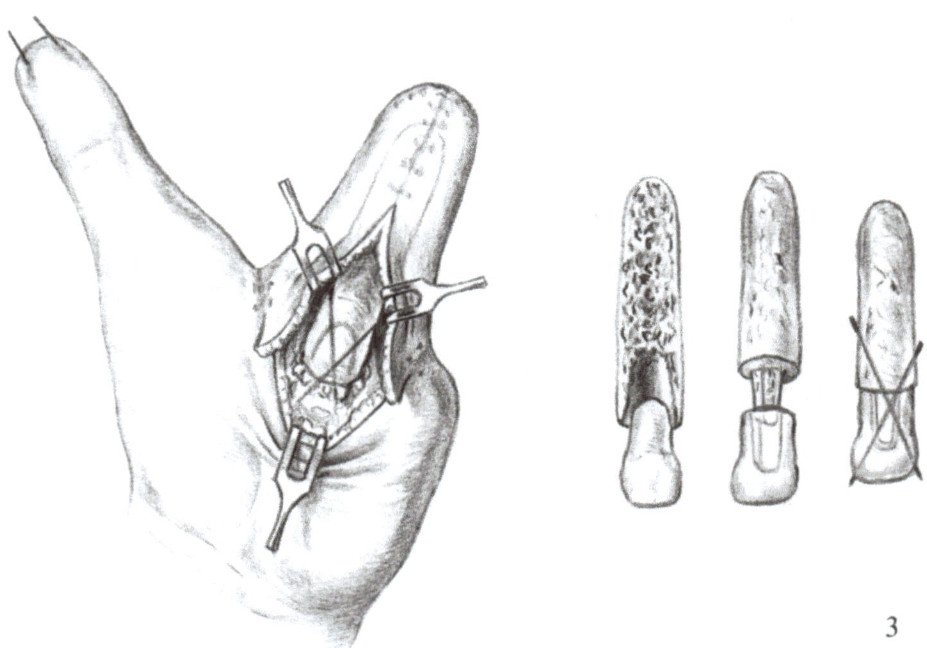

3

The position of the pelvic graft depends on the active range of mobility of the thumb (check prior to operation). Fixation with Kirschner wires and wound closure.

Fig. 4 Postoperative appearance, dorsal aspect.
The future function of the thumb is demonstrated. Sensibility of the reconstructed finger will increase to provide adequate protection.

Postoperative Care

After stages 1–3:
See general guidelines (Sects. 1.1 and 2.1) as well as Sect. 4.2.2.

After stage 4:

Wounds are covered with vaseline gauze. Slight pressure dressing using fluffs or steel wool. Padded long-arm cast keeping tip of reconstructed finger exposed so that circulation may be checked. Suture removal after ca. 2 weeks; plaster fixation for another 8 weeks. Then x-ray control and removal of Kirschner wires. Insufficient incorporation of the bone graft may require another cast for about 4 more weeks prior to physiotherapy.

Errors and Their Consequences

Tubed pedicle flap technique: See Sect. 4.2.2 and others.

E. Poor ratio between skin/soft tissue tube and size of the bone graft.
C. Loose skin cover or excessive tension of the flap inviting necrosis or secondary infections.

E. Insufficient depth of implantation of the bone graft into the metacarpal rudiment, too early institution of physiotherapy and omission of x-ray control.
C. Loosening of the graft, fatigue fractures.

E. No connection between the proximal end of the graft and the decorticated rudiment.
C. Loosening of the graft, fatigue fractures.

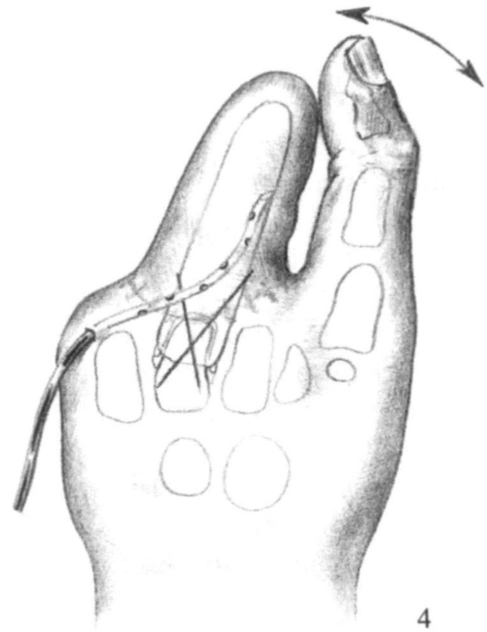

4

9 Cleft Hand

9.1 Introduction

9.1.1 General Remarks

Deformities of this nature (synonyms: Spalthand, split hand, lobster-claw hand) seem to be caused by a *wedge-shaped defect of the soft tissue blastema* of the primitive hand bud (W. MÜLLER 1937). An ectodermal defect has also been considered (WERTHEMANN 1952). Skeletal development is apparently secondarily suppressed in a wedge-shaped configuration with the basis of the wedge located peripherally. Its depth, width, and direction show marked differences. If there is a small wedge-shaped defect, the center of its base is located at the tip of the IIIrd ray and/or its adjacent interdigital spaces, taking the normal hand as a baseline. Major involvement of the radial side, which is formed during a later stage of biogenesis, results in wider defects.

Cleft hand usually occurs *bilaterally.* Both feet are frequently affected in a similar manner. *Familial increased incidence* with dominant heredity of differing degrees of penetration has been observed (LIEBENAM 1938, BIRCH-JENSEN 1949; for a review, see BAUER and BODE 1940, GREBE 1964).

According to their *presentation* one can distinguish two formal types:

The *medial type* consists of a nearly central (axial) defect. Generally, the suppression of bone development occurs most severely in the IIIrd ray. The cleft can extend to the metacarpus or the wrist joint.

Teratologic staging based on the width of the defect is possible. The slightest involvement consists of a v-shaped widening of the second or third interdigital space combined with cutaneous syndactyly of the adjacent fingers. The next stage comprises slight or more pronounced v-shaped defects of the central rays. This is followed by lobster claw-like two-finger hands with subtotal or total loss of the central rays, sometimes even with absence of corresponding carpal bones. The last stage includes cases of extreme defects of both border rays, such as adactyly (and acheiria?)

In the *medioradial type* the tip of the wedge points toward the first metacarpal. Skeletal elements of the IInd or Ist ray are mainly involved. The severity of the blastemal defect can produce deformities that no longer seem to belong to the category of "cleft" hand, but genetic investigations have shown that their assignment to this group is correct.

Teratologic staging of this entity begins with (oblique) v-shaped central ray defects, followed by increasing reductions of the Ist ray. Amputationlike shortening of the fingers is noted in wedges of little depth. The shortening increases from the IVth (IIIrd) to the IInd or Ist ray. Deep wedges result in steadily increasing suppression of the radial portion of the hand to such an extent that ulnar di- or monodactyly may occur; adactyly (the final stage) may also be possible.

In the majority of cases cleft hands are *combined with other deformities* (KLAGES and JACOB 1940) caused by lack of space in the blastema. In the case of small-based wedge defects, partial or total *cutaneous syndactylies* are rather frequently present. *Flexion contractures* and *clinodactylies* involving the PIP joints have been observed. They usually affect fingers adjacent to the defect.

Peripheral skeletal deformities may be found on the margins of the soft tissue defect if skeletal elements have not been totally suppressed. They may be shortened in an amputationlike manner or displaced. At times they are secondarily fused to neighboring bones, as in side-to-side fusion of adjacent metacarpals. It is not unusual to find two metacarpals with one common finger and MP joint.

A *transversal bone* is rather typical but not specific for cleft hand. It is observed mainly in medioradial defects and probably represents a proximal phalanx that has been forced out of its normal anatomic position. The distal phalanges of this finger ray may be missing. In the presence of a rudimentary phalanx joint one finds the metacarpal head, the basis of the proximal phalanx, and one end of the transversal bone in a common MP joint capsule (see IIIrd ray in Sect. 9.4). The other end of the transversal bone is in contact with the MP joint of the adjacent finger. Synostotic connections of the transversal bone with other skeletal elements have been occasionally described. Neither we nor BURGER (1928) found tendon or muscle insertions on the transversal bone.

Finger rays may have additional *errors of differentiation of the skeletal blastema.* They are almost always *excess deformities,* such as triphalangeal thumbs, incomplete polydactylies (particularly of the Ist ray), or transversal bones with two epiphyseal plates. *Segmental anomalies* in the form of joint hypoplasias of differing severity all the way to biphalangy have been noted.

In cases of more pronounced deformities of the medioradial type, i.e., near-complete or complete suppression of preaxial skeletal elements, one can observe *ulnar deviation* of the hand. The deviation is probably caused by muscular imbalance.

The diagnosis of a true cleft hand nearly always rests on the specific wedgelike skeletal defect and the smooth border of the soft tissue defect. Soft tissue remnants or finger stubs (atypical cleft hands) are evidence of disorders of other origins simulating cleft hand (symbrachydactylies, peripheral hypoplasias a.o.) (M. LANGE 1937, BIRCH-JENSEN 1949, BARSKY 1964, BLANKENBURG 1967).

9.2 Cleft Hand with Wide Interdigital Space

Goal of Surgery

Reduction of the interdigital space for cosmetic reasons.

Fig. 1 Preoperative appearance and incision, dorsal aspect.
This is a cleft hand of the median type. The second and the rudimentary third metacarpals are in close approximation with their adjacent rays, but do not impair their function.
An ulnar-based pedicle flap with its subcutaneous fatty layer is raised at the apex of the interdigital space. A triangular area is then excised from the dorsal and palmar sides of the interdigital space. The *hatched areas* are removed and it may be necessary to excise the *dotted area* of skin prior to wound closure.

Fig. 2 Palmar aspect.
The palmar triangular flap has been formed; the palmar neurovascular bundles are visible. Wedge resection out of m. add. poll. followed by wound closure in layers.

Fig. 3 Postoperative appearance, palmar aspect.
The thumb ray has been temporarily immobilized in position of function with two Kirschner wires (for purposes of demonstration, Fig. 3 does not show the above-mentioned position of function).

Postoperative Care

Long-arm plaster cast for ca. 2 weeks, then removal of Kirschner wires.

Errors and Their Consequences

E. Injury of palmar blood vessels and nerves.

E. Overzealous reduction of the interdigital space.
See also Sect. 9.1.4.

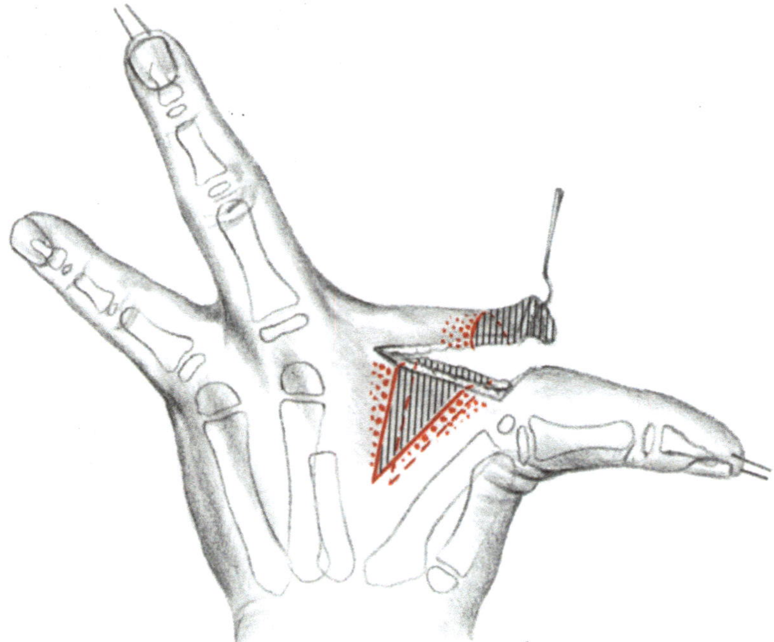

1

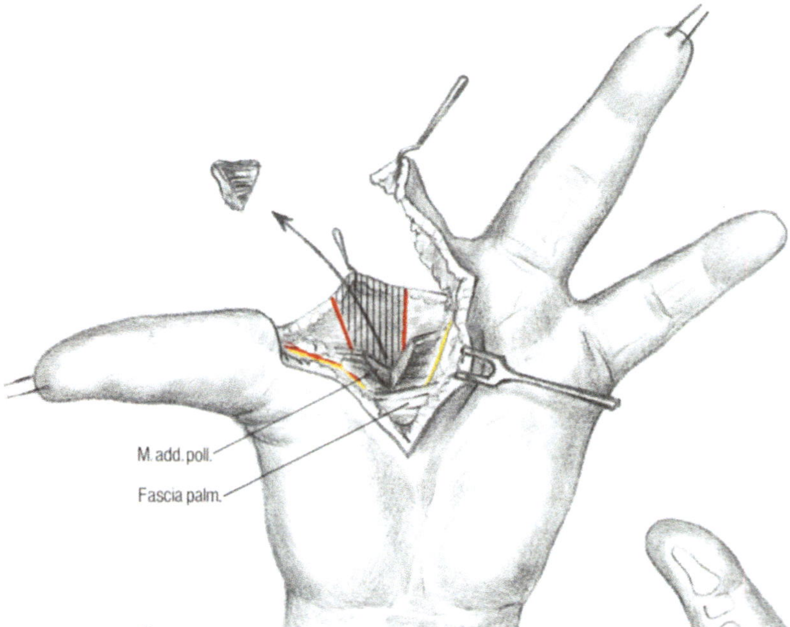

2

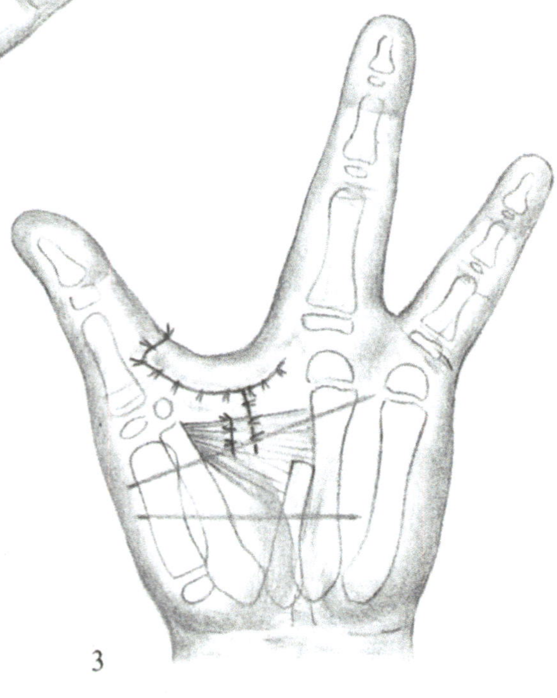

3

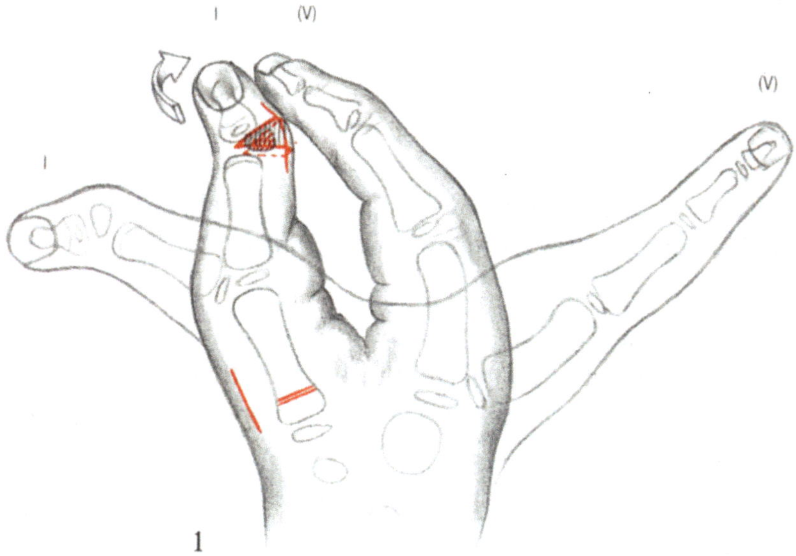

1

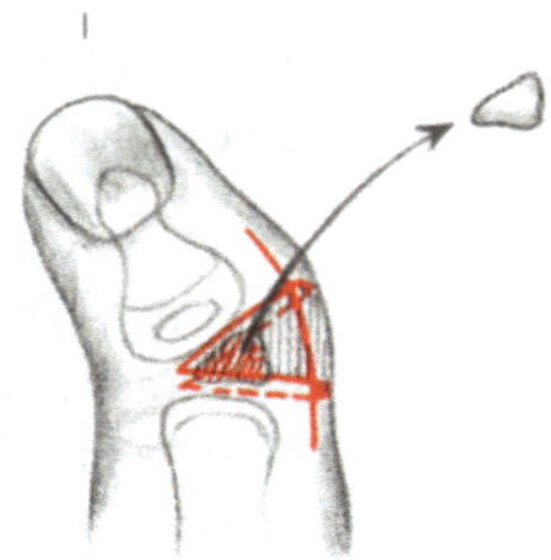

2

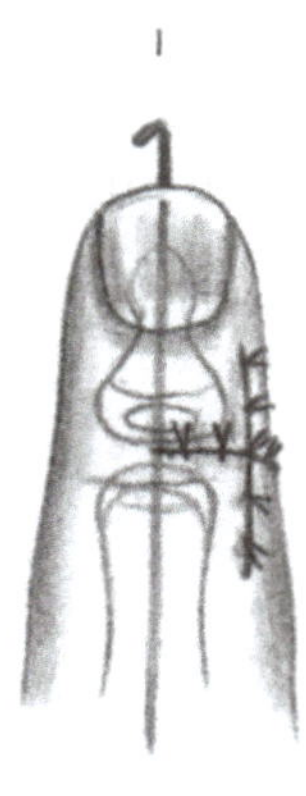

3

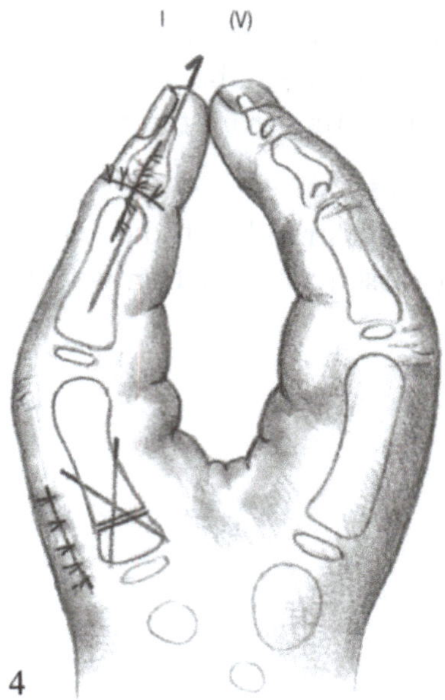

4

Goal of Surgery

Removal of the transversal bone, the third metacarpal, and the phalanx rudiment. Reduction of the interdigital space between ring and index finger.

Fig. 1 Preoperative appearance, dorsal aspect.
A transversal bone articulates with the hypoplastic third metacarpal and with the MP joint of the index finger. The skin *areas hatched in black* and the bony *parts hatched in red* will be removed.

Fig. 2 Excess skin has been removed from the dorsal and palmar sides of the hand. An extensor tendon that crosses the transversal bone and fuses with the flexor tendons of the index finger on the palmar side of the hand has been exposed. It will be freed on the dorsal side of the hand as far proximal as possible and transected at that level. A distally based periosteocapsular pedicle flap is constructed at the transversal bone and the second MP joint. The flap covers the capsular defect resulting from the removal of the transversal bone.

Fig. 3 Palmar aspect.
The distal strands of the palmar aponeurosis are transected. The tendon loop is cut close to its junction with the flexor tendons of the index finger.

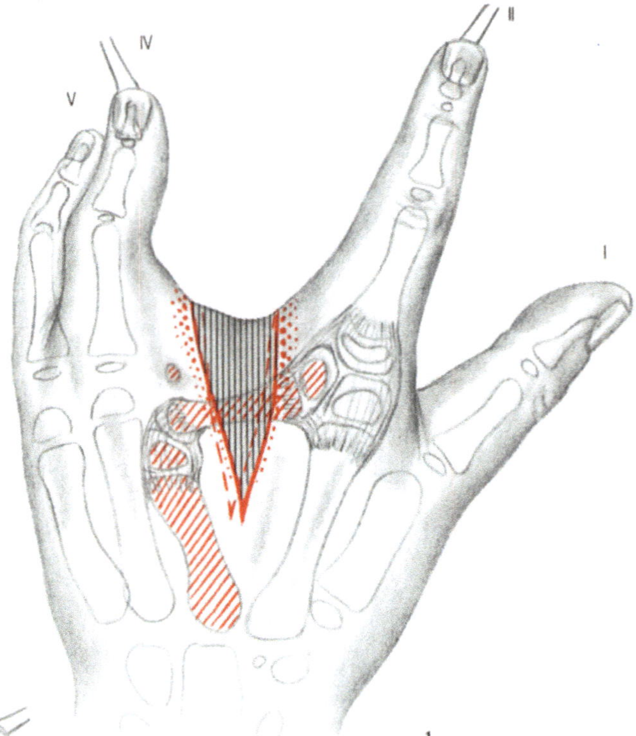

1

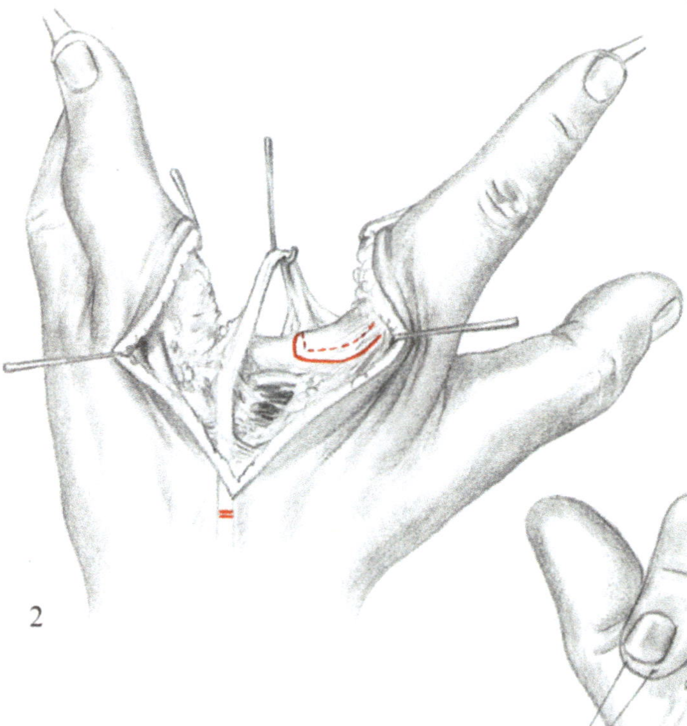

2

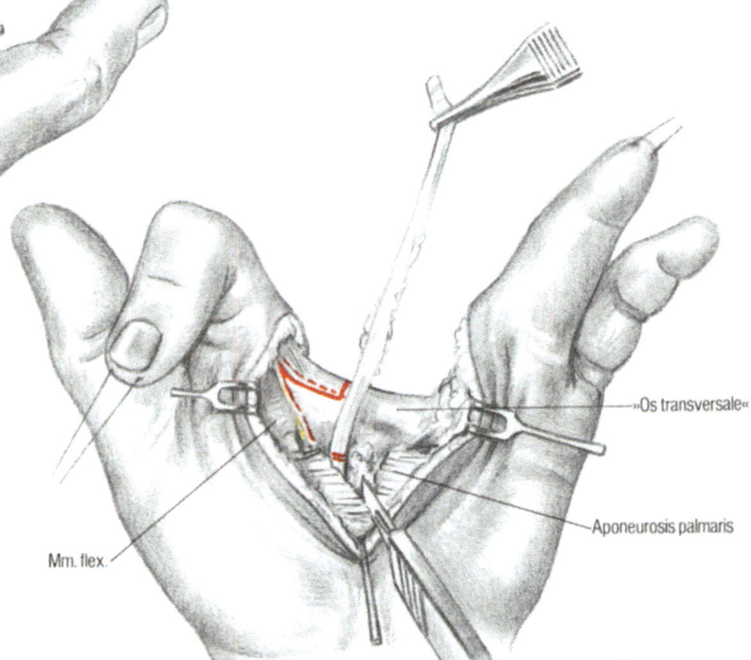

3

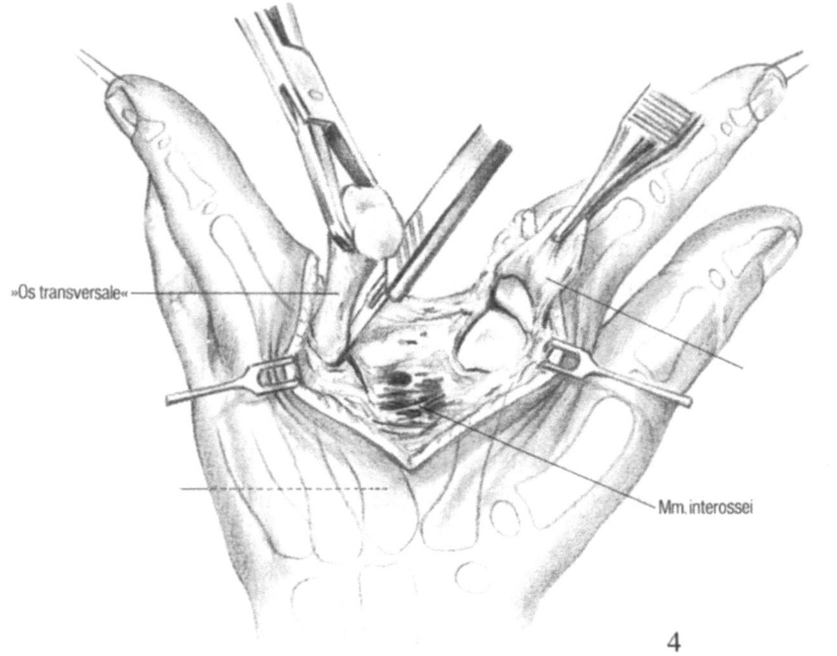

4

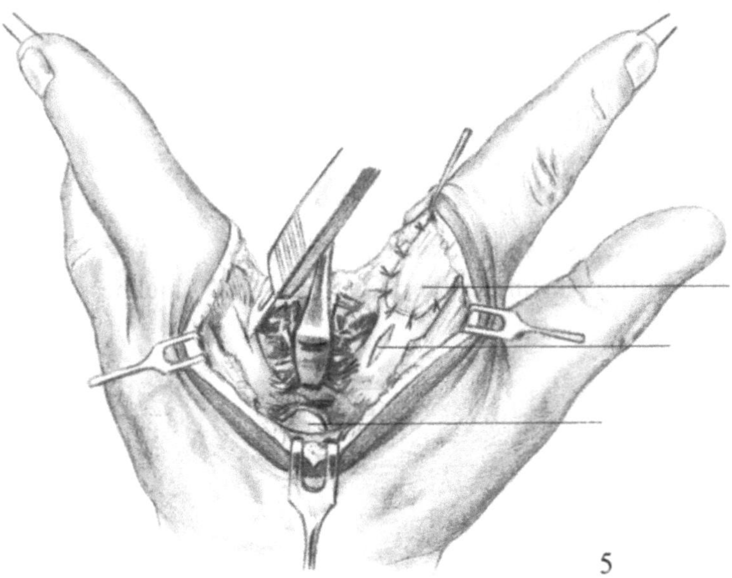

5

Fig. 6 The previously removed extensor tendon is looped subperiosteally around the second and fourth metacarpals and sutured under tension into itself.

Fig. 7 Postoperative appearance.
The tendon tethers the metacarpals; the interdigital space is reduced. The position of the metacarpals is secured with two Kirschner wires.

Postoperative Care

Fixation in a long-arm plaster cast. Removal of the Kirschner wires 4 weeks after surgery. Short-arm cast for another 4 weeks without inclusion of the fingers.

Errors and Their Consequences

E. Major blood vessels and nerves have been damaged during the removal of the transversal bone.

E. The tethering tendon loop has not been placed subperiosteally.
C. Important structures can be strangulated.

E. The tendon loop has not been sutured under tension, Kirschner wires have not been used for additional fixation.
C. The metacarpals may spread apart, too much tension is exerted on the skin suture.

E. Too much "excess" skin has been excised.
C. The skin suture is under tension, thick-split thickness skin transplants may be required.

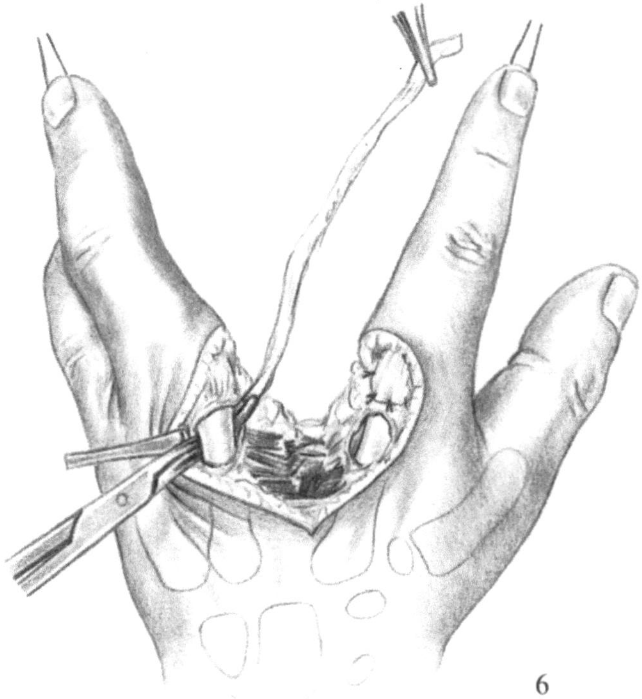

6

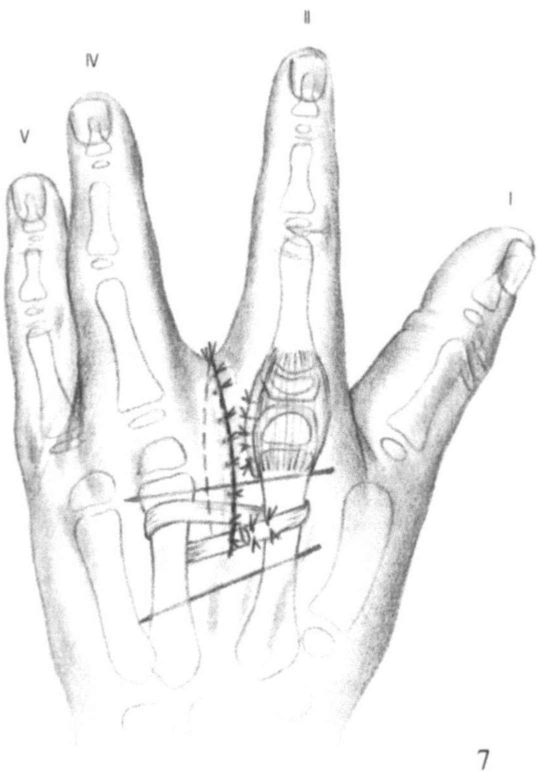

7

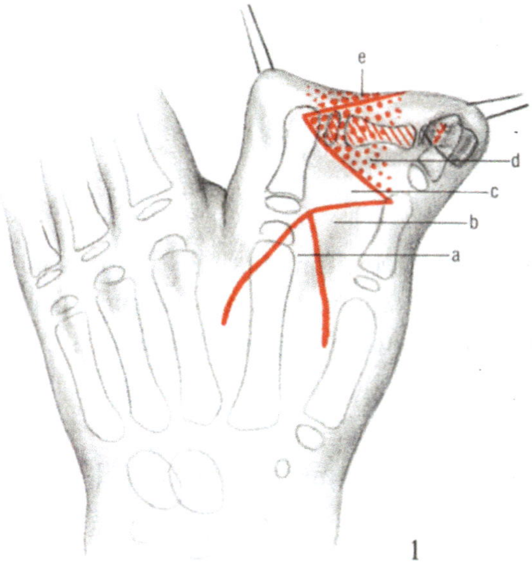

1

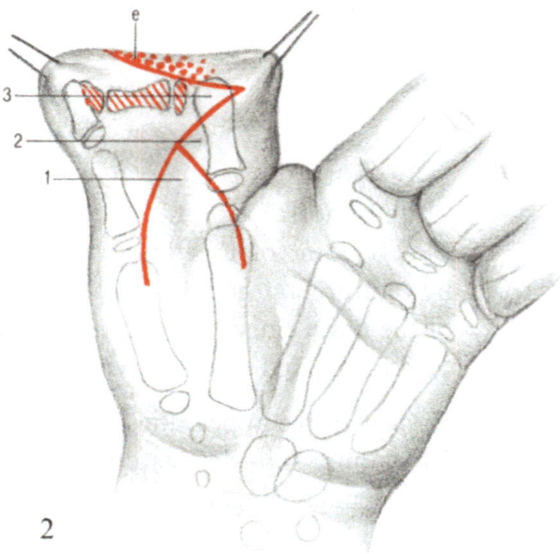

2

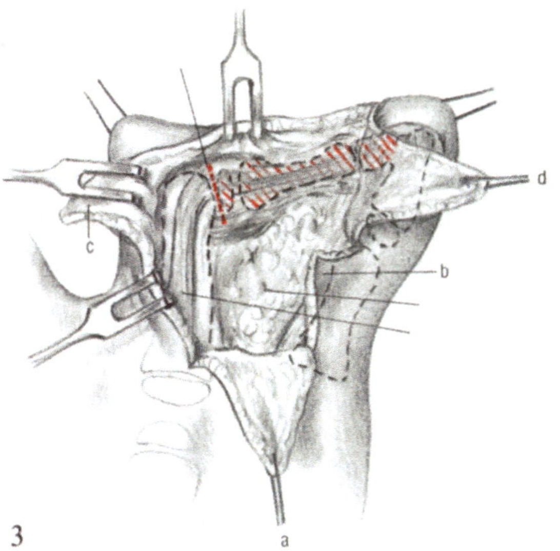

3

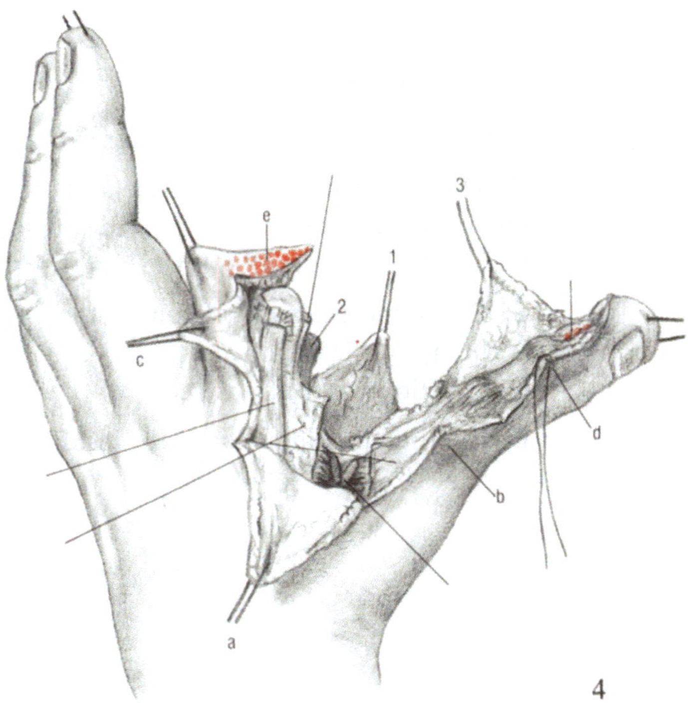

4

Fig. 5 Thumb, dorsal aspect.
The IP joint of the thumb is unstable in radial abduction. Stability is obtained by reinforcing the ulnar capsular elements with the remains of the extensor tendon of the index finger or with suitable material from adjacent structures. Transosseous, transarticular Kirschner wire fixation.

Figs. 6, 7 Postoperative appearance.
Remaining skin defects on the palmar aspect of the thumb and the radial aspect of the index finger have been covered with thick-split thickness skin transplants *(Tr)*.
One could consider amputation of the dysplastic finger at the DIP joint in older children if sufficient skin is available for closure. In such a case one would have to arthrodese the PIP joint in position of function.

Postoperative Care

Long-arm plaster cast for 2–3 weeks. First dressing change after 8–10 days if the wound heals without complications. Removal of the Kirschner and pull-out wires 3 weeks after surgery, then graduated physiotherapy with continuing night splint protection.

Errors and Their Consequences

E. Injury of important blood vessels and nerves.

E. The capsular elements have not been sufficiently reinforced, immobilization was inadequate or was terminated too soon.
C. Instability of the IP joint of the thumb.

E. Flexor and extensor tendons of the amputated finger have been sutured together at the tip of the stump.
C. Function will be impaired.

E. The thumb commissure is of insufficient depth.

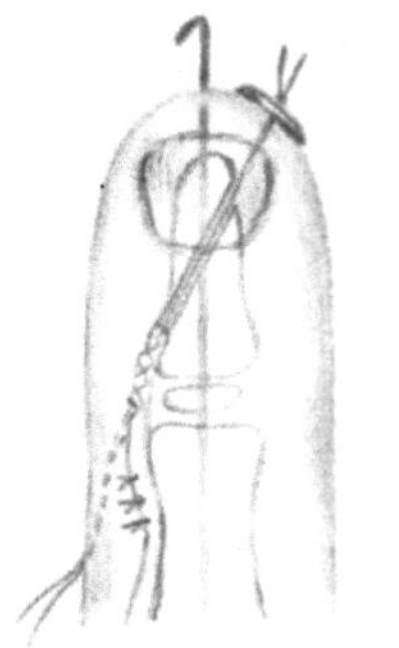

5

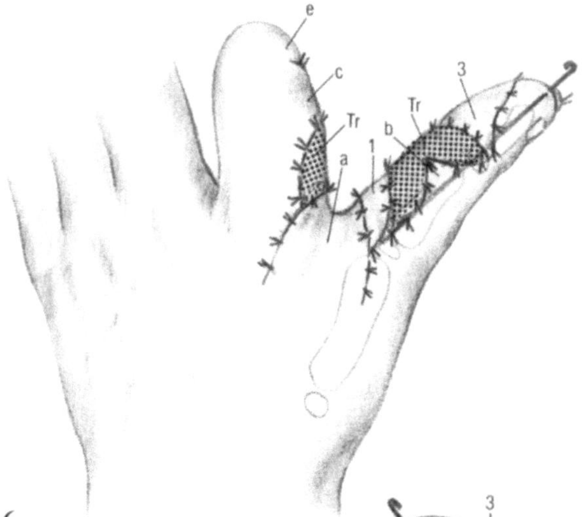

6

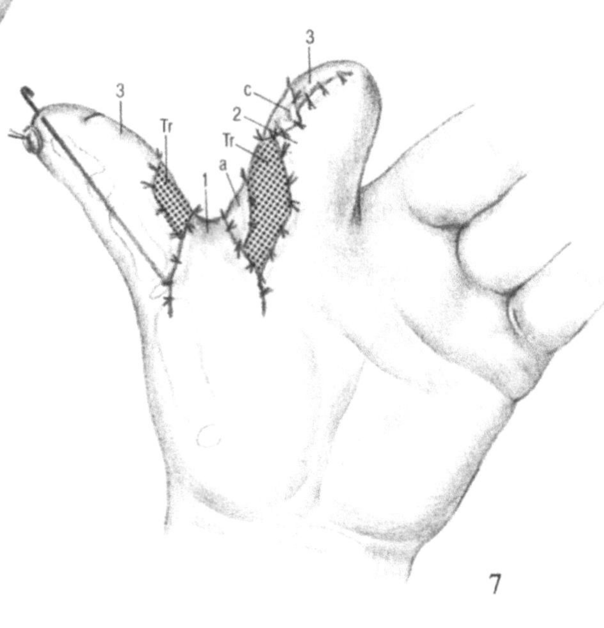

7

9.6 Cleft Hand with Flexion Contracture of the Ring Finger

Goal of Surgery

Correction of the flexion contracture of the ring finger PIP joint.

Fig. 1 Preoperative appearance and incision, palmar aspect.
The diagnosis of cleft hand has been confirmed by typical findings on the other hand and both feet.
Attempted extension results in tension of the skin at the flexor surface of the PIP joint, like a sail.
Longitudinal zig-zag skin incision over the apex of the sail-like skin.

Fig. 2 Palmar aspect of ring finger.
The skin flaps have been raised, the palmar neurovascular bundles have been exposed, and tight connective tissue strands have been transected. The flexion contracture is only slightly improved, therefore a palmar capsulotomy will be required.

Fig. 3 The tendon sheath has been incised longitudinally and the profundus tendon pulled laterally. The joint capsule has been incised in a transverse direction. Full extension is obtained only after indentation of a collateral ligament. Temporary transarticular Kirschner wire fixation, wound closure.

Fig. 4 Postoperative appearance.

Postoperative Care

Plaster cast for 2–3 weeks followed by removal of the Kirschner wire and institution of physiotherapy. Passive mobilization attempts are forbidden! Dynamic finger splints are expedient, night splints are required.

Errors and Their Consequences

E. Injuries of palmar vessels and nerves.

E. Articular cartilage damage during capsulotomy.

E. Forced extension of the contracted PIP joint.

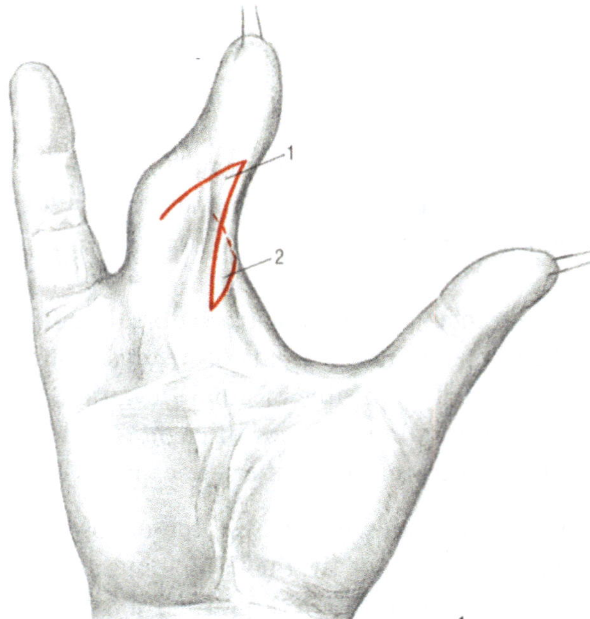
1
2

1

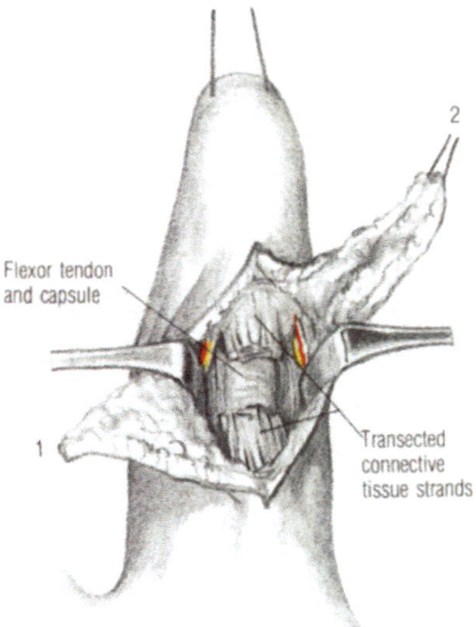
2
Flexor tendon
and capsule
1
Transected
connective
tissue strands

2

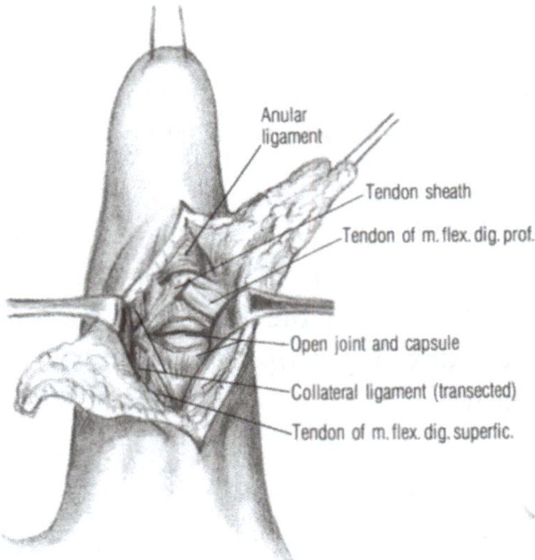
Anular
ligament
Tendon sheath
Tendon of m. flex. dig. prof.
Open joint and capsule
Collateral ligament (transected)
Tendon of m. flex. dig. superfic.

3

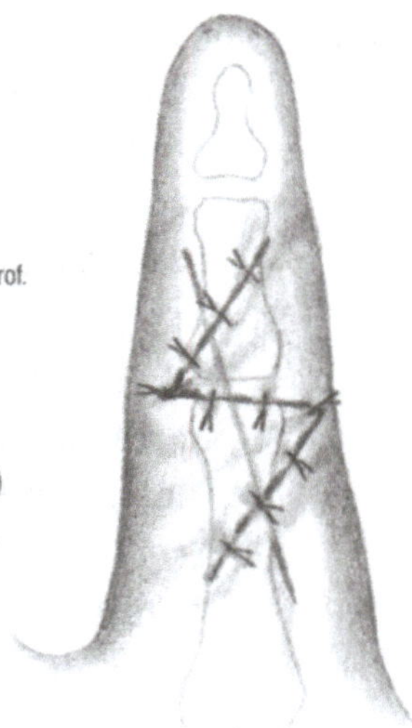

4

Goal of Surgery

Correction of the instability and abnormal position of the PIP and DIP joints of the index finger, creating a fibrous ankylosis of both joints in position of function. (Arthrodeses will be performed after cessation of bone growth.)

Figs. 1, 2 Preoperative appearance, partial view from dorsal and radial. Median type of cleft hand. The IP joints of the dysplastic index finger are markedly flexed and only partially movable. Radial deviation (clinodactyly) is present at the PIP joint. Lateral stability in insufficient, pinch between thumb and index finger is very weak. Therefore the patient does not use his index finger.

Figs. 3, 4 The radial aspect of the index finger has been exposed (composite view). A tendon anomaly is present at the PIP joint. A shortened lateral expansion (*) on the radial side is noted. The abnormal axial position of the PIP joint can be corrected in both planes after transection of the lateral expansion and semicircular incision of the joint capsule on the radial side. The malposition of the DIP joint will be corrected in a similar manner, but from the ulnar side.

Figs. 5, 6 Postoperative appearance (the skin suture of the extensor surface is not demonstrated). Proper axial position of the phalanges. The IP joints have been stabilized in functional position with transarticular Kirschner wires.

Postoperative Care

Fixation in a short-arm (if necessary, a long-arm) plaster cast for 3–4 weeks followed by removal of the Kirschner wires. Splint fixation with exclusion of an area of the index finger tip until joint stability is sufficient. Night splint for at least 6 months.

Errors and Their Consequences

E. Joint fixation in nonfunctional position.

E. Wires and plaster fixation have been removed too soon.
C. Recurrence of the deformity and joint instability.

Remarks

It is not always possible to obtain a good result. A reoperation may become necessary if thumb pressure during grasp displaces the soft tissues, resulting in ulnar deviation. A chondrodesis (parsimonious resection of the dysplastic joint surfaces to improve the position of function) and additional Kirschner wire fixation would then be indicated, but it should not be performed too soon.

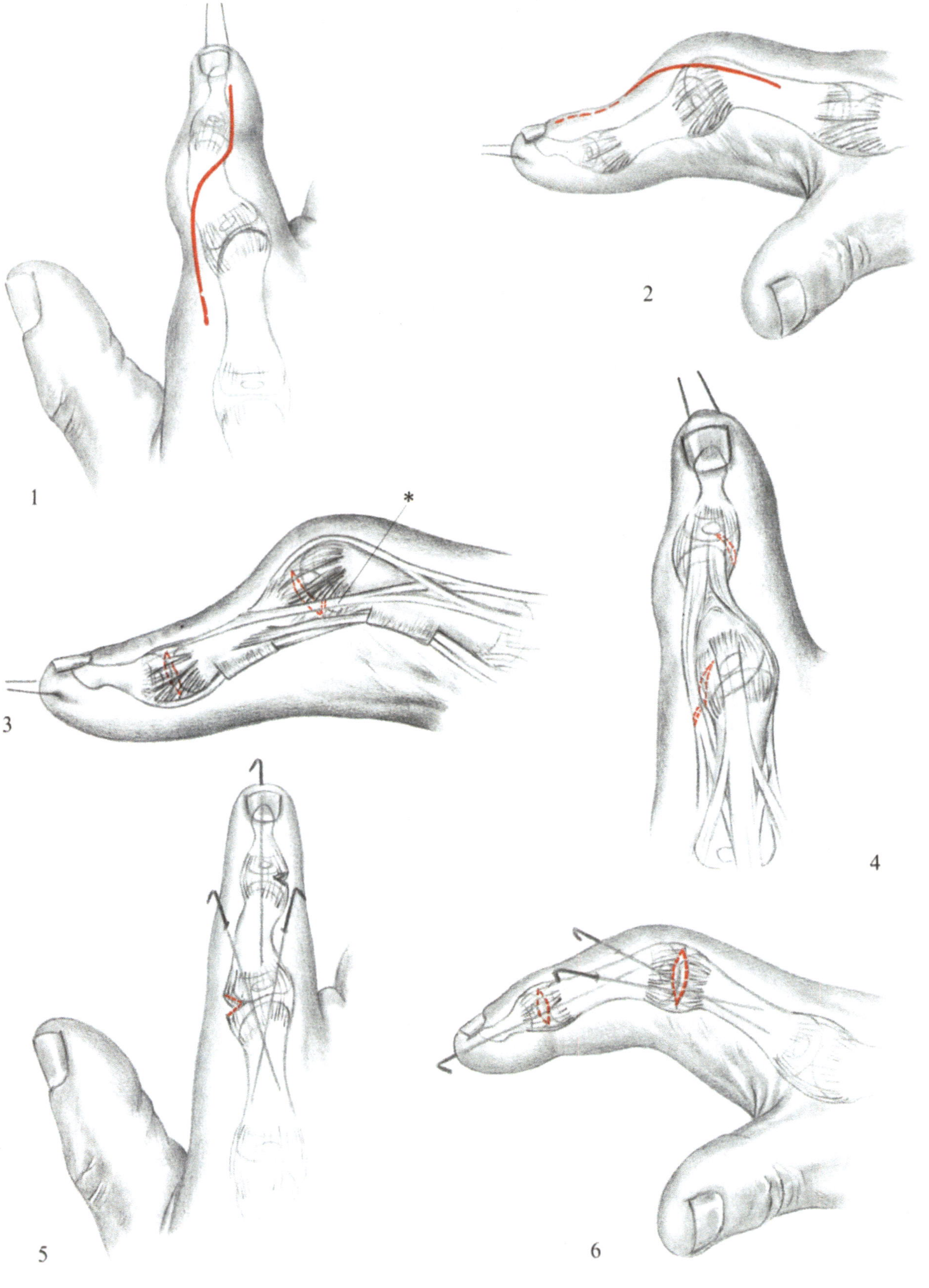
1
2
*
3
4
5
6

9.8 Duplication of the Proximal Thumb Phalanx, Thumb Hyperphalangia, and Partial Syndactyly I/II

Goal of Surgery

Removal of the accessory thumb rudiment and deepening of the thumb commissure.

Fig. 1 Preoperative appearance and lines of incisions, dorsal aspect.
Diagnosis of cleft hand confirmed by typical findings on the other hand and both feet. Total syndactyly of the IIIrd and IVth rays, combined with acrosynostosis. The triphalangeal (brachymesophalangeal) thumb articulates with an accessory dysplastic proximal phalanx. Opposition is satisfactory. The shallow commissure is displaced distally. The index finger is dysplastic.

Fig. 2 Incisions, palmar aspect.
The commissure will be formed by two local flaps *(a, 2)*. The incisions on the dorsal side are demonstrated by the *broken lines*.

Fig. 3 Dorsal aspect.
The rudimentary, supernumerary proximal phalanx has been exposed subperiosteally. A proximally based periosteal flap (*) will be used to reinforce the capsular defect of the MP joint replacing the ulnar lateral ligament. It may be necessary to indent the fascia and m. add. poll. to form a commissure of sufficient depth (see Sect. 2.2.2 a.o.).

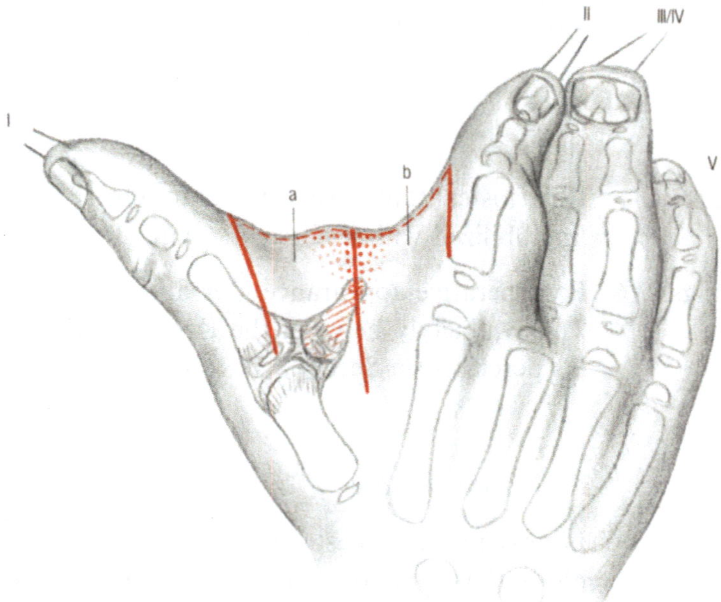

1

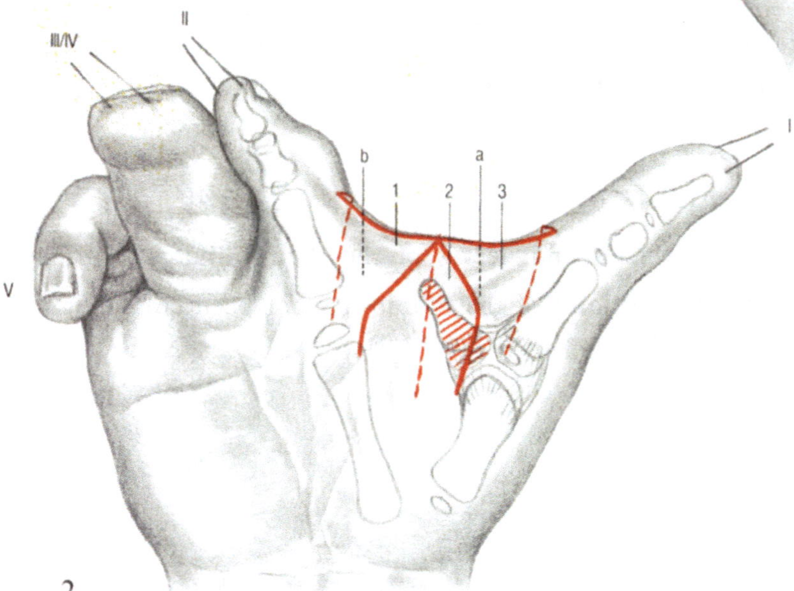

2

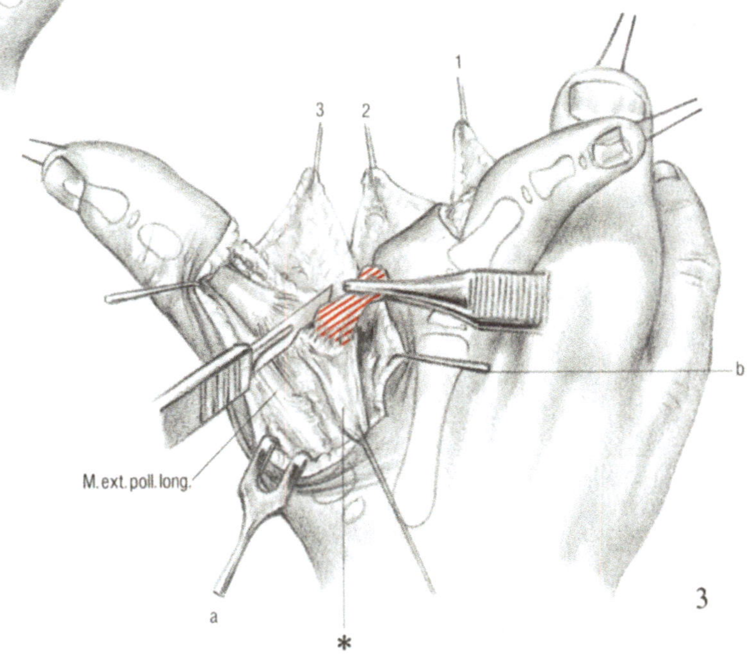

3

Fig. 4 A periosteal flap covers the joint defect. The MP joint of the thumb is temporarily immobilized with a Kirschner wire.

Figs. 5, 6 Postoperative appearance, dorsal and palmar aspects.
The syndactyly between the IIIrd and IVth rays will be corrected at a later date (as described in Sect. 4.5.7 a.o.).

Postoperative Care

Long-arm plaster cast. The Kirschner wire will be removed after 3 weeks; graduated physiotherapy and a night splint are then employed.

Errors and Their Consequences

E. Injuries of palmar blood vessels and nerves of the thumb and index finger.

E. The capsular defect of the MP joint of the thumb has not been closed tightly, the joint has not been stabilized with a Kirschner wire.
C. Instability of the joint.

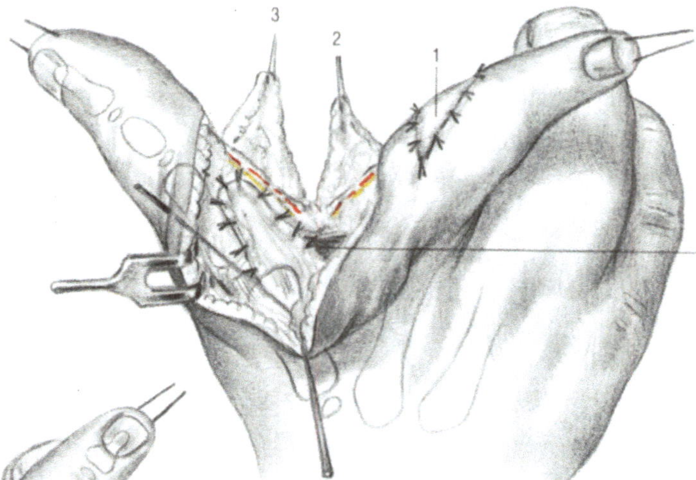

4

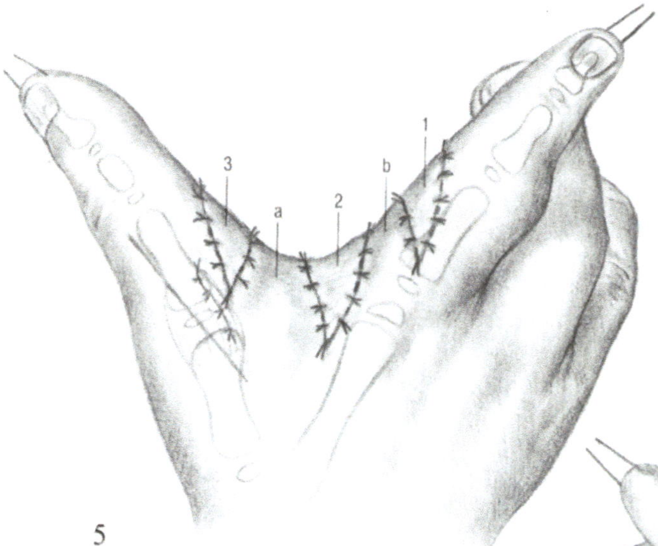

5

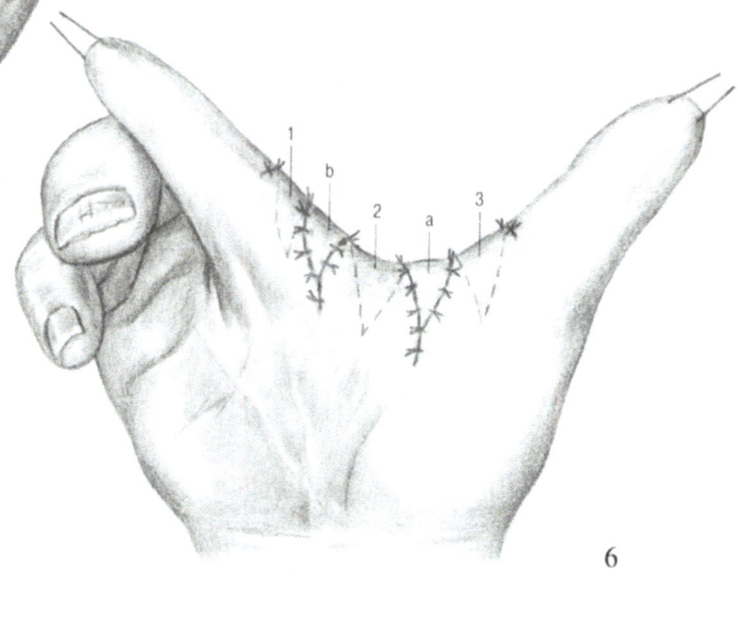

6

10 Congenital Localized Giantism of the Hand (Macrodactyly)

10.1 Introduction

10.1.1 General Remarks

Idiopathic localized giantism of the hand (synonyms: macrodactyly, megalodactyly, partial gigantocheiry, giant fingers) is characterized by a wedge-shaped enlargement of the hand with an increase in volume of at least two types of tissue (KEHRER 1948).

The wedge-shaped area with its peripheral basis seen in macrodactyly is similar to the involvement found in cleft hand deformities (W. MÜLLER 1937); central or radial sections are mainly affected in both disorders.

The *cause* of this rare anomaly is unknown; it is probably a constitutional factor (WERTHEMANN 1952), in spite of the fact that a familial incidence has hardly ever been noted (the world literature contains only four such cases). Basically an increased local tissue sensitivity to growth stimuli seems to be its cause.

A classification of this disorder has not yet been generally accepted. The question as to whether congenital localized giantism of the hand is a homogeneous malformation cannot be answered, as only a small number of cases have been carefully analyzed. Based on histologic and macroscopic examinations, heterogeneity appears to be more likely.

Earlier authors felt that an exorbitant increase of subcutaneous fatty tissue was its most striking feature (FERIZ 1926: macrodystrophia lipomatosa progressiva).

Numerous publications have suggested a *causal connection between hyperplasia of nerves and giantism* (MCCARROLL 1950; TSUGE 1967; a.o.). The involved area corresponds exactly with changes in neural tissues (JÄGER 1973; TSUGE 1967; BLAUTH 1972). KELIKIAN (1974) noted a close relationship of the most common type of macrodactyly with the median nerve innervated sections of the hand. He called this type *"nerve territory oriented macrodactyly,"* but it seems that a causal relationship of (inconstant) hyperplastic nerves and giantism can be found only in some cases.

Among others, BROOKS and LEHMAN (1924) and MOORE (1941, 1942) proposed a connection between macrodactyly and neurofibromatosis generalisata (Recklinghausen disease) because they found neurofibromatous changes in finger nerves and, in rare cases, simultaneous appearance of macrodactyly and neurofibromatosis. In such cases, POSCH (1956) and KELIKIAN (1974) spoke of a "Recklinghausen type" of macrodactyly. However, KELIKIAN himself gave a well-reasoned and comprehensive account as to why there is no reason to assume that such a connection exists – even as a forme fruste (there are more contrasts than similarities).

DELAURENZI (1962) proposed distinguishing between a *static* and a *progressive* type of macrodactyly. The former is characterized by a neonatal macrodactyly, the size of which increases proportionally with the growth of the rest of the body ("simple giantism" according to WINDHOLZ 1931). The progressive type of macrodactyly, which is clinically more important, is diagnosed by a disproportional continuous increase in size during the postnatal period. Occasionally it involves other areas, especially those proximal to its original site. The speed of growth varies from case to case and from finger to finger. Surgical intervention may on occasion stimulate progression of the deformity (FISCHER 1880; LERCH 1949; a.o.).

KELIKIAN described another type which he called the *osteoblastic* or *hyperostotic variant*. The main trunk of the median nerve and the digital nerves are not markedly involved in such cases. The disproportioned metacarpals and phalanges contain cauliflowerlike osteocartilaginous excrescences (without exostoses in the rest of the extremities). They may limit joint motion as they continue to grow (see also WIELAND 1907).

In cases of congenital localized giantism, an increase in the size of one or several fingers is mostly noted at the time of birth. In the majority of patients the macrodactyly will *develop into grotesque deformities* during childhood. *Growth usually stops at puberty* (an exception was a case cited by KAPLAN 1947). Usually one observes hyperplasia of bony and fatty tissues. A considerable thickening and lengthening of the palmar digital nerves and their common trunk in the palm is frequently noted. Giantism may increase from proximal to distal (KEHRER 1948). The IInd and IIIrd fingers are most commonly and most intensively involved; macrodactyly of the little finger is a rarity. Involvement of the metacarpal and the carpal area, of parts of the forearm, or even of the entire limb has been reported. Slight hypoplasia of the remaining parts of the hand has been described (see BERNOULLI 1944).

Rather typical for macrodactyly is an *angular or arc-like* lateral deviation of a giant finger. Its convexity points away from the wedge. Extreme deformities of up to 90° angulation have been noted in many cases. They are possibly caused by a hemilateral hypertrophy of a digit, as one may conclude from observations of concomitant unilateral hypertrophy of a corresponding palmar digital nerve (TSUGE 1967; a.o.).

KELIKIAN noted *total syndactyly* in 10% of the enlarged digits. *Other concomitant deformities* have been noted by some authors (see GRUBER and KUSS 1937; HENTSCHEN 1936; JÄGER 1967).

Macrodactyly involves *periosteal bone growth* to at least the same extent as it does endochondral development. The distal segments of a phalanx are frequently thicker and wider than the proximal parts; the processus unguiculares are often particularly involved. As a rule *maturing of bone* appears to be *accelerated;* epiphyseal nuclei appear prematurely. A similar process has been postulated for the subcutaneous fatty tissue, which even in childhood resembles that of an adult (see BARSKY 1967, a.o.): large, dark lobules and firmer fixation by adjacent connective tissue have been described. *Bone histology* is mostly uncharacteristic. BEN BASSAT et al. (1966) noted a band of fusiform cells (fibroblasts or osteoblasts) between the periosteum and the cortex. FRITZSCHE (1955) observed a case of remarkable softness of bone and markedly disturbed calcification (see also THOMAS 1936; IOVANNOVICH and BARTSCH 1971).

Several patients with *hypo- and aplasias of IP joints* have been reported.

An increase in size of the cutis, tendons, and muscles seems to correspond with the increase in bone growth. Angiomatous changes of the blood vessels have been described by only a few authors.

Palmar *digital nerves* of the involved segment are frequently of considerable thickness and length and take an irregular serpentine course. It is difficult to free them from adherent connective and fatty tissue. Their common trunk in the palm of the hand, usually the median nerve, can be involved in a similar manner. It may be enlarged two or three times.

By way of histologic examinations, MOORE (1942, 1944) discovered a remarkable increase of the endo- and perineurium and of thickened neurofibrils. Similar observations have been made by TSUGE (1967), BEN BASSAT et al. (1966), SCHÖLLNER (1973), and others. Electromicroscopic investigations by IOVANNOVICH and BARTSCH (1971) revealed an increase of all neural components and degenerative changes of the myelin sheaths. They interpreted the degenerative changes as a pressure phenomenon.

"Idiopathic" macrodactyly has to be distinguished from other forms of enlargement of the hand, in particular from elephantiasis caused by primary or secondary *lymphangiopathies*. Elephantiasic changes are in general not of a local nature and involvement of skeletal parts does not occur. Other forms of hand enlargement can be caused by some systemic diseases (e.g., generalized *neurofibromatosis*). Giant fingers have been observed in patients suffering from *Klippel-Trenaunay-Weber Syndrome*. The slight enlargement is the result of angioblastic processes. Angular deformities are unknown (see also DAMBRIN 1963). The diagnosis in cases of congenital or acquired bone *tumors* is easily made (e.g., *multiple heredity exostoses* or *Maffucci syndrome* with chondromatosis and hemangiomas) if visible changes, diffuse involvement, the absent elongation of a finger, and the histologic findings are properly considered and interpreted.

The *cosmetic appearance*, particularly in patients with the progressive type of congenital localized giantism of the hand, can result in pronounced psychological problems. The *function* of such a hand is also frequently markedly impaired. Axial deformities may restrict functions of grasp and grip, and impairment is aggravated by limited finger flexion caused by soft tissue hypertrophy, bony blocking, or occasionally joint aplasias. More intricate finger functions may even be impeded by the excessive length of a finger. Hypo- and anesthesias of the digits may increase the impairment (see DAMBRIN 1936; KELIKIAN 1974).

10.1.2 Indications for Surgery

Pronounced macrodactylies and giant fingers of the progressive type require surgical intervention for functional and cosmetic reasons.

All known operations to normalize size and length of a digit are fraught with problems. It is impossible to outline a specific procedure for each individual case. So far, results have been barely satisfactory in regard to improved function and cosmetic appearance.

10.1.3 Timing of Surgery

In general, patients with congenital localized giantism of the hand require surgery as early as possible to prevent further functional and secondary morphological impairment. BUCK-GRAMCKO (1971) recommended that operations should be performed during the 1st year of life. However, treatment of most patients is begun at a later date, after the finger enlargement has become more obvious. Follow-up examinations with x-ray control should be continued until bony maturity has occurred, as the rate of growth of giant fingers is quite variable.

10.1.4 General Surgical Directives

Type and number of surgical interventions will vary with the age of the patient.

Children and adolescents may be treated with *epiphysiodeses* to retard longitudinal growth of a finger (see MASSONNOUD 1874; TUCKER and CARPENTER 1951; CLIFFORD 1959; JONES 1963; a.o.). Proper timing of this operation is of great importance, but difficult. It does not influence progressive transverse thickening of the bone or soft tissue enlargement (see TSUGE 1967).

Another operation consists of *soft tissue excision*, mainly of the fatty tissue with careful protection of nerves, combined with removal of superfluous skin. Staging of surgery is recommended. The operation should be performed on each half of a digit with a period of 3 months between each intervention (TSUGE 1967; KELIKIAN 1964). It may be necessary to perform similar operations on the palm of the hand.

Authors who accept a causal relationship of neural hyperplasia and macrodactyly have developed their own therapeutic conclusions. TSUGE believes that *excision of involved palmar nerves* and excessive soft tissue masses results in the arrest of further growth. The restitution of sensation in children is reported to be good (MCCARROLL 1950). In cases of marked hypertrophy, reduction in size of a digit may require a segmental resection of palmar nerves with end-to-end anastomosis. The anastomosis should be carried out distal to the PIP joint. KELIKIAN reported good sensibility after this operation in six out of seven patients; we have achieved a similar result in an infant. It may be necessary to implant island flaps with proper neurovascular structures if sensibility remains insufficient. BUCK-GRAMCKO (1973) obtained very good residual sensiblity after splitting and partial resection of the median nerve.

Carpal tunnel release is occasionally necessary.

In most patients the previously mentioned operations are insufficient to reduce the length and thickness of an involved finger to normal size. For infants KELIKIAN also recommended removal of the periosteum, resection of superficial cortical strata, and cauterization of remaining cambium layers, but reported that bone growth cannot always be arrested by this procedure. Our experience with one of our patients has been the same.

BARSKY (1967) described a *resection arthrodesis* in cases of moderate finger elongation combined with other necessary surgical measures. TSUGE modified this procedure. Employing a lateral approach, he resected a distal segment of the middle phalanx and the proximal end of the distal phalanx. This was followed by soft tissue excision with careful protection of the nail bed and fusion of the DIP joint. In later operations the tendon of m. flexor superficialis was shortened and remaining excess soft tissue and skin was removed (for particulars see TSUGE 1967; similarly: BONOLA and MORELLI 1972).

Another method employed by TSUGE involved resection of the palmar portions of the distal phalanx and shortening of the nail (op. cit.). It should be pointed out that he and BUCK-GRAMCKO (1971) observed circulatory problems after such an operation.

MILLESI (1966) described a *"surgical slimming" of skeletal parts* and subsequently of the soft tissue in older children and adults. On occasion it is advisable to resect the involved processus unguiculares in combination with shortening and slimming of the nail to improve an unsightly macronychia. However, nail dystrophies have been observed as a result of this operation.

An *angulation osteotomy* with partial resection of the middle phalanx may be indicated in patients with clinodactyly. Alignment in flexion will improve function. Successive *segmental resections* of the phalanges have been suggested by KELIKIAN ("recession osteotomy"). They can be combined with joint excisions and arthrodeses, but such operations involving the distal phalanx will result in destruction of the nail matrix. Preferred treatment in cases of thumb involvement is a fusion of the MP joint.

Occasionally it is necessary to perform a partial or total *amputation* of one or several digits (see DAMBRIN 1936; TIMONEY 1944, a.o.). This operation is only indicated if a satisfactory result cannot be obtained by any other method.

The number of surgical interventions required until bony maturity has been reached, concomitant psychological problems, and the expected functional value of the finger require critical considerations.

11 Pollex Flexus Congenitus (Congenital Trigger Thumb)

11.1 Introduction

11.1.1 General Remarks

A congenital flexion contracture of the thumb at its IP joint is caused by a *constriction of the anular ligament* of the MP joint at the level of the sesamoid bones in combination with a *fusiform swelling* of the tendon of m. flex. poll. long. This *tendinous "nodule"* cannot glide through the anular ligament, and it is impossible to extend the joint even passively. Similar findings are present in patients suffering from hypo- or aplasia of this tendon. Familial appearance of this disorder is not infrequent; twins can be affected by it.

11.1.2 Timing of Surgery

The relatively small operation required for correction of this functionally disabling disorder permits surgery during the 1st year of life, as soon as the active and passive flexion impairment has been noted.

11.1.3 General Surgical Directives

Therapy consists of *transection* or partial resection of the *anular ligament.* This allows unimpaired movement of the nodular tendon. Extirpation of the nodule or slimming of the tendon is *superfluous and full of problems.* These steps can produce tendinous adhesions or reactive changes resulting in recurrence of a fusiform mass. Subcutaneous transection of the anular ligament is also inadvisable, as this "simple" method of therapy may damage the main palmar neurovascular structures (HUBENSTORF 1961).

11.1.4 Postoperative Care

A sterile dressing is usually sufficient. Immobilization only for a few days. Early active motion prevents adhesions.

11.2 Flexion Contracture of the Interphalangeal Joint of the Thumb

Goal of Surgery

Correction of the flexion contracture by transection of the anular ligament.

Fig. 1 Preoperative appearance.
Transverse skin incision in the flexor crease of the first MP joint with proper protection of vessels and nerves.

Fig. 2 The incision is spread longitudinally with scissors. Passive extension demonstrates a fusiform mass (*) in the tendon of m. flex. poll. long. proximal to the anular ligament. *Broken lines:* incision of vaginal ligament and tendon sheath.

Fig. 3 The anular ligament and tendon sheath have been split longitudinally. The distal phalanx can be fully extended. The nodular mass glides easily distally. Partial resection of the anular ligament may be required in some cases.

Fig. 4 Final appearance after skin closure.

Postoperative Care

See Sect. 11.1.4.

Errors and Their Consequences

E. The skin incision is made longitudinally and not transversely in the flexor crease of the MP joint.
C. The scar will result in a flexion contracture.

E. Vessels and nerves have been damaged by transecting the anular ligament subcutaneously.
C. Circulatory and neurologic deficits.

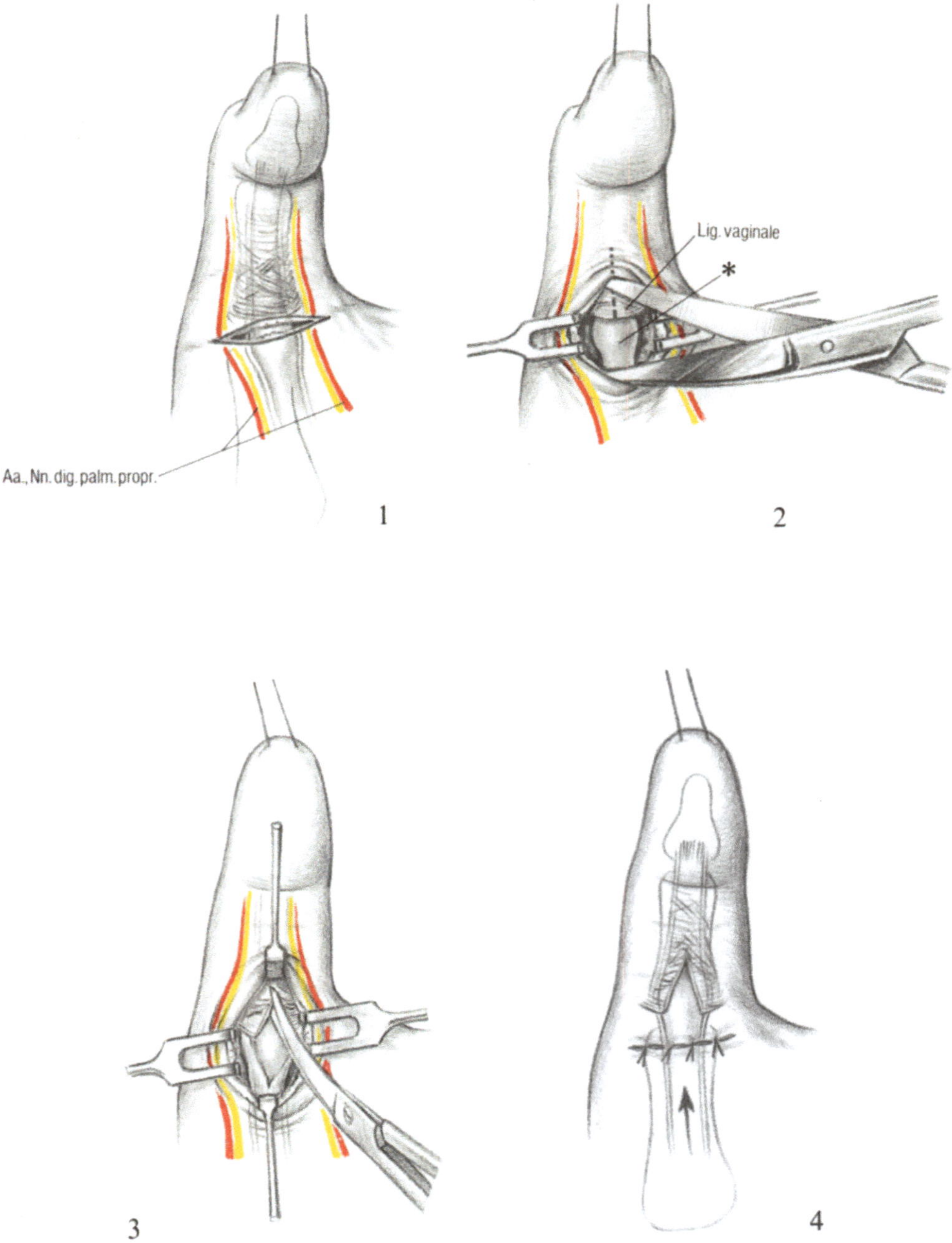
Lig. vaginale
*
Aa., Nn. dig. palm. propr.
1
2
3
4

12 Camptodactyly

12.1 Introduction

12.1.1 General Remarks

Camptodactyly (LANDOUZY 1906) [also called streblo(micro)dactyly, campylodactyly, crooked little finger, dropped finger, hammer finger, doigt crochu etc.] is a hereditary *flexion contracture of a PIP joint.*

In the vast majority of cases it affects the *little finger*. Occasionally other fingers are involved, usually in addition to the little finger. Bilaterality is prevalent. In cases of unilaterality the right hand seems to be predominantly affected (SMITH and KAPLAN 1968).

Pathogenesis of this deformity is unclear. Homogeneity does not appear to exist. Its heredity seems to be autosomal dominant with varying penetrance.

Many authors (SMITH and KAPLAN 1968; WILHELM and KLEINSCHMIDT 1968; MILLESI 1968; BRÜCHLE and MERKLING 1972; BERGER and MILLESI 1975) believe muscular imbalance to be a major factor in the development of camptodactyly. According to SMITH and KAPLAN (1968) the causative agent is a shortening or insertion anomaly of the superficial flexor tendon of the little finger. Anatomic studies by FURNAS (1965) have shown that this tendon quite often originates without a muscle belly from the superficial flexor tendon of the ring finger. Therefore adaptation of the tendon during periods of rapid bone growth is impaired, and the middle phalanx is pulled more and more into flexion.

The importance of the superficial flexor tendon in creating this deformity is supported by the impressive therapeutic success achieved by SMITH and KAPLAN (1968) by only tenotomizing this tendon.

WILHELM and KLEINSCHMIDT (1968) believe that abnormalities of the lumbrical muscles are the cause of camptodactyly. Intraoperatively they noted insertion anomalies of these muscles. The specific tendon did not insert radially into the extensor aponeurosis at the base of the proximal phalanx, but ended on the ulnar side in the para-articular tissue of the joint capsule, in the lig. capit. transversum, in the tendon sheath of the finger flexors, or even in the superficial flexor tendon. They felt that these abnormalities result in a loss of the extensor action of the lumbrical muscles on the PIP and DIP joints. The imbalance, with preponderance of a flexor potential, is thought to cause a flexion contracture in the PIP joint. BRÜCHLE and MERKLING (1972) also described an abnormal course of a duplicated lumbrical muscle inserting into the joint capsule of the little finger.

MILLESI (1968) is of the opinion that a defective development of the extensor aponeurosis over the dorsal aspect of the PIP joint produces camptodactyly. In several patients he found replacement of the extensor aponeurosis by a thin sheath of connective tissue.

A publication by BERGER and MILLESI (1975) mentions other possible pathogenetic factors.

In most cases, the deformity is recognizable even during childhood. It *progresses rapidly* during growth spurts. A mainly *tendinous* contracture exists in children and adolescents. It can be compensated by flexion of the wrist and MP joint, but compensation is reduced as tightness of the joint capsule and ligaments increases. Patients with marked deformities develop a position of internal rotation of the little finger. Isolated arthrotic involvement of the PIP joint has been reported.

Camptodactyly may occur in combination with aminoaciduria (PARISH et al. 1963), pectus excavatum, slight scoliosis, and ptosis (MAURER 1938; WELSH and TEMTAMY 1966; a.o.).

Deformities of similar appearance have been observed in patients with other hand anomalies such as cleft hand (see Sect. 9.7) or numerical variations. The term "camptodactyly" has also been used in describing all congenital digital flexion deformities [e.g., flexion deformities of the MP joints (with ulnar deviation) in cases of craniocarpotarsal dystrophy (Freeman-Sheldon syndrome)].

Differential diagnosis should include deformities caused by arthrogryposis multiplex congenita or Dupuytren disease, as well as those occurring after ulnar paresis or tendovaginitis. These conditions are usually easily recognizable.

12.1.2 Indications for Surgery

Surgical correction of camptodactyly requires critical evaluation and a high degree of conservatism. Patients should be informed that due to underlying anatomic conditions full active extension of the PIP joint may not be achieved in all situations.

Until extensive operative experience and long-term results have been obtained, cosmetic factors alone should not be considered a reason for surgical intervention. Slight limitation of extension can be readily compensated by hyperextension of the MP joint. Only marked progressive flexion contractures justify an operation.

12.1.3 Timing of Surgery

Surgery should not be performed too early in childhood. In cases of rapidly progressing flexion deformities and/or development of an additional rotatory malposition, surgery is justified between the 6th and 8th year of life. It is inadvisable to postpone it until adulthood. Tendinous contractures of juveniles will turn into capsuloligamentous deformities as the patient grows older and thereby preclude therapeutic success. BERGER and MILLESI (1975) have reported that each of their unsatisfactory long-term results were noted in patients who had undergone surgery as adults.

12.1.4 General Surgical Directives

Plastic operations involving the skin only, e.g., a Z-plasty on the flexor surface, have generally been unsuccessful (BARINKA 1964; CURRARINO and WALDMAN 1964). The therapeutic goal is *reconstitution of the impaired balance between flexors and extensors* at the PIP joint of the little finger. Several methods have been recommended:

SMITH and KAPLAN (1968) reported good results (see above) with *transection of the superficial flexor tendon* in the palm of the hand. This method can be used only in patients with strictly tendinous contractures. WILHELM and KLEINSCHMIDT (1968) also recommended tenotomy of the superficial flexor tendon and its fixation onto the extensor aponeurosis in more severe conditions. In addition they advised an *exploration of the palm* to correct possible abnormal insertions of the lumbrical muscles. MILLESI (1968) also recommended, because of good results, *transplantation of the superficial flexor tendon* onto the extensor aponeurosis. In the presence of marked deformities he advised a *Z-plasty of the flexor tendon* in the forearm, a *capsulotomy* of the PIP joint, and in cases of tight skin conditions a *swivel flap plasty* at the flexor surface. In one case we were able to correct a camptodactyly by performing a Z-plasty at the flexor surface, transecting the tight para-articular strands of connective tissue, and carrying out capsulotomy of the PIP joint (see also BONOLA and MORELLI 1972).

12.1.5 Postoperative Care

All authors stress the point that scrupulous postoperative care is of extreme importance. Elastic exercise splints are essential. To avoid recurrences, a night splint fixed in extension has to be worn for 6 months.

13 Hypoplasias and Aplasias of the Radius (Radial Club Hand)

13.1 Introduction

13.1.1 General Remarks

Hypoplasias and aplasias of the radius (synonyms: radial ray defect, radial club hand) belong to a group of inhibitory malformations in which the *radial portion of the upper limb bud* has been damaged. Their increased endemic appearance caused by the thalidomide embryopathies gave us an opportunity to advance our knowledge of the morphology and functional anatomy of these relatively rare differentiation disorders (see LENZ 1963; O. HEPP 1962; BLAUTH 1968, 1969; SCHÖLLNER 1972; WILLERT and HENKEL 1969; a.o.).

These malformations are occasionally combined with deformities of the lower limb, such as aplasias of the femur or tibia. They have been described as part of the Holt-Oram syndrome, the Fanconi panmyelopathy, the phocomelia-thrombocytopenia syndrome, the Rothmund-Thomson syndrome, and Trisomy 18. In general only in these syndrome is bilateral involvement present (LENZ 1969). Familial accumulation has been reported (see BAUER and BODE 1940).

Visually one notices shortening and often bowing of the forearm combined with club hand deformity *(manus vara et flexa)*.

The *radius* is hypoplastic or partially or totally absent. The amount of involvement forms a *teratologic progression,* beginning with hypoplasias in which the radius keeps its shape but is smaller and shorter. The distal skeletal segment including the epiphysis is missing in partial aplasias. Total aplasia can be present. It is not unusual to find concomitant more or less well developed bony bridges *(radioulnar synostoses)*. They are usually located in the proximal segment, but occasionally in the middle one; they may also appear in the proximal and distal segments of the forearm simultaneously. In extreme situations both bones may be fused into one skeletal part (BLAUTH 1969). Radioulnar synostoses result in a fixed position of supination with impaired function.

Isolated radioulnar synostoses, sometimes combined with anular grooves of the forearm, have been reported (see Sect. 3.12). Their functional and therapeutic problems correspond to those found in radius malformations (see Sect. 13.4).

The radius may be replaced by a tough band of connective tissue extending from the lateral humeral epicondyle or a proximal radial rudiment to the carpus. Muscles may originate from it (STOFFEL and STEMPEL 1909).

The degree of underdevelopment of the radius influences the shape of the *ulna*. It is usually shortened and bowed in a dorsoradial direction. Sometimes the ulna is squat and its diaphyseal cross section is flattened. The distal part of the ulna may be thickened and wider than usual. A shallow trough that articulates with the proximal carpal row may be present at its radiopalmar aspect. The trough may be covered with hyaline cartilage, but this "joint surface" frequently contains only connective tissue.

Skeletal dysplasias are also known to be present at the *proximal end of the ulna and the distal end of the humerus.* Combined with capsular and muscular anomalies they limit or inhibit elbow mobility. A bony spur resembling a processus supracondylaris humeri has been reported by SCHÖLLNER (1972). Even the *shoulder joint* may occasionally be hypoplastic.

Radial defects are always combined with *bony anomalies of the hand,* which usually involve elements of the radial rays. Hypo- and aplasias of the carpal scaphoid and the os trapezium are frequently seen, as well as many types of synostoses (the most common being between the os lunatum and os triquetrum).

The carpal bones deviate in a radial or radiopalmar fashion in relationship to the distal ulna. *Hypo- and aplasias of the Ist ray* are usually present. The amount of their involvement does not always correspond with the severity of the radius defect. *Triphalangeal syndactylous thumbs* or *thumb duplications* have been observed, as have polydactyly and oligodactyly. Further functional impairment can be caused mainly by finger joint hypoplasias involving radial rays. Maturing of the involved skeletal parts is retarded (HIPPE 1970).

Muscles and tendons show a multiplicity of anomalies (hypo- and aplasias, coalitions, or abnormal origins and insertions). Most frequently involved are the mm. brachioradialis, flexor carpi radialis, extensor carpi radialis longus and brevis, extensor pollicis longus and brevis, supinator, pronator teres and quadratus, extensor digitorum communis, and the thenar musculature. The tendon of m. extensor carpi ulnaris takes its course through a trough in the capitulum ulnae and inserts distally at the basis of the Vth metacarpal. The amount of muscular and tendon anomalies of the Ist ray corresponds in general with the degree of its bony inhibitory development (see Chap. 4).

The radial long fingers are occasionally supplied by extremely thin extensor tendons. Multiple extensor tendons may insert on the little finger with a conjoint aponeurosis. Muscular anomalies of the upper arm and shoulder girdle have been observed, particularly as aplasias of the biceps and deltoid muscle (BLAUTH 1969; SCHÖLLNER 1972).

The usually tight *capsule of the carpal joint* adheres to the radiopalmar and radiodorsal portions of the distal ulna.

Vessel anomalies are observed, mainly at the radial side (BLAUTH and SCHMIDT 1969; STOFFEL and STEMPEL 1909). The radial artery may be missing or hypoplastic. The ulnar artery is usually well developed. One or both deep palmar arches may be absent. Vessel anomalies of the index finger, mainly of its radial palmar artery, have to be expected if the Ist ray is abnormally developed. This can be of importance if one considers pollicization of the index finger. Anomalies of more proximal arteries have been observed (brachial and interosseous arteries); this may influence surgical approaches.

Neural structural and anatomic *abnormalities* occur mainly at the radial nerve. It may be hypoplastic and at times terminates at the level of the elbow joint. On one occasion we observed a hypoplastic radial nerve twisted around the tendon of m. extensor carpi radialis at the midportion of the forearm in a looplike fashion.

The median nerve is frequently found in a superficial radial position beneath the flexor crease of the wrist. It may provide sensibility to areas normally supplied by the radial nerve.

Functional impairment in cases of radial ray defects is generally severe. A combination of *extension rigidity at the elbow* and *fixed supination* of the forearm found in radioulnar synostoses is particularly disabling. Flexion contractures (claw fingers) of the PIP joints cause lesser degreees of impairment, as they are usually compensated by an ability to hyperextend the MP joints.

Patients learn to compensate quite readily. Active radial abduction of the hand in the presence of extension elbow joint rigidity permits a type of vise grip. Adduction of the ulnar long fingers results in a lateral grasping action if the thumb is malformed. Both actions are functionally of great value and are sometimes even indispensable.

13.1.2 Indications for Surgery

Surgical correction of a *club hand* should be considered only in *exceptional* circumstances. Such operations require critical evaluation of hand function and adaptive mechanisms. Considerations of functional improvement are of much greater importance than those of cosmesis. The increased surgical risk caused by concomitant malformations (e.g., cardiac involvement: Holt-Oram syndrome, kidney impairment) should be discussed preoperatively with pediatricians and anesthesiologists. Surgery may be *considered* if:

- The *range of motion of the elbow joint* is essentially within normal limits and club hand position is *not* required for compensatory reasons.
- The *club hand malposition* can be nearly or completely corrected by passive manipulation, if necessary after conservative therapy, i.e., if the axis of the hand corresponds with the longitudinal axis of the forearm. Persistent radial deviation of more than 10°, as noted regularly in cases where the carpal bones are displaced radial and proximal-palmar to the shaft of the ulna, makes surgery problematic. Such situations involve a high risk of damaging the distal ulnar epiphysis. Proper axial alignment can be obtained only with extensive additional surgery such as large-scale resection of carpal bones distal to the bases of the metacarpals or a shortening osteotomy of the ulna.
- Several days of *functional testing* does not reveal any loss of function after passive correction and fixation of the club hand in plaster. (In general one can expect an increase in power and flexion ability of the fingers in such a situation.)

The above-mentioned prerequisites apply mainly to children. Adults with club hands have learned to live with their deformity to such a degree that surgery is even less indicated. Occasionally it may be necessary to consider an arthrodesis if pain in the arthrotic wrist joint has become a major factor.

Indications for a *lengthening osteotomy* of the ulna are extremely rare. It may be indicated for unilateral club hands if fibrous ankylosis of the wrist joint is present after an otherwise successful correction. Other operations that are rarely indicated are *arthrolysis* of the elbow joint, biceps reconstruction plasty, and resection of a supracondylar spur. Long-term results of such operations are not available; consequently it is impossible to give clear directives.

Rotational malpositions of the forearm as seen in patients with *radioulnar synostosis* require surgical intervention. The marked functional impairment can only be corrected with a derotation osteotomy.

13.1.3 Timing of Surgery

Marked rotatory deformities of the forearm should be treated at an early age, preferably in the 2nd year of life. Their correction is of great functional value. It can be performed without interference with the zones of bone growth. All other operations should be postponed until functional adaptation can be better evaluated and epiphyseal plate damage limited. Surgery may be performed in cases of *lesser involvement* during preschool age if passive overcorrection can be easily obtained and if the carpus is in good apposition with the distal ulna. More severe cases should be operated on several years later. Surgery on patients with club-hands that may require an additional *pollicization* due to aplasia of the thumb should be planned for the 4th or 5th year of life. Club hand correction should be undertaken *prior* to pollicization, as we have observed that thumb activity is better after stabilization of the wrist joint in a position of function.

13.1.4 General Surgical Directives

Operations placing the distal end of the ulna in close contact with carpal bones require certain considerations (Blauth 1968):

- In every case the tendon of m. extensor carpi ulnaris has to be exposed in and removed from the groove in the capitulum ulnae.
- The extensor tendons of the fingers are mobilized en bloc, i.e., without removing them from their sheaths. Dissection begins at the carpus and is continued in a radial direction. Portions of the dorsal joint capsule remain attached to them, which prevents postoperative adhesions of the tendons.
- It is imperative to transect all capsular and ligamentous structures between ulna and carpus, including those of the palmar surface, to permit "repositioning" of the carpus. The ulnar styloid may have to be removed after parts of the carpal bones have been excised. This guarantees a better fit of the head of the ulna with these bones. Soft tissue removal from the distal ulna has to be done in a parsimonious manner and may have to be carried out with surgical telescopes. Extensive dissection or exposure of the epi- or metaphyseal area has to be avoided to prevent damage of the vessels supplying the epiphyseal plate.
- Two methods are available for proper approximation of the distal ulna with the carpal bones. One can open the proximal carpal row between the os lunatum

and os triquetrum in a booklike fashion and partially resect the os capitatum (Sect. 14.2.1) or create a cavity in the carpal bones by employing a gouge or hand-driven(!) burr (Sect. 13.2.2). The second method usually results in a better fit.

- Positioning the carpus in extension of 20° and ulnar deviation of 10–15° results in better function and limits the tendency for recurrence. The position should be secured with two crossed Kirschner wires. Kirschner wire fixation is not required if the bony adaptation is really perfect. In such a situation a row of sutures that penetrate capsule and cartilage are sufficient (Sect. 13.2.2).
- Imbalance of the muscles of the forearm and hand persists postoperatively, but to a lesser degree. Consequently shortening of the tendon of m. extensor carpi ulnaris prior to wound closure (Sect. 13.2.1) is recommended. Even with this step it is impossible to correct the muscle imbalance definitely. *Recurrences with deviation into the previous malposition have to be expected so long as bones grow.* This threatened recurrence can be held back by employing night splints, and sometimes it is even possible to prevent it.

For cosmetic reasons corrective osteotomies for *club hand recurrence* (Sect. 13.3) should be performed near the epiphyseal plate of the ulna. The size of the bony wedge should be determined radiographically. Younger patients require a higher amount of overcorrection.

Derotation osteotomies for malpositions of the forearm are always carried out within the synostotic segment (Sect. 13.4).

Hypoplasias of the radius are better treated by *shortening osteotomies of the ulna* than by lengthening osteotomies of the radius. Attempts to lengthen the radius in one step fail due to the resistance of the soft tissues (two personal observations) or result in an increase of the palmar malposition of the carpus. Proper instrumentation (distractors) for gradual lengthening osteotomies as described for lower limb discrepancies is not yet available for the bones of the forearm. At times it may be necessary to combine the shortening osteotomy of the ulna with corrective measures to change its longitudinal axis. This can be accomplished by concurrent valgus wedge osteotomies (with an ulnar basis of the wedges) of the radius and ulna followed by compression osteosynthesis with self-compressing plates. In such cases it is advisable to transfer the tendon of m. extensor carpi radialis to the ulnar side of the metacarpal region.

13.1.5 Postoperative Care

The main goal of club hand surgery is a fibrous rigidity of the "wrist joint" after the distal end of the ulna has been fitted into the carpal bones. A long-arm plaster cast is initially employed for 4 weeks. The Kirschner wires are removed at that time and an unpadded short-arm plaster cast is applied for another 4–6 weeks. Plaster cast fixation is followed by a rigid wrist joint orthosis for 6 months.

The rigid sleeve is then gradually removed and will finally be worn at night only, if satisfactory stability of the wrist joint is noted. It may be necessary to wear the orthosis even longer if instability persists.

Other pertinent measures will be discussed in the sections concerning operative examples.

13.2 Radius Aplasia

13.2.1 Correctable Club Hand (Operation According to Blauth)

Goal of Surgery

Correction of the club hand attitude and creation of a fibrous ankylosis of the "wrist joint" in a position of improved function. (We advise the reader to review the preoperative prerequisites mentioned in Sect. 13.1.2!)

Fig. 1 Preoperative appearance and incision with the hand held in the best possible amount of correction.
The radial ray defect is combined with aplasias of the os scaphoideum and the os trapezium and a fourth-degree hypoplasia of the thumb.
The skin incision begins along the longitudinal axis of the distal ulna. At the ulnar head it curves radially and ends along the longitudinal axis of the IIIrd ray. Stellate capsulotomy between the ossa lunatum, triquetrum, and capitatum is demonstrated by *red lines*. The *hatched areas* outline portions of bone that will have to be removed. Partial resection of the os capitatum is always required. A half-moon shaped resection surface permits a tighter fit of the ulna.

Fig. 2 The extensor tendons have been exposed, main veins should be protected. The tendon of m. ext. carpi uln. has been identified and exposed proximally and distally after the fascia carpi dors. has been incised over the head of the ulna.
The dorsal joint capsule is approached from the ulnar aspect of the small finger extensors. From there all extensor tendons are mobilized en bloc. For this step one holds the scalpel tangentially. In this manner one prevents damage to the paratendinous tissues (see insert, Fig. 2a).

Remarks

It is not our intention to create a movable "wrist joint." Muscle imbalance remains, even after a technically successful operation! Satisfactory motion of the "wrist joint" carries a high risk of recurrence of the deformity and the need for permanent bracing.

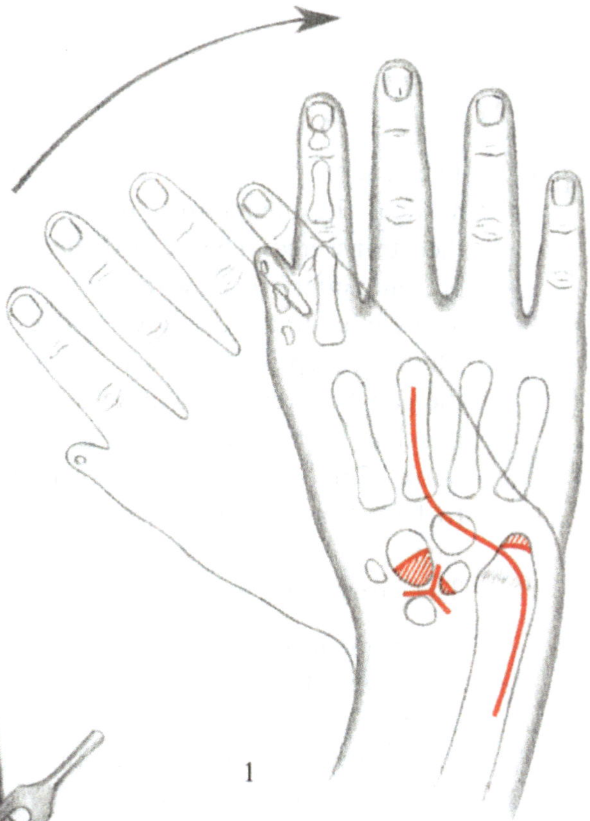

1

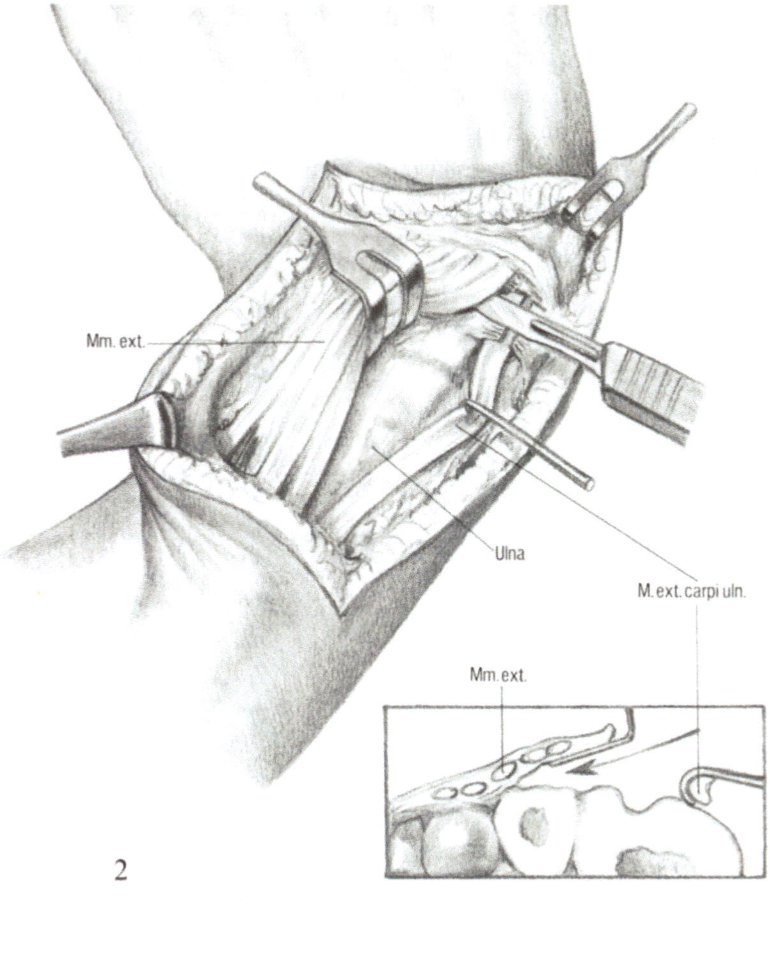

2

Fig. 3 The tendon of m. ext. carpi uln. has been pulled across the ulnar aspect of the head of the ulna into a palmar position. The dorsal capsule and ligaments are then transected. The head of the ulna should not be completely circumcised; this prevents interference with the vascular supply of the epiphyseal plate. Palmar and, if possible, ulnar soft tissue bridges should be preserved.

The next step is a complete transection of the palmar wrist joint capsule through the gap between the ulna and the carpal bones. Visualization of these structures is achieved by pulling the distal ulna away from the carpal bones with a bone hook. This permits blunt or sharp dissection of the palmar capsule. Care has to be taken to protect the median and ulnar nerves and the vessels during this step.

The capsular tissues between the os lunatum and the os triquetrum are then incised.

Fig. 4 The os lunatum and os triquetrum have been widely unfolded in a booklike fashion. The head of the os capitatum will be resected and remaining capsular elements carefully removed from the distal end of the ulna. The head of the ulna is then fitted into the gap between the os lunatum, os triquetrum, and the remaining segment of the os capitatum. It may be necessary to remove additional portions of the central carpal bones if a proper fit of the ulna is impossible.

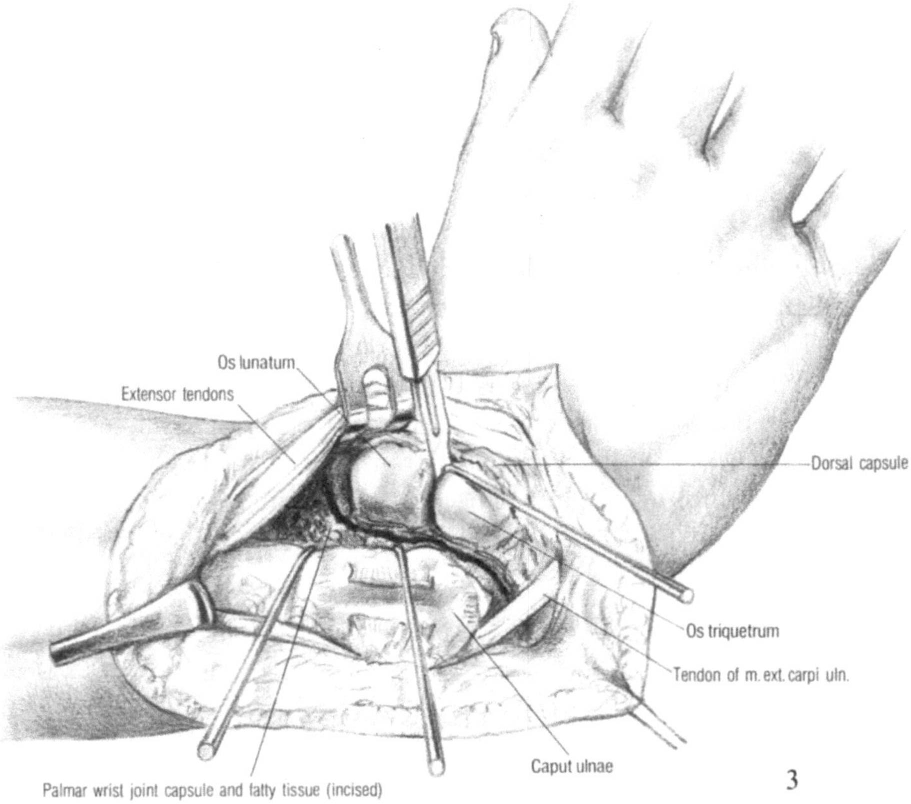
Os lunatum
Extensor tendons
Dorsal capsule
Os triquetrum
Tendon of m. ext. carpi uln.
Caput ulnae
Palmar wrist joint capsule and fatty tissue (incised)

3

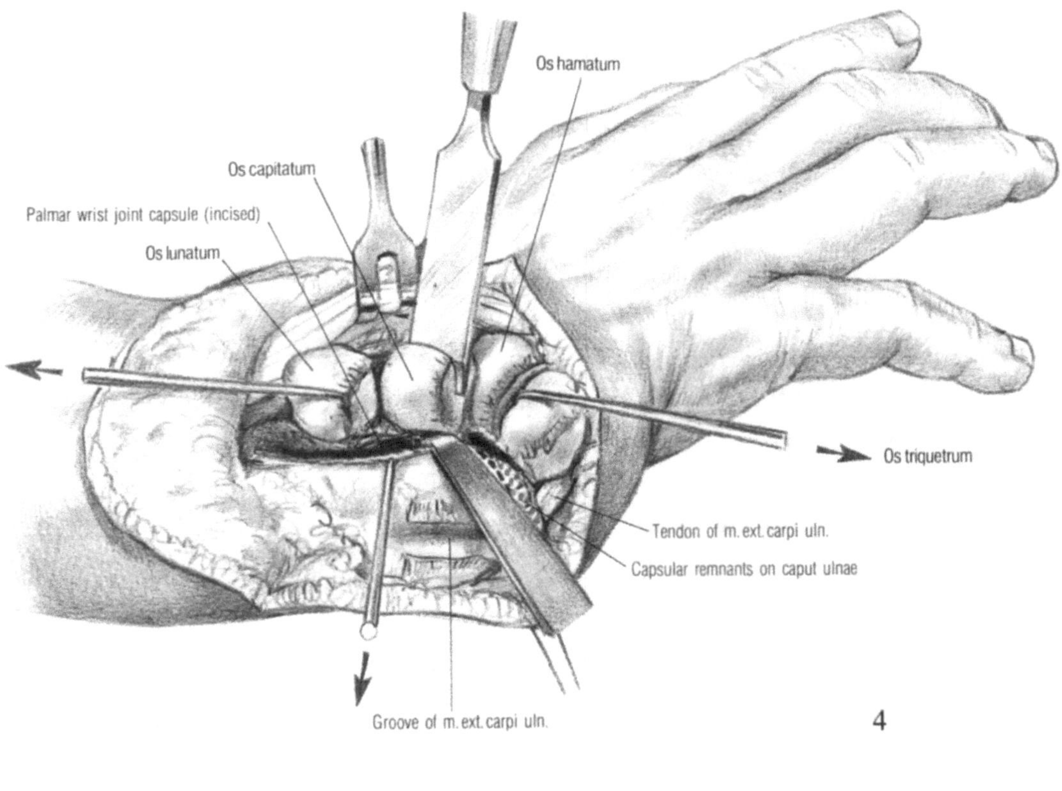
Os hamatum
Os capitatum
Palmar wrist joint capsule (incised)
Os lunatum
Os triquetrum
Tendon of m. ext. carpi uln.
Capsular remnants on caput ulnae
Groove of m. ext. carpi uln.

4

Fig. 5 The distal end of the ulna is exposed to a degree that permits apposition with the os lunatum and os triquetrum. Overexposure will result in damage to the epiphyseal plate!
The carpal bones should be fitted to the ulna *distal* to its epiphyseal plate. Inappropriate placement may lead to synostotic processes followed by severe recurrent club hand deformities. The "wrist joint" is immobilized with two crossed Kirschner wires in slight ulnar adduction and extension. The wires penetrate the os lunatum and os triquetrum. The redundant tendon of m. ext. carpi uln. is then shortened (Fig. 6). One can also transfer it to the ulnar side of the Vth metacarpal to reduce muscle imbalance. Suction drainage and wound closure.

Fig. 6 Postoperative appearance.

Postoperative Care

Long-arm cast with inclusion of the MP joints for 2 weeks, then suture removal. Reapplication of a long-arm cast for another 4 weeks, after which x-ray control is carried out and Kirschner wires are removed. Short-arm cast for another 6–8 weeks. This is followed by using a removable orthotic device which stabilizes the "wrist joint" in its corrected position for another 3–4 months. The orthotic device is then gradually discontinued, depending on the amount of fibrous ankylosis. A night splint has to be worn until bony maturity has been attained.

Errors and Their Consequences

E. The dorsal main veins have been damaged.
C. Circulatory impairment, edema.

E. The space between the distal ulna and the carpus has been mistaken for the intercarpal or metacarpal joint.
C. Impairment of the growth plate, resulting in reduced and/or crooked development of the ulna.

E. The extensor tendons have not been mobilized en bloc.
C. Adhesions, resulting in finger movement limitation.

E. The capsule of the wrist joint has not been completely transected at its palmar side.
C. Force is required to align ulna and carpus properly, rapid recurrence of the deformity is likely.

E. Dissection and shaping of the bones has been performed carelessly.
C. Nerves and vessels can be damaged.
– For further errors, see above text.

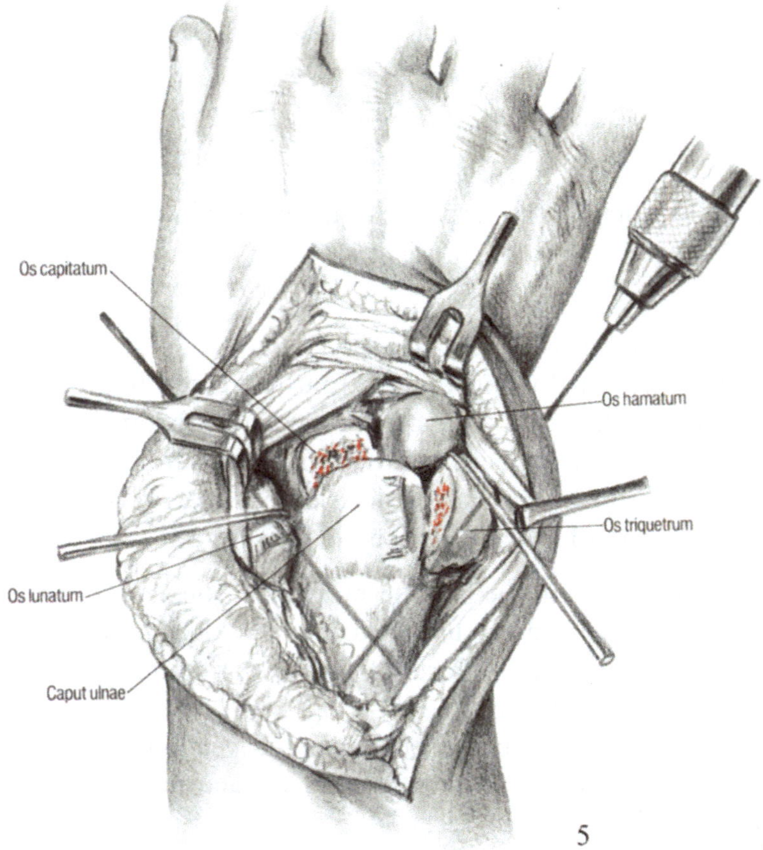
Os capitatum
Os hamatum
Os triquetrum
Os lunatum
Caput ulnae

5

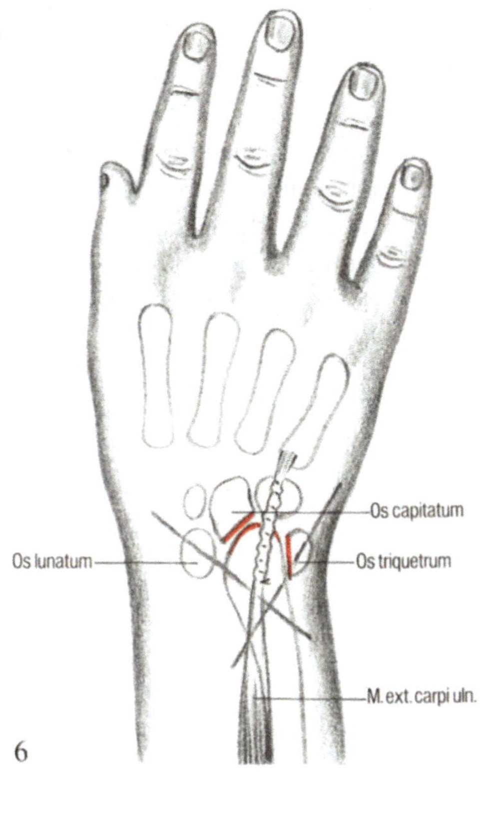
Os capitatum
Os lunatum
Os triquetrum
M. ext. carpi uln.

6

13.2.2 Correctable Club Hand (Alternative Operation According to Blauth)

Goal of Surgery

Club hand correction by aligning the carpus with the distal ulna; fibrous ankylosis of the "wrist joint".

Fig. 1 Preoperative appearance and incision, dorsal aspect.
The four finger hand with its floating thumb (fourth-degree thumb hypoplasia) can be readily aligned with the distal ulna after preoperative therapy *(arrow)*.
The *black-hatched* skin areas may be excised prior to closure if excess skin is present. Mobilization of the extensor tendons, incision of the wrist joint, and exposure of the distal ulna is carried out as described in Sect. 13.2.1.

Fig. 2 Dorsal view of the wrist joint with the hand in maximal flexion.
The os lunatum and os triquetrum are unfolded in a booklike fashion after their capsular structures have been incised. Parts of the os capitatum are removed by using a Luer-type rongeur (not shown).
The carpal bones are carefully shaped with a hand-driven burr until the head of the ulna fits into them. The position of the os triquetrum is ulnar, that of the os lunatum radial to the distal ulna.

Fig. 3 Dorsal view of the wrist joint prior to skin closure.
It was easy to position the carpus without tension in slight overcorrection (25° dorsal extension, 15° ulnar abduction). Therefore it was unnecessary to employ Kirschner wires for fixation. The capsule has been closed with heavy mattress sutures, which should grasp the periosteum as generously as possible and, if possible, the cartilaginous parts of the carpal bones. The tendon of m. ext. carpi uln. has been shortened (see diagram). The *hatched areas* of skin will be excised.

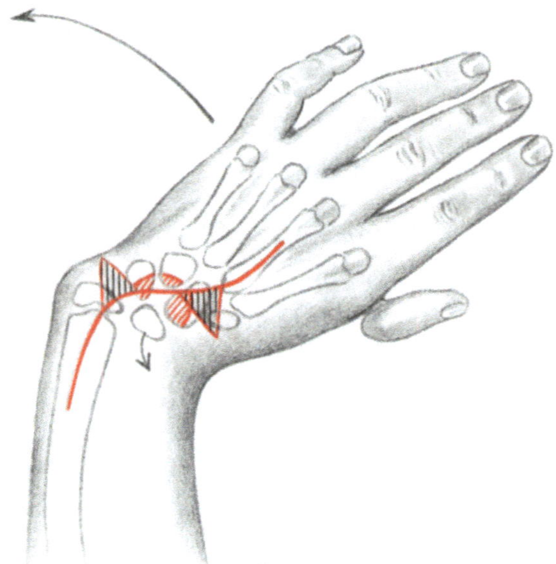

1

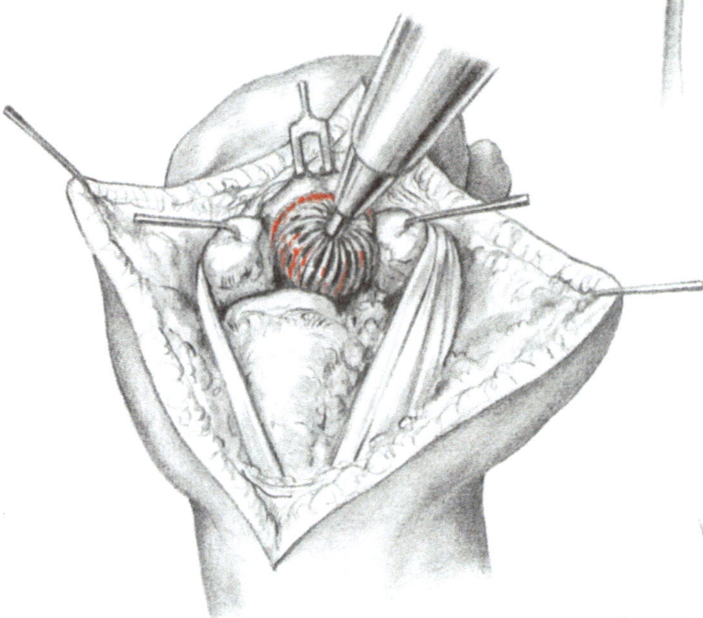

2

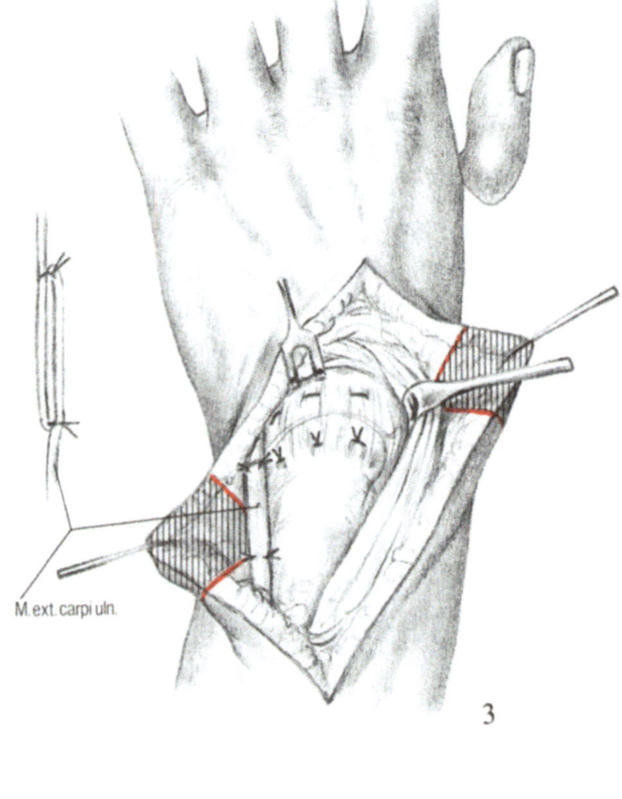

3

Fig. 4 Postoperative appearance.

Postoperative Care

See Sect. 13.2.1.
Pollicization should be performed not earlier than 6 months after the club hand operation (see Sect. 4.1).

Remarks

A small burr should be used only if the hand is relatively large and the shape of the ulna appropriate (otherwise surgery as outlined in Sect. 13.2.1).
This example of stabilizing the ulna in the carpal bones is an alternate method. It should be employed only if axial alignment can be readily obtained and if apposition of the ulna with the carpal bones is secure enough to exclude their displacement.

Errors and Their Consequences

E. Inappropriate handling of the burr.
C. Soft tissues, particularly vessels, may be traumatized or torn.

E. Mattress sutures cut out.
C. The junction of ulna and carpus remains unstable. Displacement may occur while moving the patient or during application of the plaster cast.
See also Sect. 13.2.1.

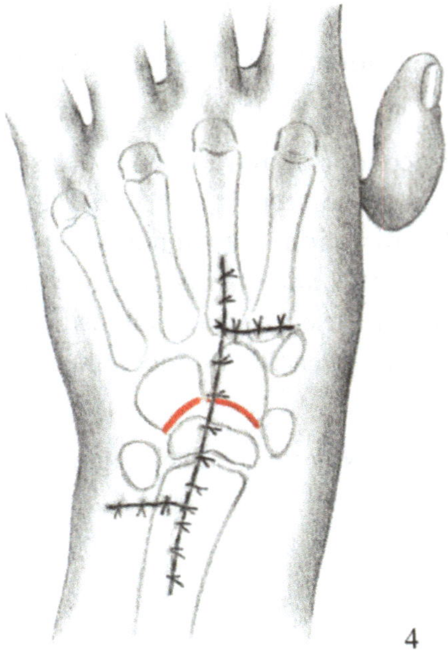

4

13.3 Recurrent Club Hand

Goal of Surgery

Correction of the malposition by wedge osteotomy of the distal ulna.

Figs. 1, 2 Preoperative appearance, dorsal and lateral aspects.
Condition after club hand correction and pollicization. The wrist joint is deviated in a palmar and radial direction. Damaging the epiphyseal plate has to be avoided during the wedge osteotomy (*hatched area*). The wedge is taken from the metaphysis. It may be advantageous to use an image intensifier for selection of the osteotomy site. Skin incision is made over the ulnodorsal aspect.

Figs. 3, 4 Postoperative appearance.
Slight overcorrection by osteotomy. The fragments are immobilized with crossed Kirschner wires.

Postoperative Care

Long-arm plaster cast with inclusion of the MP joints for 4–6 weeks. Removal of the Kirschner wires after bony union of the osteotomy site. Then, short-arm cast for another 4–6 weeks, followed by night splint protection.

Remarks

In cases of more pronounced wrist joint instability, correction can also be carried out in the carpus. The space between the distal ulna and the carpus is exposed, scar tissue is removed, and additional portions of carpal bones are excised. In this manner one obtains more space for the necessary correction. The tendon of m. ext. carpi uln. may require further shortening, or its insertion may have to be transposed onto the ulnar side of the base of the Vth metacarpal. For this the skin incision will have to be lengthened distally.

Errors and Their Consequences

E. Radical circumcision of the distal ulna or exposure of the wrong joint (see Sect. 13.2.1).
C. Impairment of the distal ulnar epiphyseal plate.
For further errors, see the text above.

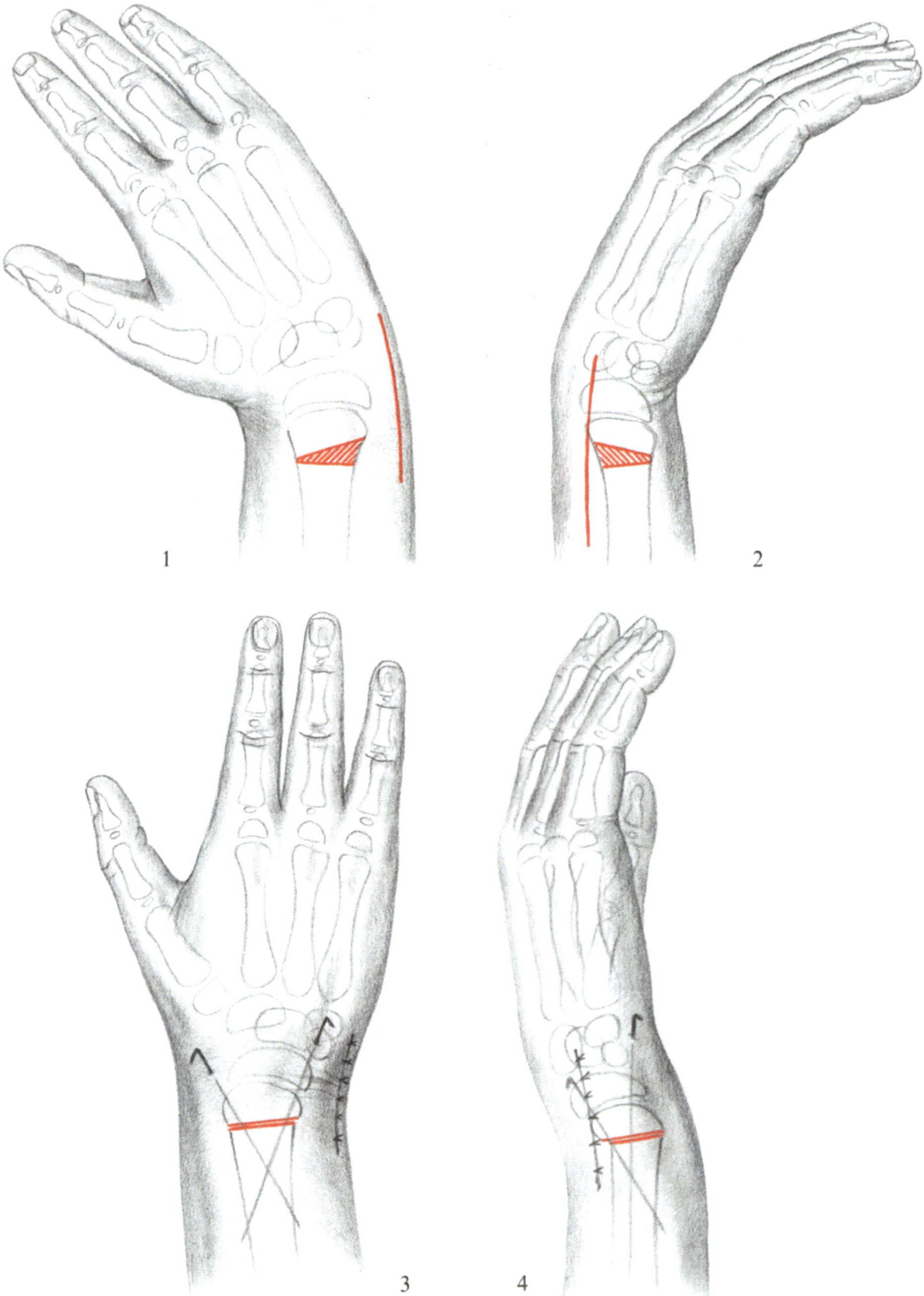

1 2 3 4

Goal of Surgery

Correction of the supination deformity by rotation osteotomy.

Fig. 1 Preoperative appearance and incision, palmar aspect.
An extensive radioulnar synostosis with fixation of forearm and hand in supination is present.
The skin incision *(red single line)* is made over the radial aspect; the osteotomy *(red double line)* is carried out in the middle third of the forearm.

Fig. 2 The synostosis has been exposed at the osteotomy site. It is approached by dissection in the interval of the border of the flexor and extensor musculature. Tendon insertions (pronator teres) are mobilized subperiosteally. A Kirschner wire is inserted proximal and distal to the osteotomy site, which has been exposed subperiosteally. The position of the wires corresponds with the necessary degree of derotation. Osteotomy is followed by pronation of the distal fragment. Correct position is obtained when the Kirschner wires are parallel to each other. This step requires sufficient freeing of the periosteum at its ulnar site.

Fig. 3 Appearance after rotation of the distal fragment.
The Kirschner wires are parallel. The hand is slightly pronated in optimal position of function. The osteotomy site is secured with crossed Kirschner wires (see Fig. 4).
Wound closure.

Fig. 4 Diagram of the position of the Kirschner wires.

Remarks: Osteosynthesis with a well-fitting compression plate is possible if the fragments are properly prepared.

Postoperative Care

Long-arm plaster cast for 4–6 weeks if Kirschner wires have been used. At that time, removal of wires and introduction of active exercises. The osteotomy site should be protected by a removable plaster splint for another 3–4 weeks. Active exercises may be started when postoperative pain has subsided if one uses compression plate fixation. The arm should be protected with a removable plaster splint during this period. Its use may be discontinued when radiologic evidence of bony union is present.

Errors and Their Consequences

E. Careless exposure. *C.* Vessels and nerves can be damaged.
E. Insufficient adaptation of the osteotomy surfaces. *C.* Delayed bony union.

E. The Kirschner wires have not been cut subcutaneously.
C. Skin necrosis, danger of infection.

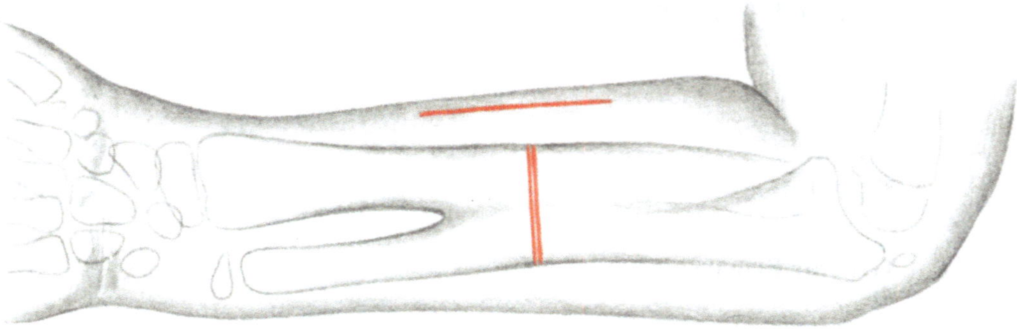

1

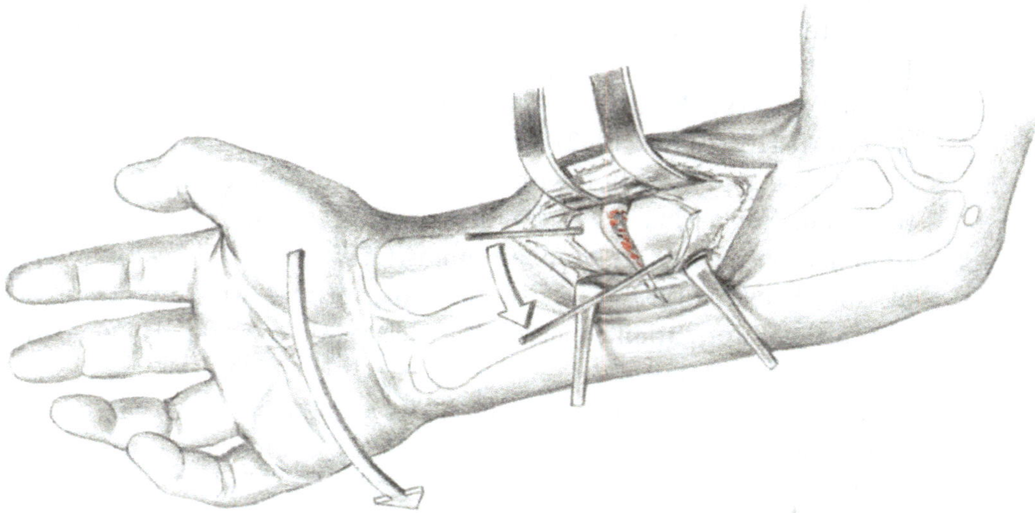

2

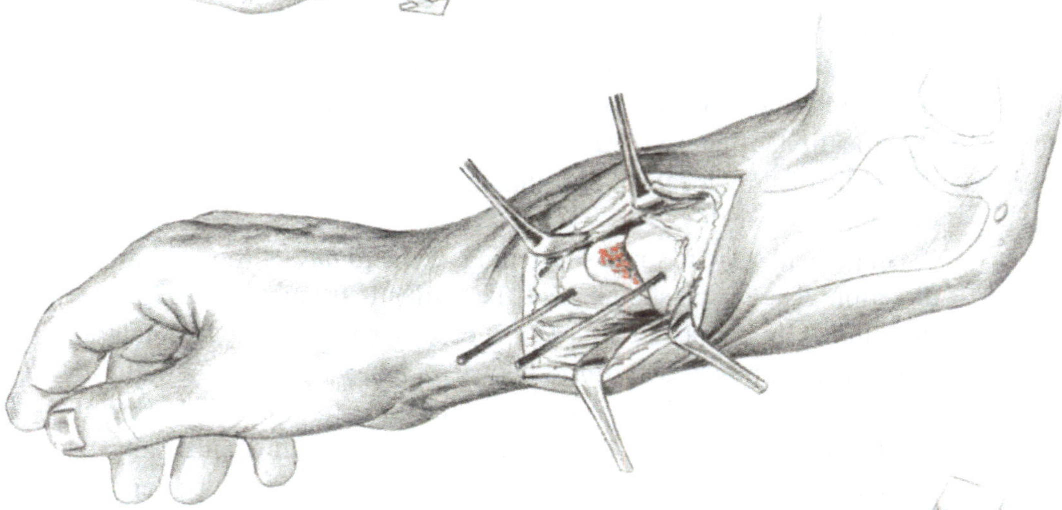

3

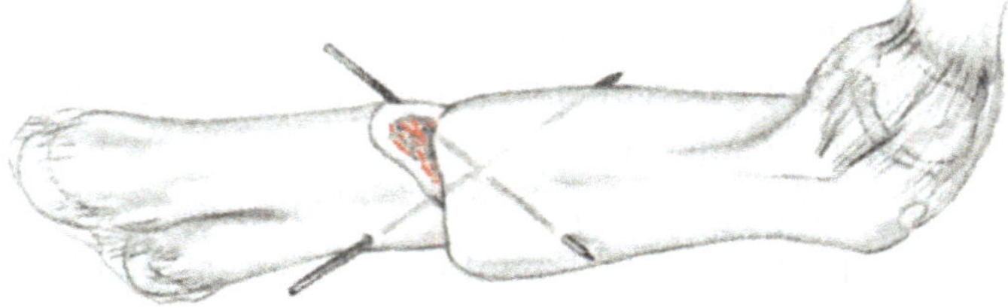

4

14 Hypoplasias and Aplasias of the Ulna (Ulnar Club Hand)

14.1 Introduction

14.1.1 General Remarks

Ulnar dysplasias (synonyms: ulnar ray defect, ulnar club hand) are the result of an *inhibitory malformation that mainly affects the ulnar parts of the upper limb.* They are much less common than radial ray defects (Chap. 13). Usually one limb only is deformed. Sporadic appearance is well-known, heredity has been considered in some cases (see KELIKIAN 1974). Preponderance of the male sex has been suggested (REIMANN-HUNZICKER 1942).

A striking combination with dysplasias of the femur and fibula has been noted, the femur-fibula-ulna (FFU) syndrome (KÜHNE et al. 1967; BLAUTH 1967). Other combination defects are double thumbs (KÜMMEL 1895; KAJON 1921) and aplasia of the tibia (KE 1937; see also the experimental study by DEGENHARDT 1967). For further information concerning associated defects and also ulnar-fibular dysplasia, see KELIKIAN (1974).

Typical for an ulnar ray defect is *shortening of the forearm,* often with *bowing in a dorsoradial direction.* The hand deviates in an ulnar direction (manus valga, ulnar club hand). The deviation is caused partly by the bowing, partly by the insufficient or absent buttressing on its ulnar aspect.

Teratologic staging seems to be present, encompassing hypoplasias, partial aplasias, and total aplasias (see, among others, BONOLA and MORELLI 1972; other classification attempts: PINGEL and ROMPE 1971). In partial aplasias the defect is usually distally located. The ulna may be replaced by a strand of tight connective tissue.

In general there is some shortening of the *radius.* It too is bowed in a dorsoradial direction. The dysplastic head of the radius is frequently *displaced,* especially when the ulna is hypoplastic. In such a case it can be palpated lateral to the lateral humeral epicondyle. *Synostoses* between humerus and the hypoplastic radius, either in a position of flexion or of extension, are likewise well-known; radiologically it may be impossible to distinguish between humeral and radial elements. Cases of bizarre *bifurcation of the distal humerus* have been reported. They seem to be the result of a synostosis between humerus and ulna. Longitudinal growth of the *humerus* is frequently impaired too, particularly in the presence of more severe types of ulnar dysplasia.

Hypo- and aplasias of ulnar ray *carpal bones* are common (os triquetrum, os pisiforme, os hamatum, and occasionally os capitatum). Synostoses of extant carpal bones, (in addition and simultaneously), have been described.

Aplasia of the ulnar digits (oligodactyly) is nearly always observed. The ring and little fingers are most frequently missing, absence of the Vth ray alone is rare. Concomitant differentiation anomalies of the radial border ray may be present, i.e., thumb hypoplasia with partial syndactyly. Also fully developed fingers are sometimes misshapen; cutaneous and osseous syndactylies, spoon hands, brachydactylies, joint aplasias, finger duplications, camptodactylies and other anomalies have been reported. In extreme cases of ray reduction only *one* tri- or biphalangeal finger may be present (monodactyly).

Soft tissue anomalies, especially of the ulnar part, are found in addition to the bony changes. The literature (see WIERZEJEWSKI 1910) contains reports of aplasias and insertion anomalies of m. triceps, m. biceps, and the ulnar wrist joint flexors and extensors, as well as aplasias of m. palmaris longus, m. extensor digiti quinti, m. supinator, and m. anconeus. The ulnar nerve and artery are frequently missing or take an abnormal course.

14.1.2 Indications for Surgery

Functional disability is quite severe in most cases of ulnar dysplasia. Surgery on the other hand is indicated only if marked improvement of function may be expected.

Surgery may be considered in the presence of the following deformities:

– *Aplasias of the elbow joint* with the joint in extension or hyperextension or in marked flexion. The most satisfactory position of function is an angle of about 90°, (depending on the amount of shortening of the forearm). It can be obtained with an angulation osteotomy.

– *Radial head dislocations* may result in marked limitation of motion or malposition. The protruding head can be a source of local irritation. Therapeutically it may be necessary to resect the radial head.

– *Shortening of the ulna and bowing of the radius* with ulnar deviation of the hand require surgery if the axial deviation results in markedly impaired function and if neutral position of the hand may be obtained by corrective osteotomy of the radius, or if by an (additional) lengthening osteotomy of the ulna buttressing of the hand can be improved, or by a radius-pro-ulna operation (see BONOLA and MORELLI 1972; KELIKIAN 1974). A derotation osteotomy may be required in cases of fixed supination of the forearm.

– *Malformations of the hand* if marked functional improvement can be expected by correction of partial finger duplications or of syndactylies, or by creation of a post in cases of monodactyly, if a metacarpus is present (see also Chaps. 2, 4, 8.7).

14.1.3 Timing of Surgery

The optimal time for surgical intervention depends partially on the number of operations needed to create a functional hand. Patients with bilateral involvement (especially those with pronounced manus valga) require surgical measures at an earlier age.

Soft tissue surgery, such as finger separations, may be considered during the 2nd and 3rd years of life (see Chap. 2). Axial corrections should be performed during preschool age. All other operations should be postponed until the second decade of life. This prevents pronounced postoperative growth disturbances and permits better evaluation of possible adaptive mechanisms and of success attainable by surgery. Early resection of the radial head diminishes longitudinal growth.

Prostheses should be considered in more severe cases.

14.1.4 General Surgical Directives

Surgery of the *elbow region,* e.g., *angulation osteotomies* or *radial head resections,* carries a high risk of damage to important nerves (above all the n. radialis) and blood vessels. Incisions and exposures have to be carefully planned. Osteosyntheses between humerus and radius require Kirschner wire or ventral tension band fixation. We do not show figures of such operations as we have little personal long-term experience with them; furthermore, similar operations have been described for trauma patients. *Arthroplasties* of synostotic elbow joints have not been successful. The above-mentioned muscle anomalies (irregular insertions, hypolasias and aplasias of, for example, m. biceps or m. triceps) prevent effective elbow motion. Interposition arthroplasties can result in marked functional instability.

Corrective osteotomies of the shaft of the radius have to be planned with care. We recommend the use of preoperative diagrams to determine the size and proper placement of the wedge osteotomy. Osteosynthesis is carried out with compression plates of proper shape and diameter (see Sects. 14.3, 14.4).

In the presence of only a proximal ulnar portion in combination with a dislocation of the head of the radius and acceptable motion of the elbow joint one may consider a *fusion between radius and ulna* after resection of the proximal radius. This operation will improve stability and position of the forearm.

Hypoplasia of the ulna combined with marked bowing of the radius is best treated with a corrective osteotomy of the radius with a *synchronous lengthening osteotomy of the ulna* (see Sect. 14.2). Treatment of *concomitant finger and hand deformities* is discussed in the pertinent sections.

14.1.5 Postoperative Care

Corrective osteotomies of synostotic elbow joints require a thorax-arm cast for a period of 4–6 weeks if two Kirschner wires had been employed as a (minimal) osteosynthetic device. The wires are removed after x-ray control and the limb immobilized in a long-arm cast for another 3–4 weeks.

Tension band osteosyntheses require a posterior long-arm plaster splint for 4–6 weeks until bony union is clinically and radiologically established.

"Exercise stable" osteosyntheses of the forearm are treated without additional plaster fixation.

14.2 Ulnar Hypoplasia with Bowing of the Radius

Goal of Surgery

Correction of the ulnar deviation of the wrist joint by lengthening osteotomy of the ulna and wedge osteotomy of the radius.

Fig. 1 Preoperative appearance; incision and bone resections are indicated (schema). This is a case of ulnar hypoplasia combined with aplasia of several carpal bones and of the two ulnar finger rays.
Longitudinal skin incision over the ulnar and radial aspects. The ulnar portion of the ulnar diaphysis is osteotomized subperiosteally as outlined. A wedge with a radial base is then removed from the radial shaft. The size and position of the wedge had been determined preoperatively by employing diagrams and x-rays. Osteosynthesis of the radius by means of a self-compressing plate (see *Fig. 2*). The soft tissues between the distal end of the ulna and the proximal carpal row are spread with dissecting scissors and the osteotomized ulnar portion of the ulna advanced as close to the carpus as possible. The ulnar artery and nerve have to be carefully protected during this step. Next, compression osteosynthesis of the ulnar fragments. The proximal defect of the ulnar shaft will be filled with bone chips (partially obtained from the bony wedge of the radius). Wound closure.

Fig. 2 Postoperative appearance.

Postoperative Care

As for all "exercise stable" osteosyntheses.

Errors and Their Consequences

See Chap. 13.

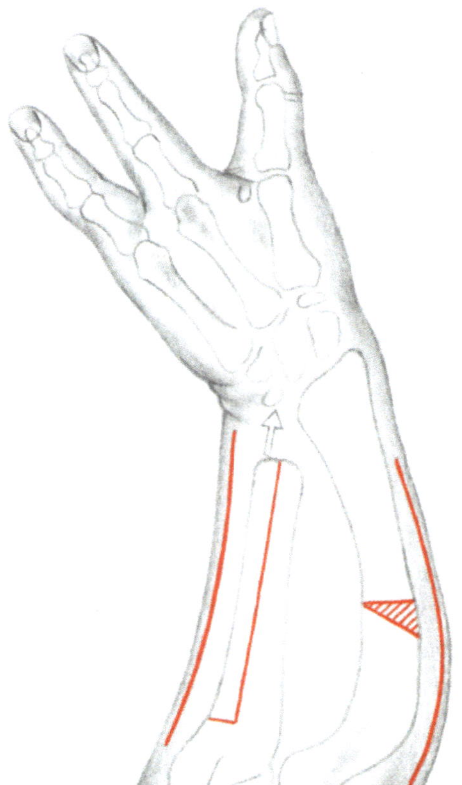

1

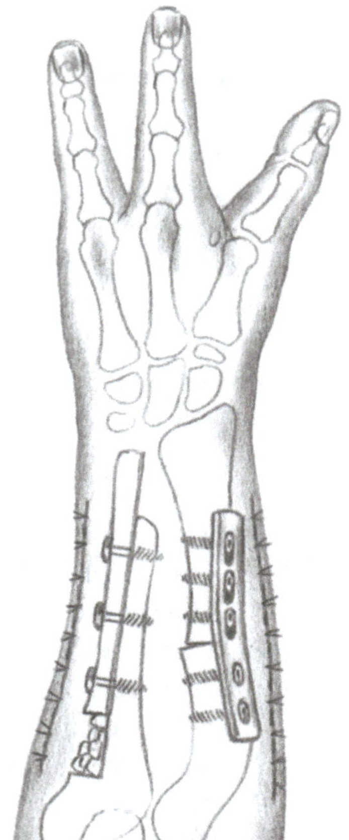

2

15 Hereditary Multiple Exostoses

15.1 Introduction

15.1.1 General Remarks

The cause of hereditary multiple exostoses (synonyms: multiple osteocartilaginous exostoses, multiple osteochondromas, diaphyseal aclasis etc.) is a *congenital developmental differentiation error of bone*. Different opinions exist as to their *pathogenesis* (BETHGE 1963; SOLOMON 1963; COCCHI 1952; WITT et al. 1966; a.o.). The disease is characterized by many exostoses of different sizes and shapes. They originate primarily from the *metaphyseal areas of cartilage preformed bones*. They can be "palpated under the nonadherent skin as firm tumors with an irregular, bossy, or smooth surface" (BETHGE 1963).

Autosomal dominant heredity of this systemic disease has been established (STOCKS and BARRINGTON 1925; a.o.). Relatively less frequent manifestations and frequent latency in females are thought to be the reasons for a much higher incidence of observations in males.

Multiple exostoses are frequently detected in adolescents and adults, but they are present since infancy. They have even been reported in neonates. Multiple exostoses *cease growing with, or in some cases shortly before, puberty*. Involution processes in later life have been described occasionally (SOLOMON 1961; a.o.). Formation of multiple exostoses in adulthood has not been reported.

Multiple exostoses are frequently bilateral and to a certain degree may have symmetrical configurations. They arise as sessile or pedunculated structures from metaphyses. The cortex and spongiosa of the bone continues into the exostosis, which is covered with a cartilaginous cap, the zone of growth. This cap may calcify. Typically, exostoses on the metaphyses with high growth tendencies *point toward the diaphysis*. Tubulation of the epiphysis is retarded (BETHGE 1963; SOLOMON 1961, 1963). The pedicles of exostoses wander from the metaphysis to the diaphysis as the bone matures. *Longitudinal growth* of involved bones is reduced. This is most pronounced in bones with epiphyseal plates of small diameter, i.e., the *fibula and ulna* (SOLOMON 1961). This disseminated decrease in length causes bony deformities. Certain x-ray projections may simulate pictures suggestive of enchondromas (no simultaneous incidences with multiple exostoses!) or solitary bone cysts (BETHGE 1963; SOLOMON 1961). The *histologic* appearance of multiple exostoses has been described by JAFFE (1964), BETHGE (1963), SPJUT et al. (1971), and many others. JAFFE recognized foci of cartilaginous metaplasias in the inner periosteal zone of the exostoses. Blood chemistry is normal.

Multiple exostoses arising from radius, ulna, metacarpals, and phalanges are of importance for the hand surgeon. Secondary *deformities of one or both forearms* are frequently noted (BETHGE found involvement of these structures in 30% of his patients). A preferred site is the *distal ulna,* which is markedly shortened; the radius is bowed in a radial direction and its joint surface is angled toward the ulnar side. The deformity (manus valga) resembles that of an ulnar hypoplasia. Dorsal bayonetlike deformities have also been observed, as have dislocations of the *head of the radius* in a radiodorsal direction.

Extensive growth of the exostoses may result in pressure deformities of the adjacent bone; the bones may be pushed apart, but (distal) radioulnar *synostoses* have also been noted. Pronation and supination of the forearm are frequently limited.

Exostoses involving the tubular bones of the *hand* may result in *growth disturbances* (brachydactyly), *pressure phenomena,* and *crooked growth* (clinodactyly). Multiple exostoses of the phalanges point *toward* the joint and may deform it. They may displace tendons, blood vessels, or nerves. Exostoses localized on the palmar side may act as a source of pain when the patient tries to perform a powerful grip. Other exostoses are more of a cosmetic than a functional problem.

The cartilaginous caps of one or several of the multiple exostoses occasionally have a tendency to develop into a so-called *epiexostotic chondroma.* These chondromas may secondarily turn into chondrosarcomas. Malignant degeneration usually affects only one exostosis, usually located at the hip, pelvis, or shoulder girdle. The figures for *incidence of malignant degeneration* differ, probably due to the small numbers of cases reported in the literature (JAFFE 2%–11%; DAHLIN more than 10%; LICHTENSTEIN less than 1%–2%, but incidence increases with the number of exostoses). LICHTENSTEIN (1972) recommends regular x-ray controls in adults suffering from multiple exostoses.

15.1.2 Indications for Surgery

Due to the multiplicity of exostoses in an individual it is advisable to *observe* them by repeating functional tests and by serial x-rays. This will help in deciding whether surgery is necessary.

Surgery may be indicated if:

- Exostoses exert pressure on blood vessels or nerves or lead to spontaneous rupture of tendons.
- An exostosis of the distal ulna has resulted in a marked shortening of this bone, in a bowing of the radius, in a dislocation of the distal radioulnar joint, or in impaired function due to ulnar deviation of the hand.
- A radioulnar synostosis or a divergence of the forearm bones combined with functional limitation has developed.
- Large exostoses are cosmetically unsightly.

Even relatively small exostoses of the metacarpals and phalanges may require surgical intervention, particularly if growth impairment, compression syndromes, increasing axial deviations, or functional limitations are present.

15.1.3 Timing of Surgery

Multiple exostoses usually become apparent toward the end of the first decade of life or even later. Surgery should be performed only after a sufficient period of observation. The proper time for surgical intervention will depend on growth tendencies, the amount of functional impairment, and cosmetic factors. The number of multiple exostoses that may require surgical correction may also influence its timing.

15.1.4 General Surgical Directives

While exposing exostoses one should keep in mind that important anatomic structures may have been displaced from their normal position, e.g., the ulnar artery and nerve at the distal end of the ulna.

Incomplete removal of an exostosis may result in its recurrence. LICHTENSTEIN (1972) considers remaining periosteal caps to be foci for reappearing exostoses. Therefore, it is advisable to *saucerize* the basis of an exostosis (see WITT et al. 1966; H. MAU and SIGUDA 1974). Extensive excisions carry the risk of postoperative *fractures* as well as impairment of the growth plate. *Segmental resections* may be indicated if the exostosis involves a large portion of the meta- or diaphysis.

More pronounced bowing of the radius is best treated with a diaphyseal *corrective osteotomy* combined with a *lengthening osteotomy* of the ulna (BLAUTH 1972). Prerequisites are preoperative (x-ray) diagrams. Fixation plates of proper diameter guarantee stable osteosynthesis. Soft tissue tightness between the distal ulna and the carpus may create technical difficulties. Rigid strands of connective tissue will have to be transected for axial alignment. The shortened ulna can be lengthened by a bony Z-plasty, straightened, and its distal end brought into close proximity with the carpus (Sect. 15.4). In cases where the distal ulnar epiphyseal plate is closed, we recommend excision of the distal ulna and bridging of the defect with an autologous bone graft (Sect. 15.3). A second lengthening operation will become necessary at a later date if the progression of the deformity requires surgery prior to the end of puberty. Patients with exostoses require periodic follow-up examination until they have reached full bony maturity.

Similar surgical directives pertain to operations involving *metacarpals and phalanges*. Of special interest are exostoses *growing intra-articularly and* their tendency to deform the joint. The resulting crookedness is more a problem of cosmesis than of limited function. A *wedge osteotomy* in cases of clinodactyly performed prior to cessation of bone growth gives only temporary improvement. Total removal of the exostosis may be possible only after opening the joint and partial resection of a joint surface, resulting in *instability* and axial malposition. Partial joint rigidity may occur. We experienced these complications in a 12-year-old female patient who required a second operation at a later date. We inserted a small, properly shaped corticospongiotic graft into the joint defect, but mobility remained impaired.

15.1.5 Postoperative Care

Stable osteosyntheses of the forearm without lengthening or bridging procedures require a posterior long-arm plaster splint for 3–4 weeks. If lengthening osteotomies or bony bridging of defects are indicated one has to apply a circular long-arm cast for 6–8 weeks before bone healing is sufficient. Postoperative care has to be adjusted according to the individual case. This includes the use of night and exercise splints.

15.2 Exostosis of a Phalanx

Goal of Surgery

Removal of the exostosis.

Figs. 1, 2 Preoperative appearance, dorsal and radial aspects.
Large exostosis arising from a middle phalanx and "involving" the epiphyseal plate, but without axis deformity.
Lateral skin incision in a steplike manner. A curvilinear incision could be employed.

Fig. 3 Periosteum and the insertions of the collateral ligament have been incised and mobilized in a double-T fashion. The exostosis will be removed with an osteotome. Due to epiphyseal involvement it is necessary to open the joint and to remove the epiphyseal component of the exostosis.

Fig. 4 The exostosis has been removed and the normal contour of the phalanx has been reconstituted. The opened joint is visible.

Fig. 5 Appearance during closure.
The periosteum is closed with interrupted sutures over the smoothed resection surface. The collateral ligament has been sutured to the periosteumm.

Postoperative Care

Immobilization with a finger plaster splint in position of function for 3 weeks. Next, graduated active physiotherapy, which may require continuing effort and persistence from the patient and the physio- or occupational therapist. The use of a dynamic splint may become necessary.
Follow-up examination at intervals of 6 months to observe epiphyseal growth. Corrective osteotomies may have to be considered if axial deviation develops due to epiphyseal impairment.

Errors and Their Consequences

E. The tension on the incised collateral ligament was insufficient during its resuture to the periosteum, postoperative immobilization was too short.
C. Instability of the joint.

– See also Sect. 15.1.4.

Remarks

Careful preoperative evaluation of each individual case will determine if total removal of an exostosis with possible damage of the epiphyseal plate will result in less deformity than its incomplete removal with the probability of a second exostosectomy near the end of the period of bone growth.

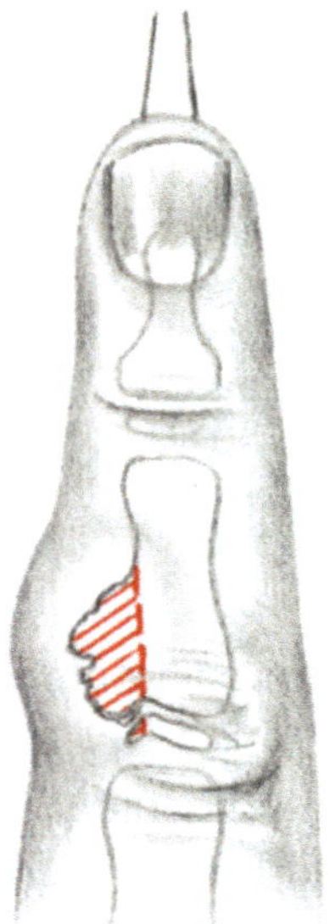

1

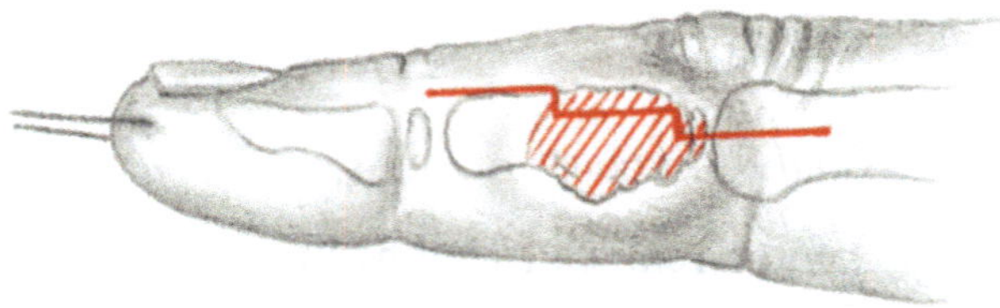

2

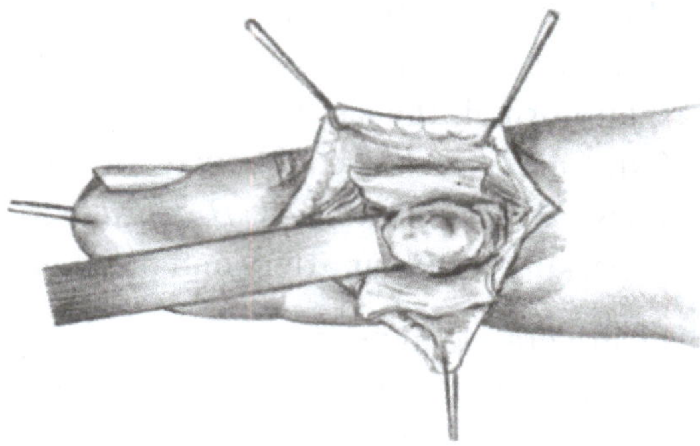

3

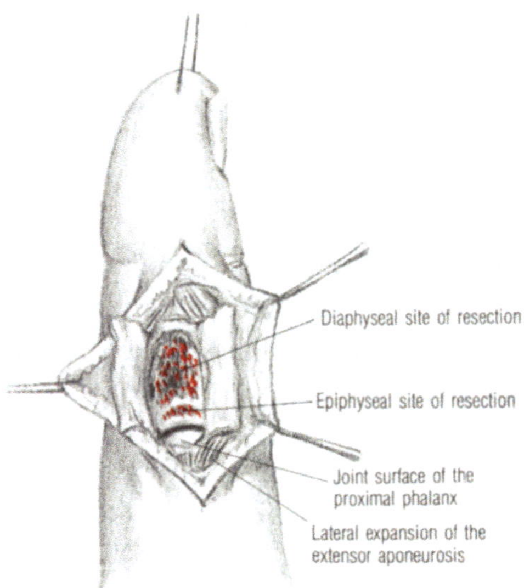
Diaphyseal site of resection
Epiphyseal site of resection
Joint surface of the proximal phalanx
Lateral expansion of the extensor aponeurosis

4

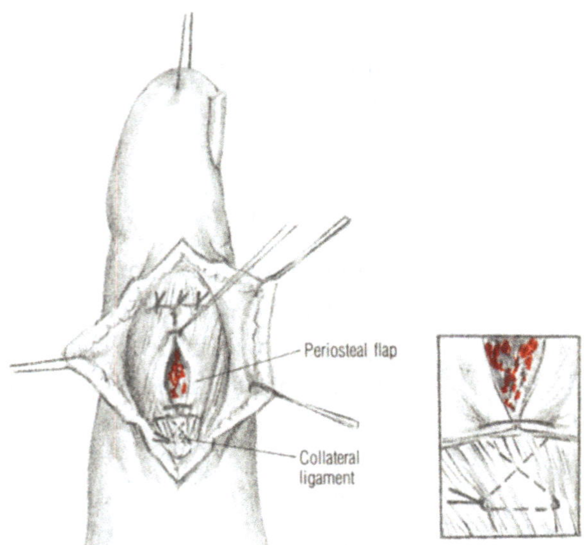
Periosteal flap
Collateral ligament

5

15.3 Manus Vara and Bowing of the Radius Caused by an Exostosis of the Distal Ulnar Epiphysis

Goal of Surgery

Tumor removal, lengthening osteotomy of the remaining ulna, and correction of the deformed radius.

Fig. 1 Preoperative appearance and incision, dorsal aspect.
The exostosis involves the entire epiphysis of the distal ulna. The ulna is shorter than normal, the shaft of the radius is bowed radially.
Exposure is achieved by way of longitudinal incisions at the radial and ulnar sides (*unbroken red lines*). *Hatched areas* of the exostosis and bone require removal. Especially the ulnar artery and nerve have to be carefully protected during dissection.

Fig. 2 Postoperative appearance.
The radius deformity has been corrected by a wedge resection after subperiosteal exposure of the ulna and distal radius. The latter has been stabilized with a compression plate. The ulna has been lengthened by a Z-plasty (see Fig. 1), and its fragments secured with three spongiosa screws. The remaining defects have been filled with autologous spongiosa chips. The ulna has been attached to the radius by means of a periosteofascial sling, the material for which has been obtained from adjacent tissues.

Postoperative Care

Immobilization in a long-arm cast for 6 weeks in medium pronation. Graduated physiotherapy after bony union of the osteotomy site and incorporation of the spongiosa chips. Immobilization is still required during physiotherapy-free periods. A plaster splint is used at night for at least another 3 months.

Errors and Their Consequences

E. Insufficient lenghtening of the ulna.
C. Recurrence of malposition.

E. Stabilization and postoperative immobilization is insufficient.
C. Marked tendency for malalignment.

E. Radial and ulnar nerves and blood vessels have been damaged.
C. Neurologic and circulatory deficits.

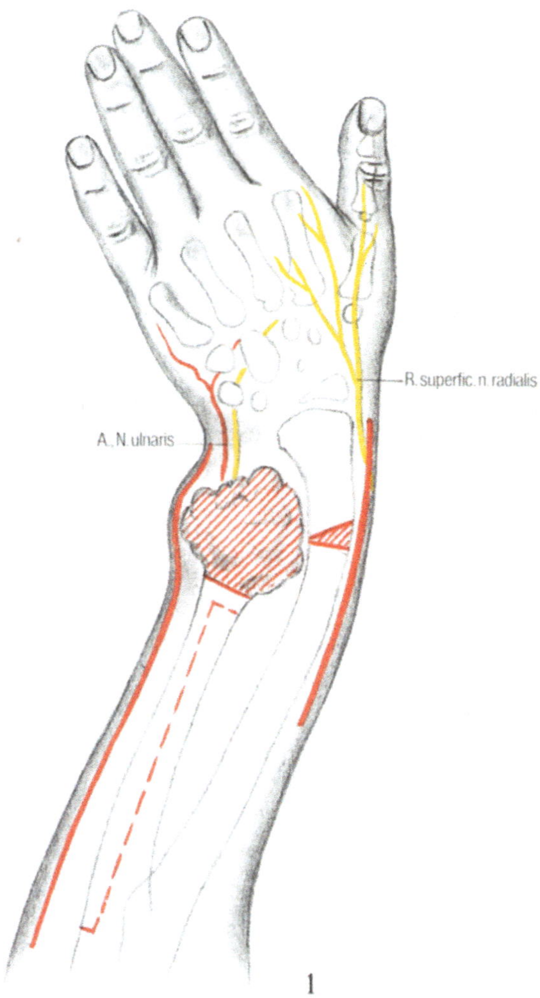

1

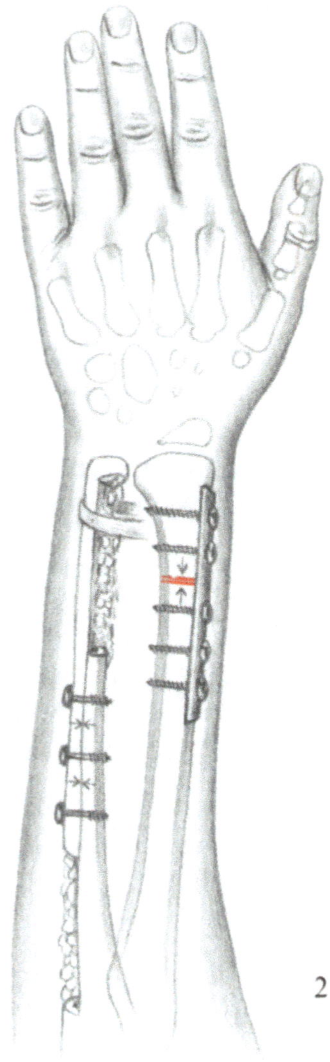

2

Remarks

Regular follow-up examinations are required until bone growth ceases. Recurrent deviation caused by loss of ulnar development has to be expected in younger patients; this makes a second operation highly probable.

Second Operation

Fig. 3 Preoperative appearance 2 yers after the first operation.
Cessation of ulnar growth requires another lengthening operation by employing an iliac crest graft. Skin incision at the ulnar side. The ulnar nerve and artery have to be carefully protected during dissection (see *Fig. 4*). The distal ulna is shaped as outlined (*hatched area*). Fatty and connective tissue has to be partially excised distally to the proximal carpal row.

Fig. 4 Ulnar aspect.
The distal ulna has been properly shaped; one end of the bone graft has been hollowed out in a cylindrical fashion. The soft tissues proximal to the carpal bones are spread with dissecting scissors to permit positioning of the bone graft as far distal as possible. Additional fixation is unnecessary if the graft fits tightly onto the ulna. Kirschner wires are required for stabilization if the fit is suboptimal.

Fig. 5 Postoperative appearance.
Additional spongiosa chips have been inserted between the graft and the remains of the ulna.

Postoperative Care and Errors and Their Consequences

As described earlier in this section.

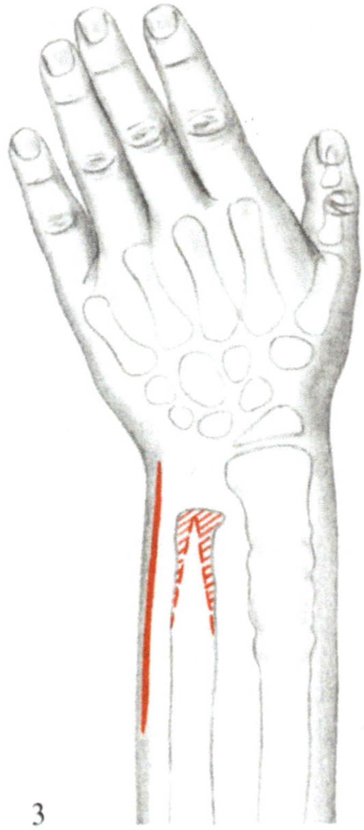

3

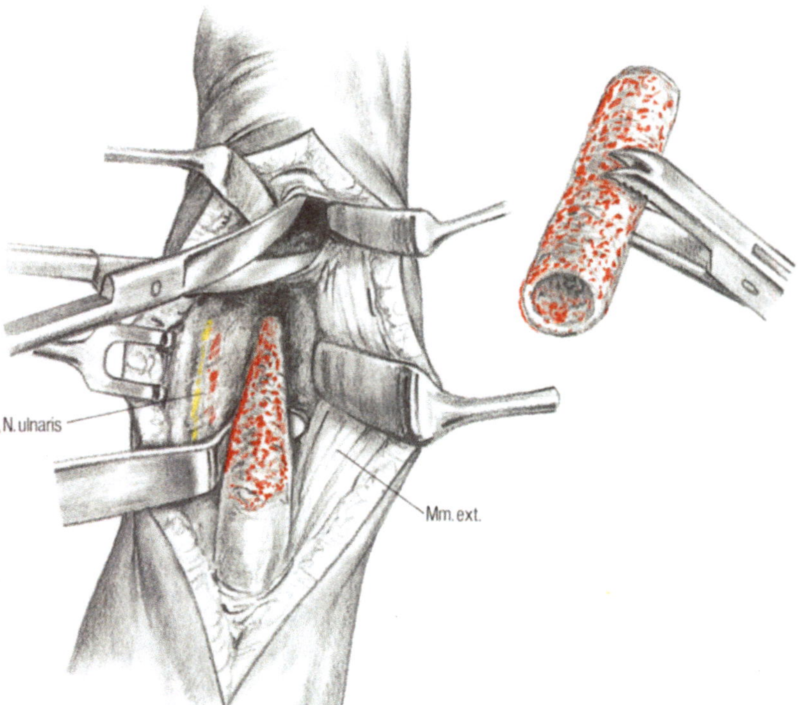

4

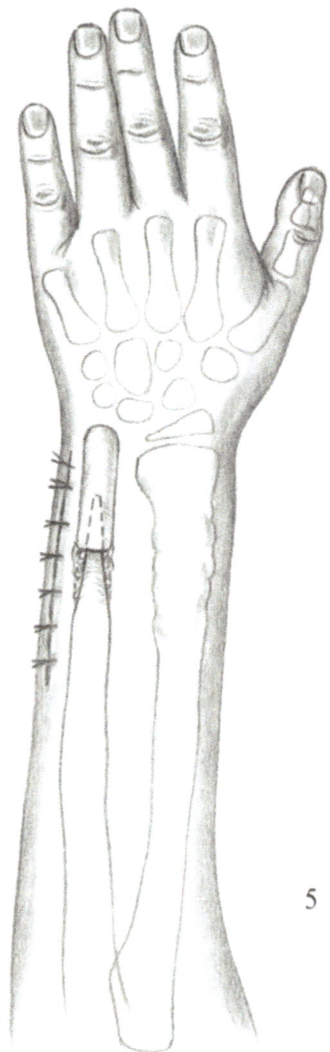

5

15.4 Bowing of the Radius Caused by an Exostosis of the Metadiaphyseal Segment of the Ulna

Goal of Surgery

Removal of the exostosis, lengthening of the ulna, and correction of the bowing of the radius.

Fig. 1 Preoperative appearance and incision, dorsal aspect.
The exostosis has caused a decrease in length of the ulna and, secondarily, a bowing of the radius.
Exposure of radius and ulna as outlined in Sect. 15.3.

Fig. 2 Postoperative appearance.
The corrective osteotomy of the radius has been stabilized with a compression plate. The exostosis has been removed, the ulna has been lengthened by a Z-plasty. The defect of the distal ulna has been filled with a long spongiosa graft and additional spongiosa chips.

Postoperative Care and Errors and Their Consequences

See Sect. 15.2.

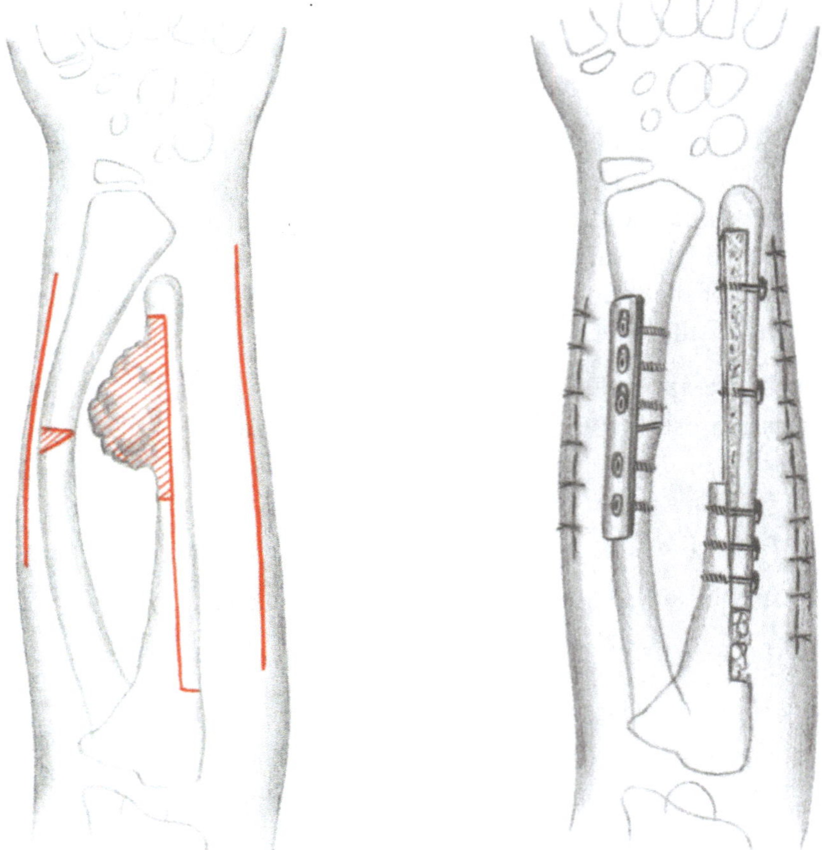

1 2

15.5 Radius Shaft Exostosis (with Relative Overgrowth of the Ulna)

Goal of Surgery

Removal of the exostosis and shortening osteotomy of the ulna.

Fig. 1 Preoperative appearance and incision, dorsal aspect.
Skin incisions as described previously (see Sect. 15.4); the superficial branch of the radial nerve and the radial artery has to be protected.
Subperiosteal removal of the dorsoulnar located tumor, superficial saucerization of the shaft of the radius at the site of the exostosis. This is followed by a shortening osteotomy of the ulna.

Fig. 2 Postoperative appearance.
Compression osteosynthesis of the shortened ulna.

Postoperative Care

Short-arm plaster cast until the incisions have healed.

Errors and Their Consequences

See Sect. 15.2.

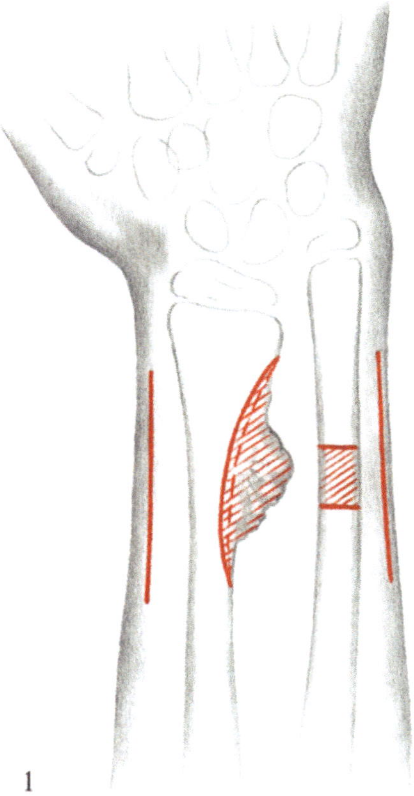

1

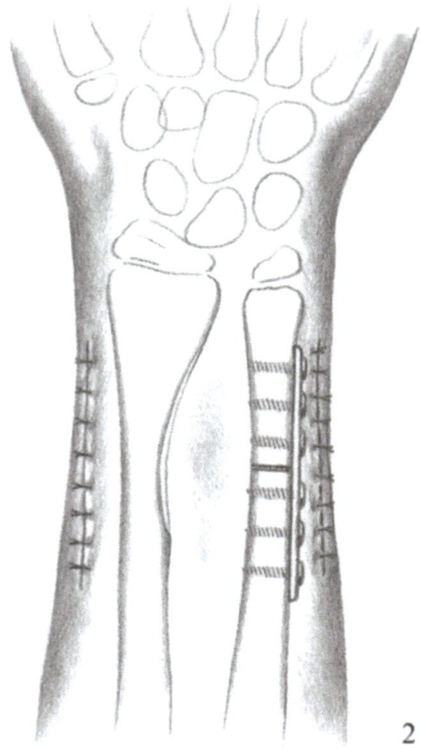

2

16 Enchondromatosis

16.1 Introduction

16.1.1 General Remarks

Nowadays these multiple, polyostotic cartilaginous tumors are considered to be *hamartomas*.

Opinions still differ on certain aspects of their *etiology* and *pathogenesis* (see LANGENSKIÖLD 1947; BETHGE 1962; SPRANGER et al. 1974; WITT et al. 1966; a.o.). Frequently used synonyms are: chondromatosis of bones, skeletal enchondromatosis, and chondromatous dysplasia; also used are: osteochondromatosis, growth disturbance of Ollier, Ollier disease, dyschondroplasia, and chondromatosis. We also refer the reader to JAFFE's critical remarks concerning terminology (1961).

Heredity of this condition has not yet been proven. In spite of numerous common factors in regard to localization, histology, therapy, and prognosis, pathogenesis is considered to be different for *multiple* and *solitary chondromas*. Some authors suggest close relationships to the multiple hereditary exostoses, while others oppose this point of view. Different opinions are also held in regard to their simultaneous occurrence.

It is generally accepted that enchondromas develop from scattered cartilaginous islands (HELLNER 1950; GESCHICKTER and COPELAND 1936) that originate from growing epiphyseal cartilage (BETHGE 1962; LANGENSKIÖLD 1947; a.o.) or also from perichondrium and articular cartilage (SPEISER 1925). During growth these islands come to rest in the diaphysis and do not ossify. Disturbance of blood flow in metaphyseal vessels has been discussed as a causative agent (BETHGE 1962). This theory, based on experiments by TRUETA (1957), is supported by the shape of some cartilaginous foci, which are elongated and correspond with the area of supply of metaphyseal vessels, and by the fact that the tumors develop only during the period of enchondral bone growth. The close proximity of enchondromas and the growth plates also supports their pathogenetic relevance.

A *classification* of enchondromatosis has been attempted on clinical grounds due to relatively frequent types of involvement (see S. WEIL 1957; COCCHI 1952; a.o.). Of interest are the type of *widespread dissemination* involving all skeletal regions, and the *acro-type*, involving hands and feet only. Nowadays many authors doubt that it is possible to classify the *hemi-type* (Ollier disease) as a separate entity (GÄDE 1938; CHRYSOSPATHES 1929; BETHGE 1962; HELLNER 1950; FRANGENHEIM 1913; HERZOG 1944; EXNER 1950). The *Maffucci-Kast syndrome* represents a different entity. It combines multiple enchondromas with subcutaneous hemangiomas, and x-rays will also reveal multiple phleboliths.

Sites of predilection of enchondromas are the small bones of hands and feet, where they, together with solitary chondromas, account for over 90% of all tumors

(NARAKAS and VERDAN 1970; a.o.). But the long bones, ribs, vertebral bodies, and pelvis are also frequent areas of involvement. Tumors of these parts can result in monstrous deformities that are partially caused by additional growth disturbances.

Multiple enchondromas are painless (TAKIGAWA 1971 a). Therefore the disease is discovered after visible enlargement of bones, joint deviation (particularly at the hand), or pathologic fractures are present. These changes are seldom noted during the first few months of life (CLEVELAND and FIELDING 1959; TAKIGAWA 1971 a). Most cases are discovered during infancy; patients with lesser involvement may not be diagnosed until they have reached adulthood.

Histologically the semihard grayish-white tumor tissue consists of hyaline cartilage with typical chondrocytes embedded in a homogenous ground substance (BETHGE 1962). It has been reported that the number of cells, particularly in older individuals, is larger when compared to solitary chondromas, and double nuclei are more frequently found (SPJUT et al. 1971).

On *x-rays* the enchondromas appear as longitudinal or ovoid, striated or cylindrical, sharply demarcated radiolucencies. They are located centrally or excentrically. Most enchondromas are found in the metaphyseal area.

During the period of bone growth the foci move away from the epiphyseal plate toward the cortex and diaphysis and can completely lose their connection with the area of growth (LANGENSKIÖLD 1947). The cortex of the meta- and diaphysis is frequently expanded. Pressure may result in thinning and perforation of the cortex. Additional tumor growth causes bulbous excrescences that can result in bizarre malformations of the hand combined with deformities of the adjacent structures. Bone spurs form at the diaphyseal border of the perforated cortex. Contrary to the spurs seen in multiple hereditary exostoses they point *toward the epiphysis,* not toward the diaphysis. Affected bones may be shortened and malformed. *Spontaneous fractures* resulting from pressure osteolysis are not uncommon.

Opinions differ in regard to further increase in size of enchondromas after puberty. Consensus exists that new foci do not appear after bone growth has ended (SPRANGER et al. 1974; SHARRARD 1971). *Malignant degeneration* has to be suspected if single tumors show an increase in size during adulthood. This is more frequently observed in tumors of the long bones. A higher incidence of malignant degeneration has to be expected in patients suffering from Maffucci-Kast syndrome (LEWIS et al. 1973: 15%; personal observation). Calcifications, ossifications, and myxomatous changes in the enchondromas are evidence of regressive processes.

The *bones of the hand* most frequently affected by enchondromas are the proximal phalanges and the metacarpals; the distal phalanges are less frequently involved (TAKIGAWA 1971 a). Enchondromas of carpal bones have been reported sporadically (NARAKAS and VERDAN 1970; TAKIGAWA 1971 b). Tumors are usually localized in the diaphyseal third next to the epiphysis. Their proximity to a joint may result in limitation of motion. Cortical expansions and bulbous excrescences of the fingers can create marked cosmetic impairment (BLAUTH and HIPPE 1973). For clinicotherapeutic reasons, TAKIGAWA (1971 a) divides the enchondromas of the short bones of the finger into *five forms.* He classifies them as central, excentric, joint juxtaposed, polycentric, and giant-sized.

Involvement of the forearm shows shortening of the ulna and a radially convex curvature of the radius with proximal dislocation of the radial head. This may result in a bayonet-type ulnar-palmar displacement of the hand, similar to the changes seen in patients with multiple hereditary exostoses. This deformity causes limitation of rotatory movements of the forearm and of motion of the wrist joint.

16.1.2 Indications for Surgery

The primary goal is the removal of *all enchondromas*. The possibility of malignant degeneration is small but always present. Due to the multiplicity of the cartilaginous tumors it is frequently impractical to attain this goal. Indications for surgery in individual cases will therefore depend on the *size* and *localization* of the tumors and the *loss of function* caused by them. Resection of *rapidly enlarging* tumors is of utmost importance and priority, particularly if they have penetrated the cortex or if compression phenomena or spontaneous fractures are judged to be imminent. Cosmetic considerations may influence the decision to operate if grotesque deformities are present.

16.1.3 Timing of Surgery

Most enchondromas are localized adjacent to the epiphysis; all such tumors should be excised close to the end of the period of bone growth. At that time only is it possible to perform a radical resection without risk of damaging the growth plate. In exceptional cases an experienced surgeon may want to operate prior to this time, i.e., if he is dealing with very large, quickly growing, or markedly deforming tumors. These interventions require extreme caution (surgical telescopes!). It is expedient to excise tumor tissue incompletely if it is difficult to find a line of demarcation between the tumor and the epiphyseal plate. A tumor recurrence can always be removed by a second operation.

The less frequently seen tumors located in the diaphysis should be excised during preschool or school age.

16.1.4 General Surgical Directives

Preoperatively it is not always possible to determine what type of surgical intervention will have to be employed.

In general one should perform the least extensive operation that still guarantees safe and complete removal of the tumor, as a long period of postoperative immobilization may impair joint mobility permanently.

The following surgical possibilities should be considered:

a) *Curettage through a window in the cortex* (Sect. 16.3).

This method is adequate in cases of slight involvement in the presence of a generally intact cortex. Depending on the location and size of the tumor, dorsoulnar, dorsoradial, curved, or s-shaped incisions will have to be employed. Tumors of the long fingers are best approached by incisions on their ulnar aspect. All these incisions allow satisfactory exposure of the fine structures of the extensor apparatus, which can be displaced by the expansion of the cortex. In the rare cases of enchondromas tending to grow in a palmar direction, one can be sure to encounter displacement of vessels and nerves. To allow removal of the tumor the thinned cortex is fenestrated with a narrow osteotome or Luer rongeur. Straight and angled curettes of different sizes are employed after the window in the cortex has been sufficiently enlarged. Some enchondromas have small bubblelike expansions which tend to indent the bone. Removal of these portions requires very fine curettes or small burrs. The fenestration has to be large enough to permit full visibility of the tumor and its total excision. Thorough and frequent irrigation will remove residual particles. The defect should be filled with small pieces of autologous spongiosa.

b) *Local resection and curettage* (Sect. 16.4).

Even larger intra- and extraosseous tumors can frequently be removed by resecting parts of the cortex. In this manner it is possible to extirpate the tumor and to remodel bulbous bony segments. These bones can be stabilized by employing autologous spongiosa (BLAUTH 1972; BLAUTH and HIPPE 1973). If possible bony remnants found within the cartilage mass should be preserved.

c) *Segmental resection and defect bridging with iliac crest bone* (Sect. 16.4, 16.5, 16.6).

Situations resulting in insufficient stability after cortical resection require diaphyseal excision of the phalanx. Such defects have to be bridged with autologous iliac crest grafts (BLAUTH 1971, 1972; BLAUTH and HIPPE 1973). The junction between graft and phalanx should consist of spongiosa to permit quicker bony fusion. Fine Kirschner wires are required to stabilize the graft and the phalangeal remnant. Only for bridging of very short distances is transarticular wire fixation recommended. Some loss of joint function has to be expected in cases of segmental resection, as postoperative immobilization has to be of long duration.

d) Occasionally one has to *fuse a joint* if safe intersegmental fixation cannot be guaranteed (see diagram in Sect. 16.2).

Redundant skin will be present after excision of larger tumors. It should be trimmed prior to wound closure. Reconstructive measures concerning the extensor apparatus are only seldom required, e.g., after rupture of or damage to the dorsal expansion.

16.1.5 Postoperative Care

Postoperative care depends on the type of surgical intervention, particularly in regard to the remaining stability of the involved bone.

In satisfactory bony stability after curettage, postoperative immobilization with a removable finger splint in the position of function is sufficient. It is worn for 2–4 weeks. Between 1 and 2 days postoperatively the patient should remove the splint three to five times daily and exercise the involved finger actively.

Curettage of a metacarpal or proximal phalanx requires additional immobilization of the wrist joint in the splint. This is not necessary if the operation was carried out at the middle or distal phalanx.

After resection of a larger portion of a phalanx, the inherent bony instability requires fixation with a finger splint or plaster cast for 4 weeks postoperatively. The next step will depend on the radiologic evidence concerning stability. Active finger movements should be started as soon as bone healing is adequate.

Segmental resection with bone grafting to replace a dia- or metaphysis requires postoperative immobilization for 5–6 weeks. X-rays indicate whether the Kirschner wires can be removed and whether careful active exercises may be instituted. These patients may require dynamic splints in addition to physio- and occupational therapy to remobilize their finger joint.

Goal of Surgery

Tumor excisions in several stages employing spongiosa as filling material and bone grafts to bridge the bony defects.

Fig. 1 Schematic view of different methods in a single case.

The hand is grotesquely deformed by enchondromas involving metacarpals, all proximal phalanges, and all middle phalanges. Finger movements are limited. The different size of the tumors necessitates different surgical procedures.

- The proximal phalanx of the thumb contains a tumor extending to the cartilaginous joint surface. Surgical intervention must consist of *segmental resection* and *arthrodesis* of the MP joint in 10° flexion.

  Operations not depicted:

  Radiolateral skin incision over the proximal phalanx. Subperiosteal exposure of the tumor with protection of the extensor aponeurosis of m. ext. poll. long. and the ventrolateral vessels and nerves. The tumor is excised through a cortical window. A paper-thin piece of cortex remains distal to the articular cartilage; this necessitates resection of the joint and fusion with a properly prepared autologous iliac crest graft (see Sect. 16.5). Fixation with two thin crossed Kirschner wires. Closure of periosteum and skin, which may need some trimming. Watch out for rotational malalignment!
- The joint-bearing portions of the middle phalanx of the index finger and the proximal phalanx of the middle finger are still intact. The diaphyses are extensively involved. Surgery consists of segmental resection and bridging of the defect with a bone graft (see Sect. 16.4).
- The other metacarpals and phalanges are only partially involved. Removal of the expanded and thinned portions of the diaphyses and careful excochleation of the tumor masses is sufficient. Bony ridges remain and guarantee satisfactory stability. The defects are filled with pieces of spongiosa (see Sect. 16.3, 16.4).

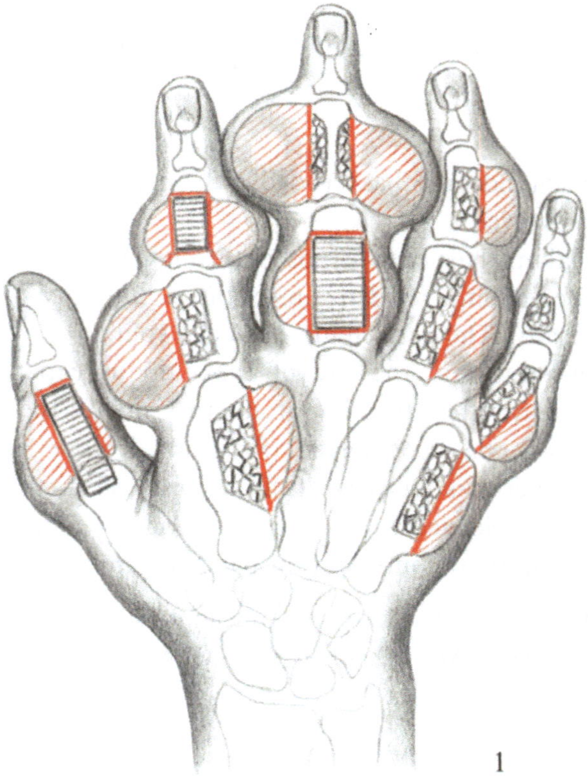

1

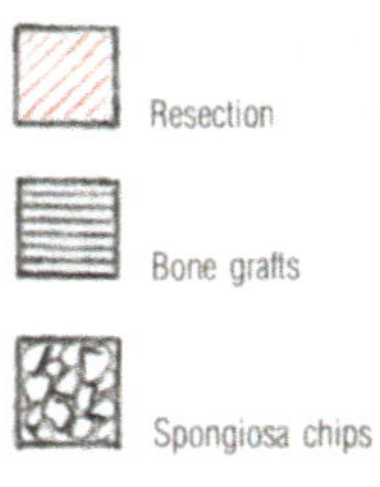

Goal of Surgery

Removal of the tumor and filling of the bone defect with autologous spongiosa pieces.

Fig. 1 The expanding enchondroma has eroded only parts of the cortex; joint-bearing portions are not involved.
The proximal phalanx has been exposed through a dorsoradial skin incision at the tumor site. The tendinous expansions of the m. lumbricalis and the mm. interossei are pulled dorsally. The periosteum has been split.
The cortex is fenestrated at the site of the bulbous expansion, and the tumor mass removed with curettes. It is important to visualize the defect cavity in toto, the entire tumor has to be excochleated. (Surgical telescopes required!) When doubt exists as to a whether this has been fully accomplished, the inner border of the cortex may have to be cleaned with a burr. Expanded paper-thin portions of cortex can be shaped to a normal configuration by slight pressure.

Fig. 2 The bony defect has been packed with autologous pieces of spongiosa (from the olecranon or iliac crest). After this the periosteum and skin are closed.

Postoperative care

A plaster splint in the position of function suffices for postoperative immobilization, if bony stability of the phalanx is sufficient. Fixation is required for 2–3 weeks. In cases of doubtful stability plaster fixation is necessary for 4–6 weeks.

Errors and Their Consequences

E. The tumor is excised without adequate visualization. Tumor tissue at the metaphyseal border is left behind.
C. Tumor recurrence has to be expected.

E. Pieces of tumor tissue adherent to the periosteum have not been completely removed.
C. Tumor recurrence has to be expected.

E. The tumor is larger than it appears on the radiograph.
C. A bone graft may be required from the iliac crest. (Does the operative permit include this part of the operation?)

– Paper-thin portions of the cortex require extremely careful manipulation after extensive excochleations.

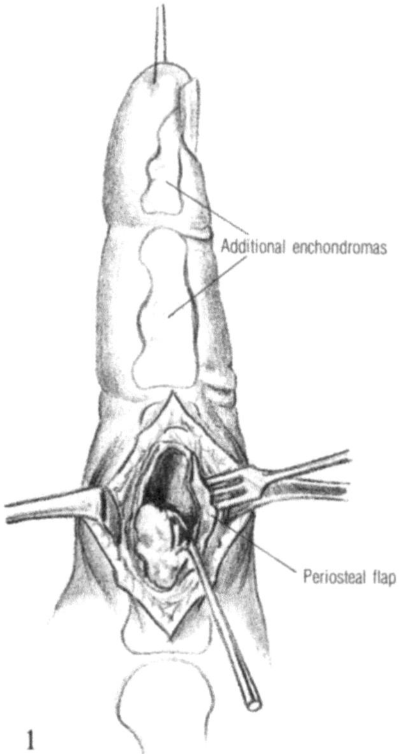
Additional enchondromas
Periosteal flap

1

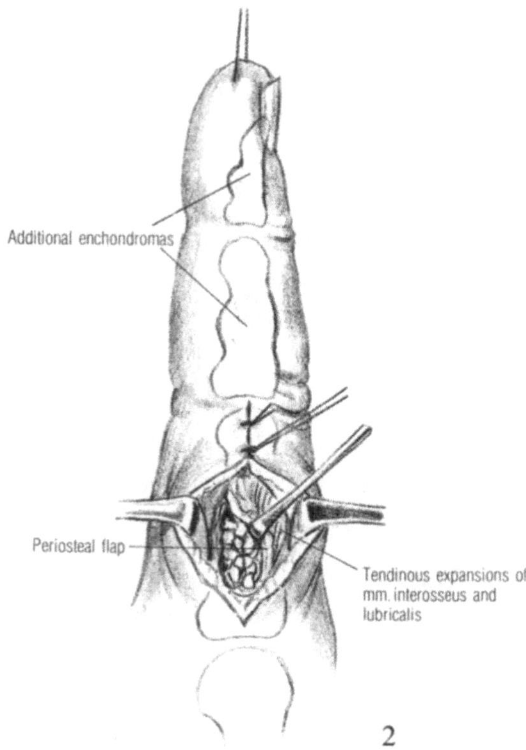
Additional enchondromas
Periosteal flap
Tendinous expansions of
mm. interosseus and
lubricalis

2

16.4 Large Enchondromas of the Proximal and Middle Phalanges (One-Stage Operation)

Goal of Surgery

Excision of tumors, reshaping of two phalanges to normal appearance (segmental resection with bridging bone grafting, partial resection with spongiosa packing).

Fig. 1 Preoperative appearance and incision. Radiodorsal aspect.
Extensive tumors of the proximal and middle phalanges of the index finger, resulting in marked deformity.
The *hatched areas* of skin will be excised at the end of the operation, the *dotted* wound edges will require additional trimming (see *Fig. 6*).

Fig. 2 The areas of tumorous enlargement have been exposed subperiosteally. The extensor aponeurosis and particularly the lateral expansions are carefully retracted.
The cortex over each tumor will be fenestrated. (Area of fenestration of the proximal phalanx is outlined by the *broken line*.)

Fig. 3 The tumor masses are carefully removed with straight and angled curettes, and the projecting and very thin cortical parts are resected using a Luer rongeur. Only with good visualization is complete removal of the usually loculated tumor possible.
The involvement of the middle phalanx is so extensive that stability of the cortex is no longer guaranteed. For this reason it is necessary to resect nearly the entire diaphysis. Its ends are prepared for insertion of a bone graft. The entire periosteum should be retained if at all possible. The area of insertion of the dorsal expansion of the extensor aponeurosis at the basis of the middle phalanx has to be retained.

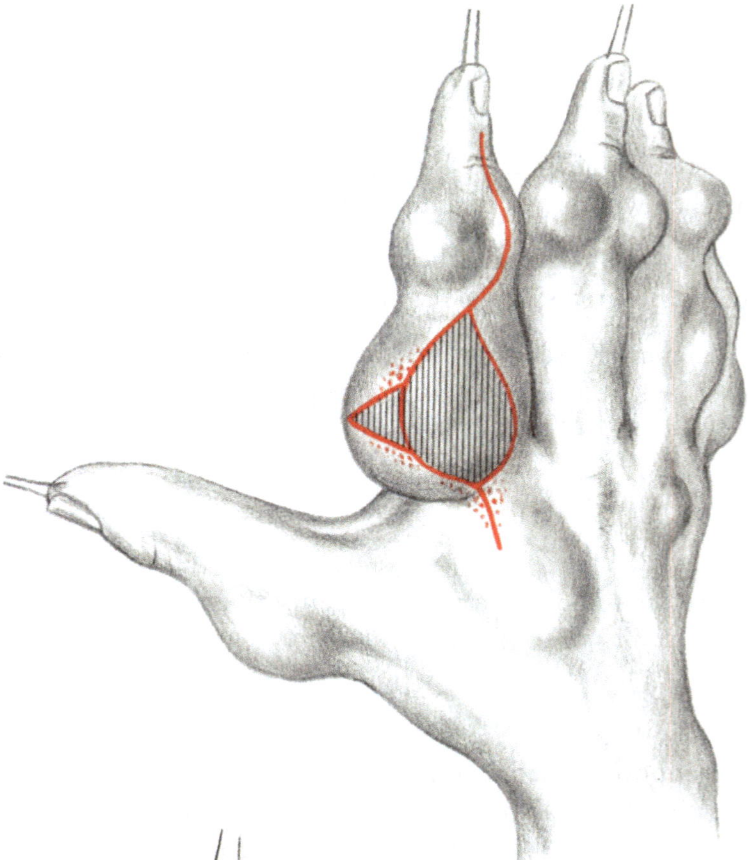

1

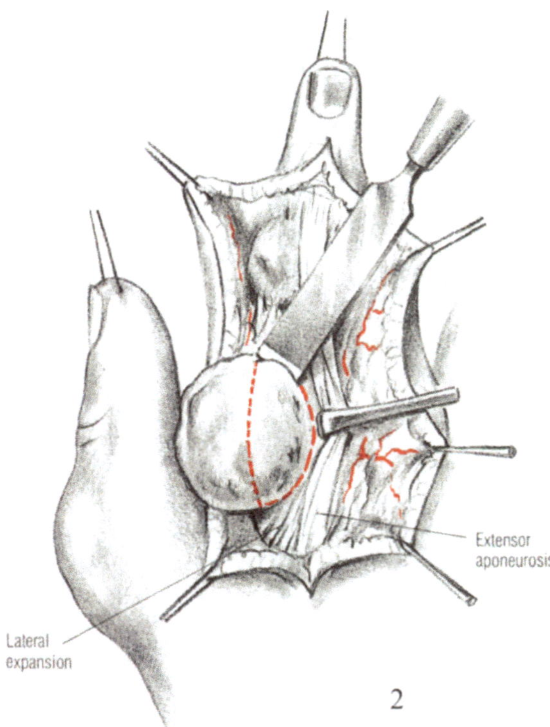

2

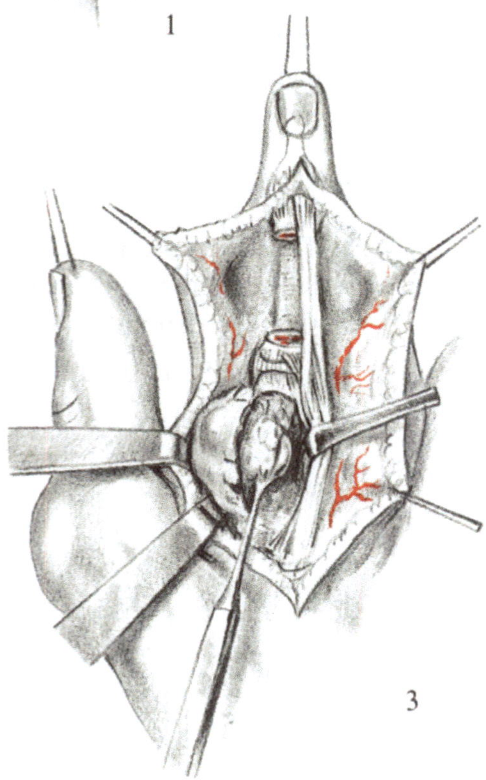

3

Fig. 4 A stable cortical bridge at the ulnar aspect of the proximal phalanx can be retained. The defect will be packed with pieces of autologous spongiosa.

Fig. 5 The defect in the proximal phalanx has been filled. The middle phalanx will be treated with a properly prepared spongiosa graft.

Fig. 6 Two pairs of thin (0.5 mm) Kirschner wires transfix the sites of resection of the middle phalanx. After closure of the periosteum superfluous skin is removed and the wound is closed.

Remarks

It is possible to remove the tumors of another finger during this operation.

Postoperative Care

Plaster fixation in position of function for 6 weeks. Removal of Kirschner wires at that time if x-rays show satisfactory healing. Careful active exercises may now be started. Therapy consists of exercises for 10 min in warm water 3–5 times daily. A night splint is worn for an additional 6 weeks. X-ray controls are imperative.

Errors and Their Consequences

E. The spongiosa graft is insufficiently prepared.
It does not fit snugly against the phalangeal remains.
C. Graft incorporation is delayed.

– Also see Sect. 16.3.

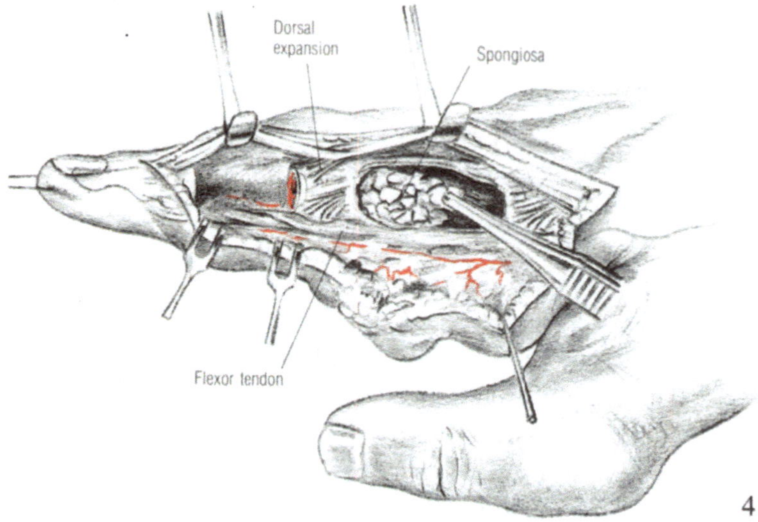

4

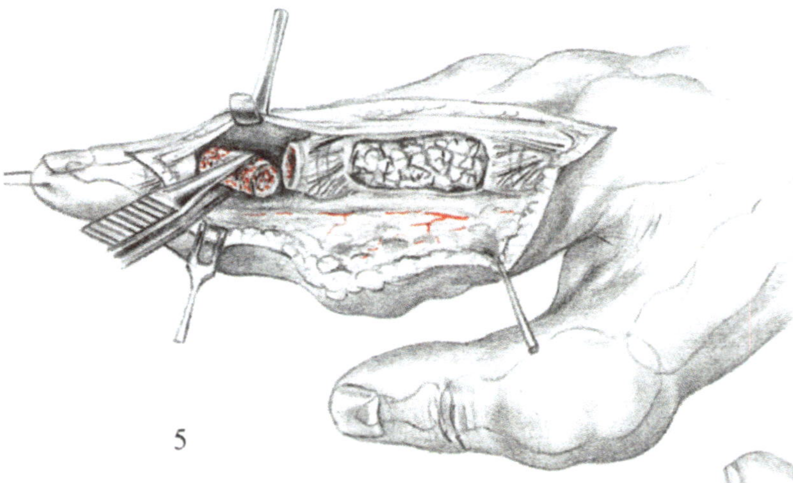

5

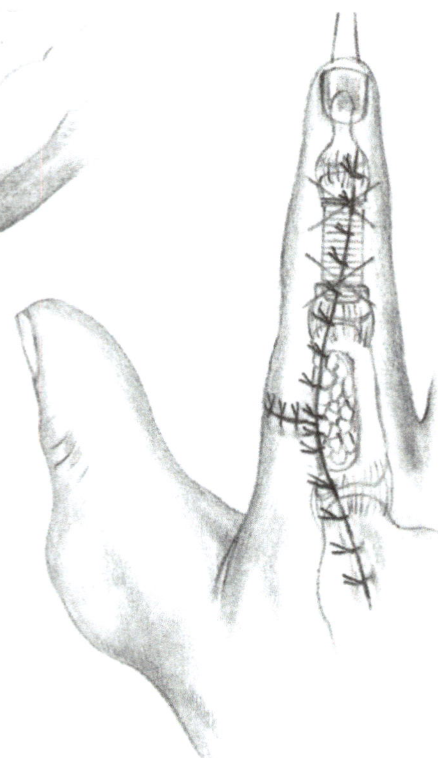

6

16.5 Enchondroma of a Middle Phalanx

Goal of Surgery

Removal of tumor by segmental resection and bridging of the defect with an autologous iliac crest graft.

Fig. 1 Preoperative appearance and incision. Ulnar aspects.
The diaphysis has been expanded by the enchondroma. The cortex has become paper thin. This case represents a recurrence after insufficient previous tumor removal. A smaller tumor is located in the distal phalanx.
The *hatched area* of bone will be excised after subperiosteal exposure.

Fig. 2 The area of insertion of the dorsal expansion is not disturbed. The remaining phalangeal ends are excavated and a properly prepared iliac crest graft is inserted.

Fig. 3 Postoperative appearance.
The bone graft is secured with two pairs of thin Kirschner wires. The wires should not penetrate the joints.

Postoperative Care and Errors and Their Consequences

See Sect. 16.4.

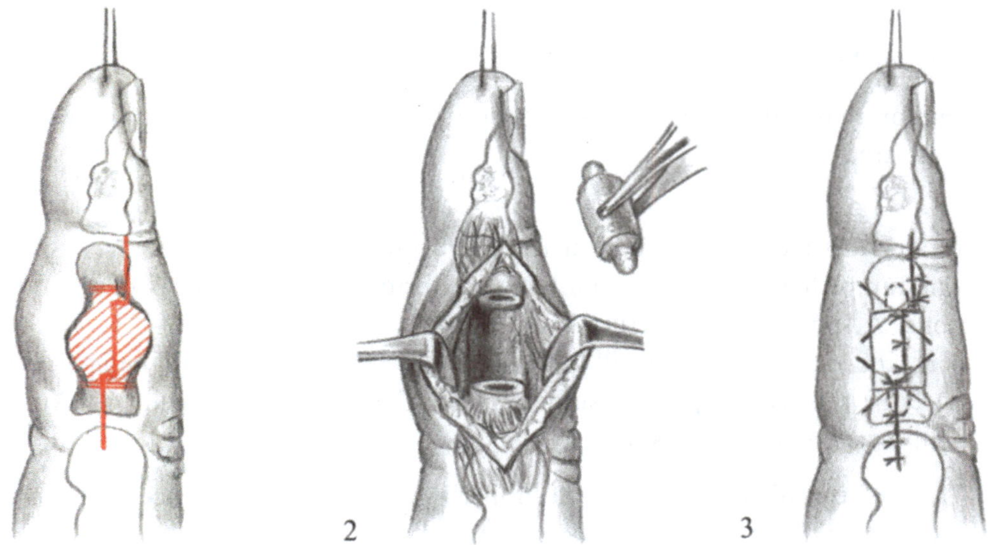

1 2 3

16.6 Metacarpal Enchondroma with Pathologic Fracture

Goal of Surgery

Tumor removal by segmental resection and bridging of the defect with an iliac crest graft.

Fig. 1 Preoperative appearance and incision. Dorsal aspect.
The tumor has resulted in a bulbous expansion of the diaphysis of the metacarpal bone. A spontaneous fracture has occurred.
The *hatched area* of bone will be excised. The periosteum should be incised dorsoulnarly as this avoids placing sutures under the extensor aponeurosis. An alternate skin incision is shown as a *broken line*.

Fig. 2 The metacarpal has been exposed subperiosteally. The extensor tendons are retracted laterally. A large window is made by using an osteotome.

Fig. 3 The tumor is removed with curettes. Every bit of the involved cortex is excised subperiosteally. Only healthy bone remains. It is better to excise portions of the periosteum than to leave tumor particles attached to it!

Figs. 4, 5 The site of the proximal resection has been smoothed; the distal site has been hollowed out to permit a more secure fit of the graft. An autologous iliac crest graft has been properly shaped and inserted. It is secured with two pairs of crossed Kirschner wires (Fig. 5: radial view). It is necessary to immobilize the MP joint temporarily as the remaining distal metacarpal portion is very short. Fixation of the joint is carried out in 30–40° of flexion. Finally the periosteum and skin are resutured.

Postoperative Care

Short-arm plaster cast with inclusion of the wrist joint, the first MP joint, and the MP and PIP joints of the index and middle fingers. Cast change and x-ray control after 4 weeks without further fixation of the PIP joints. Additional x-ray control 6–8 weeks after surgery, followed by care as outlined in Sect. 16.4.

Errors and Their Consequences

See Sects. 16.3 and 16.4.

Remarks

It will be necessary to arthrodese the MP joint if, due to the tumor size the distal metacarpal portion is so small that adequate stabilization appears impossible (see Sect. 16.2).

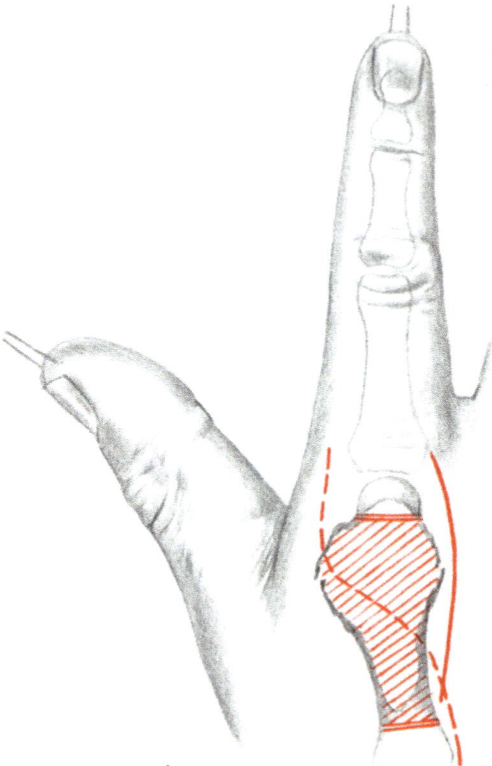

1

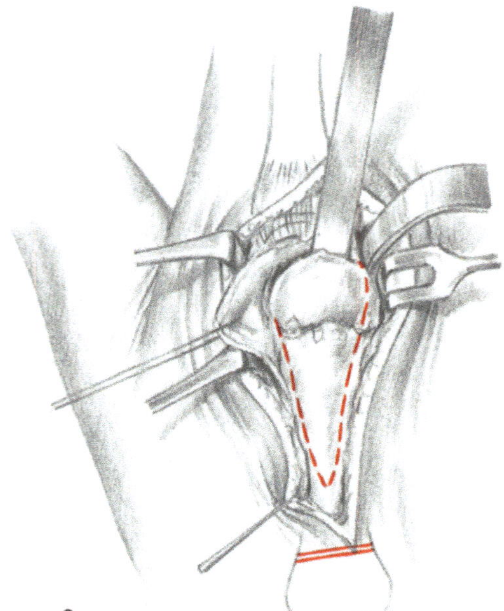

2

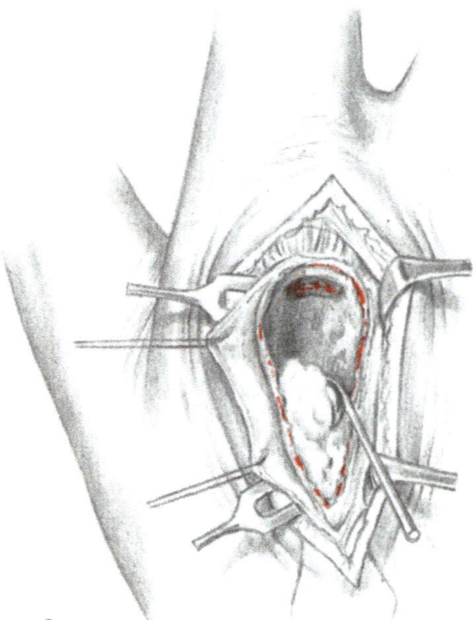

3

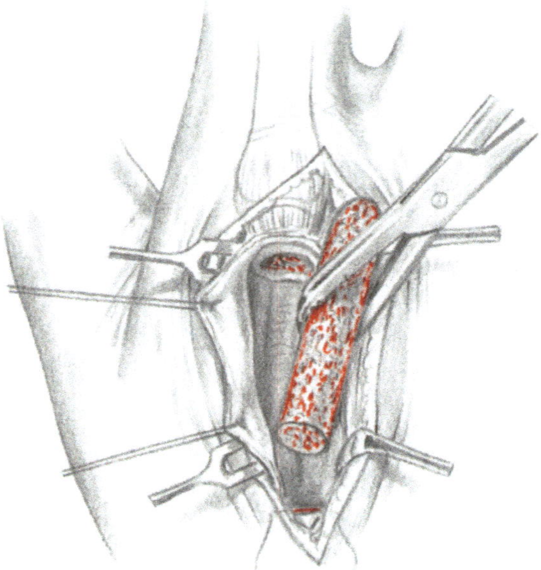

4

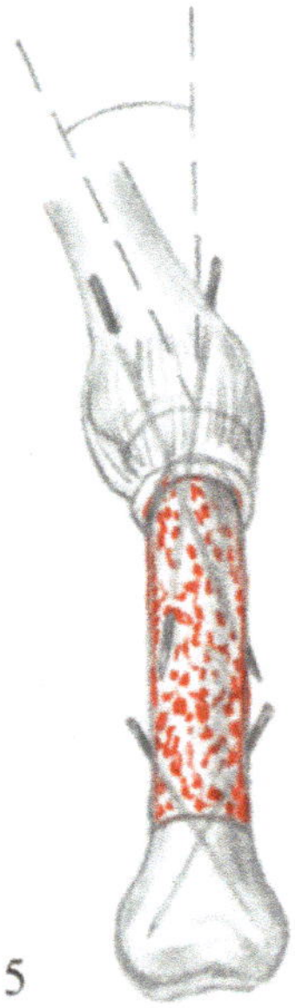

5

References

General Surgical Suggestions (Sect. 1.2) and *Review of Frequent Errors of Therapy and their Consequences* (Sect. 1.3)

Andina F (1970) Die freien Hauttransplantationen. Springer, Berlin Heidelberg New York
Bonola A, Morelli E (1972) Le deformitá congenite delle mani ed il loro trattamento. Piccin Editore, Padova
Buck-Gramcko D, Epping W (1974) Der Leistenlappen in der Handchirurgie. Handchirurgie 6:55–63
Frey R, Hügin W, Mayrhofer O (1972) Lehrbuch der Anesthesiologie und Wiederbelebung. Springer, Berlin Heidelberg New York
Iselin M (1959) Chirurgie der Hand. Atlas der Operationstechnik. Thieme, Stuttgart
Killian H (1973) Lokalanästhesie und Lokalanästhetika Thieme, Stuttgart
Koob E Personal communication
McGregor IA, Jackson JT (1972) The groin flap. Br J Plast Surg 25:3–16
Moore DC (1971) Regional Block. Thomas, Springfield, Ill
Padgett EL (1939) Calibrated intermediate skin grafts. Surg Gynecol Obstet 69:779–793; (cited by Andina)
Wilhelm A (1972) Die Schmerzverhütung bei Eingriffen an der Hand. In: Wachsmuth W Wilhelm A (eds) Allgemeine und spezielle chirurgische Operationslehre, vol X/3. Springer, Berlin Heidelberg New York, pp 38–72

Syndactylies (Chap. 2) and *Cutaneous Syndactylies* (Sect. 2.1)

Azzolini A (1975) The angiographic aspects of the syndactylies with their surgical and etiopathogenetic significance. Congr. de la Confédération Internat. de Chir. plast. et reconstruct., Paris, 25–30. 8. 1975 (unpublished work)
Barsky AJ (1958) Congenital anomalies of the hand and their surgical treatment. Thomas, Springfield, Ill.
Blauth W (1969) Die operative Behandlung der angeborenen Fehlbildungen der Hand. Verh. dtsch. Ges. Orthop. Traum., 55. Kongr. (Kassel): Z Orthop 106:Suppl. 386–402
Blauth W (1972) Möglichkeiten und Grenzen der operativen Behandlung angeborener Handfehlbildungen. In: Blauth W, Koob E (eds) Praktische Orthopädie, vol 3: Die Hand. Vordruckverlag, Bruchsal, pp 243–269
Blauth W (1972) Syndaktylien der Hand. Dtsch Ärztebl 69:2013–2021
Blauth W (1976) Zur Behandlung der verengten Daumenkommisur mit der "erweiterten Schwenklappenplastik". Handchirurgie 8:71–74
Bonola A, Morelli E (1972) Le deformitá congenite delle mani ed il loro trattamento. Piccin Editore, Padova
Buck-Gramcko D (1975) Operative Behandlung angeborener Fehlbildungen der Hand. Handchirurgie 7:53–67
Bunnell S (1959) Die Chirurgie der Hand. Maudrich, Vienna Bonn Bern
Cleeland I (1878) On the cutaneous ligaments of the phalanges. J Anat Physiol (Lond) 12:526; (cited by Lösch)
Cronin Th D (1956) Syndactylism: Results of zigzag incision to prevent postoperative contracture. Plast Reconstr Surg 18:400–468
Davis JS, German WJ (1930) Syndactylism. Arch Surg 21:32–75; (cited by Kelikian)
Ebskov B, Zachariae L (1966) Surgical methods in syndactylism. Evaluation of 208 operations. Acta Chir Scand 131:258–268
Grebe H (1964) Mißbildungen der Gliedmaßen. In: Bekker PE (ed) Humangenetik, vol. II. Thieme, Stuttgart, pp 179–343
Iselin F (1960) Traitement chirurgical des syndactylies congénitales. Résultats d'après 42 observations. Rev Prat (Paris) 10:2611–2620
Kelikian H (1974) Congenital deformities of the hand and forearm. Saunders, Philadelphia London Toronto
Kinmoth MH Syndactyly – surgical procedures. Congr. de la Confederation Internat de Chir. plast. et reconstruct., Paris, 25.–30. 8. 1975 (unpublished work)
Lösch GM (1970) Syndaktylien. Anatomie, Enwicklung, therapeutische Aspekte. In: Bargmann W, Doerr W (eds) Normale und Pathologische Anatomie, vol 23. Thieme, Stuttgart
McKusick VA (1975) Mendelian inheritance in man. Catalogs of autosomal dominant, autosomal recessive, and x-linked phenotypes. Johns Hopkins, Baltimore
Meissl G, Millesi H, Piza-Katzer H (1975) Kritische Betrachtungen verschiedener Operationsmethoden zur operativen Korrektur der Syndaktylie. (Bericht über einen Beobachtungszeitraum von 10–20 Jahren.) Handchirurgie 7:69–73
Meves H (1975) Postoperative Behandlung der kutanen Syndaktylie. Z Orthop 113:418–420
Millesi H (1961) Wachstumsbedingte Narbenkontrakturen und ihre Bedeutung für die Handchirurgie. Langenbecks Arch Klin Chir 229:112–117
Millesi H (1964) Spätresultate der plastischen Korrektur der Syndaktylie. 14th Bienn. Congress of the Internat. College of Surg. Vienna pp 293–311
Millesi H (1970) Kritische Betrachtungen zur Syndaktylie-Operation. Chir Plast Reconstr 7:99
Millesi H (1971) Plastische Chirurgie bei Fehlbildungen der Hand. Chirurg 42:60–67
Müller W (1937) Die angeborenen Fehlbildungen der menschlichen Hand. Thieme, Leipzig
Nylén B (1957) Repair of congenital finger syndactyly. Acta Chir Scand 113:310–319
Petersen D (1968) Zur Pathogenese der Syndaktylie. Verh. dtsch. Ges. Orthop. Traum., 54. Kongr. (Cologne): Z Orthop 104:Suppl. 448–451
Stucke K, Helbig D (1958) Syndaktylie. In: Schwalbe

E, Gruber GB (eds) Die Morphologie der Mißbildungen des Menschen und der Tiere, Part III. Fischer, Jena, pp 809–843

Witt AN, Cotta H, Jäger M (1966) Die angeborenen Fehlbildungen der Hand und ihre operative Behandlung. Thieme, Stuttgart

Osseous Syndactylies (Sect. 2.2) ("Apert Hand")

Apert HE (1906) De l'acrocéphalosyndactylie. Bull et Mém Soc Méd Hôp Paris 23:1310–1330

Blauth W (1969) Die operative Behandlung der angeborenen Fehlbildungen der Hand. Verh. dtsch. Ges. Orthop. Traum., 55. Kongr. (Kassel): Z Orthop 106:Suppl. 386–402

Blauth W (1972) Syndaktylien der Hand. Dtsch Ärztebl 69:2012–2021

Grebe H (1944) Die Akrocephalosyndaktylie. Eine klinisch-ätiologische Studie. Z menschl Vererb- u Konstit-Lehre 28:209–261

Hoover GH, Flatt AE, Weiss MW (1970) The hand and Apert's syndrome J Bone Joint Surg 52-A:878–894

Lösch GM (1970) Syndaktylien. Anatomie, Enwicklung, therapeutische Aspekte. In: Bargmann W, Doerr W (eds) Normale und Pathologische Anatomie, vol. 23. Thieme, Stuttgart

McKusick VA (1975) Mendelian inheritance in man. Catalogs of autosomal dominant, autosomal recessive, and x-linked phenotypes. Johns Hopkins, Baltimore

Pfeiffer RA (1964) Dominant erbliche Akrocephalosyndaktylie. Z Kinderheilk 90:301–320

Pfeiffer RA (1969) Associated deformities of the head and hands. (In: Bergsma D (ed) Clinical delineation of birth defects, Part III: Limb malformations) Birth Defects: Original article series, vol V/3. The National Foundation, New York, pp 18–34

Temtamy SA (1966) Carpenter's syndrome; Acrocephalopolysyndactyly. An autosomal recessive syndrome. J Pediatr 69:111–120

Valentin B (1938) Die Korrelation (Koppelung) von Mißbildungen, erläutert am Beispiel der Acrocephalosyndaktylie. Acta Orthop Scand 9:235–316

Recurrent Syndactylies (Sect. 2.3)

Blauth W (1970) Das Syndaktylie-Rezidiv. Handchirurgie 2:95–101

Blauth W, Hippe P (1973) Schnittführungen bei Syndaktylie-Rezidiven. Arch Orthop Unfallchir 77:97–107

Buck-Gramcko D (1975) Operative Behandlung angeborener Fehlbildungen der Hand. Handchirurgie 7:53–67

Iselin J (1959) Chirurgie der Hand, Atlas der Operationstechnik. Thieme, Stuttgart

Millesi H (1961) Wachstumsbedingte Narbenkontrakturen und ihre Bedeutung für die Handchirurgie. Langenbecks Arch Klin Chir 299:112–117

Peripheral Hypoplasias (Chap. 3)

Blauth W (1969) Die operative Behandlung der angeborenen Fehlbildungen der Hand. Verh. dtsch. Ges. Orthop. Traum., 55. Kongr. (Kassel): Z Orthop 106:Suppl. 386–402

Grebe H (1964) Mißbildungen der Gliedmaßen. In: Bekker PE (ed) Humangenetik, vol. II. Thieme, Stuttgart, pp 179–343 (esp 230–232)

Gruber GB (1937) Gliedmaßenfehler aus plazentärer Beeinträchtigung. In: Schwalbe E, Gruber GB (eds) Die Morphologie der Mißbildungen des Menschen und der Tiere, Part III. Fischer, Jena, pp 278–299 and 329–332

Gruber GB (1937) Hypoplasie, Makromelie, Phokomelie, Amelie, Peromelie (einschl. der sog. „Spontanamputationen"). In: Schwalbe E, Gruber GB (eds) Die Morphologie der Mißbildungen des Menschen und der Tiere, Part III. Fischer, Jena, pp 300–328

Kelikian H (1974) Congenital deformities of the hand and forearm. Saunders, Philadelphia London Toronto

Kino Y (1975) Clinical and experimental studies of the congenital constriction band syndrome with an emphasis on its etiology. J Bone Joint Surg 57-A:636–643

MacArthur JW, McCullough E (1932) Apical dystrophy as inherited defect of hands and feet. Hum Biol 4:179–207 (cited by Grebe a.o.)

Müller W (1937) Die angeborenen Fehlbildungen der menschlichen Hand. Thieme, Leipzig

Schade H (1937) Zur endogenen Entstehung von Gliedmaßendefekten. Z Morph Anthrop 36:375–391

Schade H (1940) Untersuchungen zur Frage der Erblichkeit von Mangel- und Fehlbildungen der Gliedmaßen. Erbarzt 8:239–256

Werthemann A (1952) Periphere Hypoplasie der Gliedmaßen (quere Stummelbildungen), Fingerenddefekte. In: Lubarsch O, Henke F, Rössle R (eds) Handbuch für Spezielle Pathologische Anatomie und Histologie, vol. IX/6. Springer, Berlin Göttingen Heidelberg, pp 119–128

Witt AN, Cotta H, Jäger M (1966) Die angeborenen Fehlbildungen der Hand und ihre operative Behandlung. Thieme, Stuttgart

Witt AN, Jäger M (1968) Die operative Behandlung der peripheren Hypoplasie der Hand. Arch Orthop Unfallchir 64:52–63

Numerical Variations (Chap. 4)

Bilhaut (M) (1890) Guérison d'un pouce bifide par un nouveau procédé opératoire. Congr. franç. de Chir. (Paris, 1889) 4:576–580

Blauth W (1967) Der hypoplastische Daumen. Arch Orthop Unfallchir 62:225–246

Blauth W (1969) Indikation und Technik des „Zeigefinger-Daumens" bei Daumenaplasien. Handchirurgie 1:28–33

Blauth W (1970) Prinzipien der Pollizisation unter besonderer Berücksichtigung einer neuen Schnittführung. Handchirurgie 2:117–121

Blauth W (1972) Die Aplasie und Hypoplasie am Daumenstrahl. In: Wachsmuth W, Wilhelm A (eds) Allgemeine und spezielle chirurgische Operationslehre, vol. X/3. Springer, Berlin Heidelberg New York, pp 579–610

Blauth W, Schmidt H (1969) Über die Bedeutung arteriographischer Befunde bei Fehlbildungen am radialen Randstrahl (radiale Dysplasie). Z Orthop 106:102–110

Blauth W, Schneider-Sickert F (1975) Die operative Behandlung der Mißbildungen im Bereich der Mittelhand. 35. Kongr. Schweiz. Ges. Orthop., (Solothurn)

Bonola A, Morelli E (1972) Le deformitá congenite delle mani ed il loro trattamento. Piccin Editore, Padova
Buck-Gramcko D (1966) Daumenrekonstruktion bei Aplasie und Hypoplasie. Klin Med (Vienna) 21:325–329
Buck-Gramcko D (1968) Indikation und Technik der Daumenbildung bei Aplasie und Hypoplasie. Chir Plast Reconstr 5:46–51
Buck-Gramcko D (1971) Pollicisation of the index finger. Method and results in aplasia and hypoplasia of the thumb. J Bone Joint Surg 53-A:1605–1616
Buck-Gramcko D, Epping W (1974) Der Leistenlappen in der Handchirurgie. Handchirurgie 6:55–63
Bunnell S (1959) Die Chirurgie der Hand. Maudrich, Vienna Bonn Bern
Edgerton MT, Snyder GB, Webb WL (1965) Surgical treatment of congenital thumb deformities (including psychological impact of correction). J Bone Joint Surg 47-A:1453–1474
Fritz G, Deutschmann W (1974) Der Leistenlappen zur Versorgung komplizierter Handverletzungen. Handchirurgie 6:51–54
Kelikian H (1974) Congenital deformities of the hand and forearm. Saunders, Philadelphia London Toronto
McGregor IA, Jackson JT (1972) The groin flap. Br J Plast Surg 25:3–16
Mellin GW (1963) The frequency of birth defects. In: Fishbein M (ed). Birth defects. Lippincott, Philadelphia, pp 1–17; (cited by Kelikian)
Müller W (1937) Die angeborenen Fehlbildungen der menschlichen Hand. Thieme, Leipzig
Schneider-Sickert F, Blauth W (1975) Die Morphologie der Mittelhandfehlbildungen. 35. Kongr. Schweiz. Ges. Orthop., (Solothurn)
Smith PJ, Foley B, McGregor IA, Jackson JT (1972) The anatomical basis of the groin flap. Plast Reconstr Surg 49:41–47
Thompson TC (1942) A modified operation for opponens paralysis. J Bone Joint Surg 24:632–640

Metrical Variations (Chap. 5)

v. Andrian-Werburg H (1975) Verbesserung der Greiffunktion durch MC-Verlängerungsosteotomie bei Brachymetacarpie. 35. Kongr. Schweiz. Ges. Orthop., (Solothurn) (unpublished work)
Bell J (1951) On brachydactyly and symphalangism. In: Penrose LS (ed) The treasury of human inheritance, vol. V/1. University Press, Cambridge, pp 1–31
Blauth W (1976) Zur Behandlung der verengten Daumenkommissur mit der „erweiterten Schenklappenplastik". 16. Symposium d. Deutschspr. Arbeitsgem. Handchir., Handchirurgie 8:71–74
Cocchi U (1952) Erbschäden mit Knochenveränderungen. In: Schinz HR, Baensch WE, Friedl E, Uehlinger E (eds) Lehrbuch der Röntgendiagnostik, 5th edn, vol I. Thieme, Stuttgart, pp 621–873 (esp 727–742)
Cotta H, Jäger M (1965) Die familiäre Triphalangie des Daumens und ihre operative Behandlung. Arch Orthop Unfallchir 58:282–290
Fürst N (1900) Ein Fall von verkürzten und zweigliedrigen Fingern, begleitet von Brustmuskeldefekten und anderen Mißbildungen. Z Morph Anthrop 2:56; (cited by W Müller)
Grebe H (1964) Mißbildungen der Gliedmaßen. In: Becker PE (ed) Humangenetik, vol II. Thieme, Stuttgart, pp 179–343
Hopf A (1959) Der dreigliedrige Daumen. In: Hohmann G, Hackenbroch M, Lindemann K (eds) Handuch der Orthopädie,vol III. Thieme, Stuttgart, pp 450–454
Joachimsthal G (1900) Verdoppelung des linken Zeigefingers und Dreigliederung des rechten Daumens. Berl Klin Wschr 1900:835–838
Jones GB (1964) Deltaphalanx. J Bone Joint Surg 46-B:226–229
Kelikian H (1974) Congenital deformities of the hand and forearm. Saunders, Philadelphia London Toronto
McKusick VA (1975) Mendelian inheritance in man. Catalogs of autosomal dominant, autosomal recessive, and x-linked phenotypes. Johns Hopkins, Baltimore
Müller W (1937) Die angeborenen Fehlbildungen der menschlichen Hand. Thieme, Stuttgart
Nauck ETh (1938) Extremitätenskelett der Tetrapoden. In: Bolck L, Göppert E, Kallius E, Lubosch W (eds) Handbuch der Vergleichenden Anatomie der Wirbeltiere, vol V. Urban & Schwarzenberg, Berlin, pp 71–248
Pfitzner W (1898) Über Brachydaktylie und Verwandtes. Anat Anz 14, Erg-Heft (12. Verh. Anat. Ges., Kiel), 18–23
Pol R (1921) „Brachydaktylie" – „Klinodaktylie" – „Hyperphalangie" und ihre Grundlagen: Form und Entstehung der meist unter dem Bild der Brachydaktylie auftretenden Varietäten, Anomalien und Mißbildungen der Hand und des Fußes. Virchows Arch Path Anat 229:388–530
Pol R (1937a) Hyperphalangie des Daumens, Klinodaktylie des Daumens (Pollex varus, valgus). In: Schwalbe E, Gruber GB (eds) Die Morphologie der Mißbildungen des Menschen und der Tiere, Part III. Fischer, Jena, pp 646–654
Pol R (1937b) Brachydaktylie (Acrochondrodysplasie). In: Schwalbe E, Gruber GB (eds) Die Morphologie der Mißbildungen des Menschen und der Tiere, Part III. Fischer, Jena, pp 597–645
Rochlin DG, Zeitler E (1968) Röntgendiagnostik der Hand und Handwurzel. In: Diethelm L et al (eds) Handbuch der medizinischen Radiologie, vol IV/2. Springer, Berlin Heidelberg New York, pp 62–65
Schinz HR (1943) Erbtypen und Formen bei Brachydaktylie. (Kurzfinger, Kurzzehen.) Arch Klaus-Stift Vererb-Forsch 18:361–404
Schneider-Sickert F (1975) Beitrag zur familiären Brachyhyperphalangie. 16. Symposium of Deutschspr. Arbeitsgem. f. Handchir., (Vienna)
Schneider-Sickert F, Hippe P Zum Problem des dreigliedrigen radialrandständigen Fingers (Sul problema del dito del margine radiale a tre falangi). 13. Congr. Naz., Soc. Italiana di Chir della Mano, (Merano) (unpublished work)
Temtamy S, McKusick VA (1969) Synopsis of hand malformations with particular emphasis on genetic factors. In: Bergsma D (ed) Clinical delineation of birth defects, Part III: Limb malformations Birth Defects: Original article series, vol V/3. National Foundation New York, pp 125–184
Verdan C (1975) Diskussionsbeitrag zum Thema Mittelhandfehlbildungen. 35. Kongr. Schweiz. Ges. Orthop., (Solothurn) (unpublished work)
Werthemann A (1952) Allgemeines über Störungen der Epiphysenentwicklung. In: Lubarsch O, Henke F,

Rössle R (eds) Handbuch für Spezielle Pathologische Anatomie und Histologie, vol IX/6. Springer, Berlin Göttingen Heidelberg, pp 160–185
Witt AN, Cotta H, Jäger M (1966) Die angeborenen Fehlbildungen der Hand und ihre operative Behandlung. Thieme, Stuttgart,

Hypoplasias and Aplasias of Finger Joints (Chap. 6)

Barsky AJ (1958) Congenital anomalies of the hand and their surgical treatment. Thomas, Springfield, Ill.
Blechschmidt E (1961) Die vorgeburtlichen Entwicklungsstadien des Menschen. Karger, Basel New York
Blechschmidt E, Petersen D (1967) Die frühembryonalen Entwicklungsbewegungen des menschlichen Armes als Faktor möglicher Mißbildungen. Ergeb Chir Orthop 49:62–111
Cushing H (1916) Hereditary anchylosis of the proximal phalangeal joints (Symphalangism). Genetics 1:90–106
Drinkwater H (1917) Phalangeal anarthrosis (Synostosis, Ankylosis) transmitted through fourteen generations. Proc Roy Soc Med, Section Pathology 10:60–68
Duken J (1921) Über die Beziehungen zwischen Assimilationshypophalangie und Aplasie der Interphalangealgelenke. Virchows Arch Path Anat 233:204–225
Fischel A (1909/10) Über Anomalien des Knochensystems, insbesondere des Extremitätenskeletts. Anat Hefte 40:1–45; (cited by Pol)
Kelikian H (1974) Congenital deformities of the hand and forearm. Saunders, Philadelphia London Toronto
Mestern J (1934) Erbliche Aplasie der Interphalangealgelenke (erbliche Phalanxsynostose). Z Orthop Chir 61:421–422
Pfitzner W (1898) Über Brachydaktylie und Verwandtes. Anat Anz 14:Suppl. (12. Verh. anat. Ges., Kiel), 18–23
Pol R (1921) „Brachydaktylie" – „Klinodaktylie" – „Hyperphalangie" und ihre Grundlagen: Form und Entstehung der meist unter dem Bild der Brachydaktylien auftretenden Varietäten, Anomalien und Mißbildungen der Hand und des Fußes. Virchows Arch Path Anat 229:388–530
Pol R (1937) Aplasie der Finger- und Zehengelenke. („Angeborene steife Finger", „Geradfingrigkeit".) In: Schwalbe E, Gruber GB (eds) Die Morphologie der Mißbildungen des Menschen und der Tiere, Part III. Fischer, Jena, pp 655–582
Werthemann A (1952) Erbliche Aplasie der Interphalangealgelenke. In: Lubarsch O, Henke F, Rössle R (eds) Handbuch für Spezielle Pathologische Anatomie und Histologie, vol IX/6. Springer, Berlin Göttingen Heidelberg, pp 325–331
Weyers H (1968) Erbliche Gelenkleiden. In: Diethelm L et al (eds) Handbuch der medizinischen Radiologie, vol V/3. Springer, Berlin Heidelberg New York, pp 407–511
Witt AN, Cotta H, Jäger M (1966) Die angeborenen Fehlbildungen der Hand und ihre operative Behandlung. Thieme, Stuttgart

Joint Dysplasias (Chap. 7)

Blauth W (1967) Der hypoplastische Daumen. Arch Orthop Unfallchir 62:225–256
Blauth W (1972) Die Aplasie und Hypoplasie am Daumenstrahl. In: Wachsmuth W, Wilhelm A (eds) Allgemeine und spezielle chirurgische Operationslehre, vol X/3. Springer, Berlin Heidelberg New York, pp 579–610
Bunnell S (1959) Die Chirurgie der Hand. Maudrich, Vienna Bonn Bern
Edgerton MT, Snyder GB, Webb WL (1965) Surgical treatment of congenital thumb deformities (including psychological impact of correction). J Bone Joint Surg 47-A:1453–1474
Goldthwait JE (1914) Über Handgewölbe und „Platthand". Z Orthop Chir 34:377–389
Hohmann G (1949) Hand und Arm, ihre Erkrankungen und deren Behandlung. Bergmann, Munich
Hopf A (1959) Die Platthand. Habituelle Subluxationen im I. Carpometacarpalgelenk. In: Hohmann G, Hakkenbroch M, Lindemann K (eds) Handbuch der Orthopädie, vol III. Thieme, Stuttgart, pp 485–486
Kelikian H (1974) Congenital deformities of the hand and forearm. Saunders, Philadelphia London Toronto
Volkmann J (1953) Über die sogenannte Platthand. Verh. dtsch. orthop. Ges., 40. Kongr. (Wiesbaden). Beih zu Z Orthop 83:Suppl. 284–285
Weckesser EC Convention reports (abstracts): J Bone Joint Surg 36-A:663–664 (1954) and 27-A:619 (1955)
Witt AN (1957) Funktionsverbessernde Eingriffe an den Fingergelenken. Langenbecks Arch Klin Chir 287:541–546
Witt AN, Cotta H, Jäger M (1966) Die angeborenen Fehlbildungen der Hand und ihre operative Behandlung. Thieme, Stuttgart

Symbrachydactylies (Chap. 8)

Barsky AJ (1964) Cleft hand: Classification, incidence, and treatment. Review of the literature and report of nineteen cases. J Bone Joint Surg 46-A:1707–1720
Blauth W (1972) Möglichkeiten und Grenzen der operativen Behandlung angeborener Handfehlbildungen. In: Blauth W, Koob E (eds) Praktische Orthopädie, vol 3: Die Hand. Vordruckverlag, Bruchsal, pp 243–269
Blauth W, Gekeler J (1971) Zur Morphologie und Klassifikation der Symbrachydaktylie. Handchirurgie 3:123–128
Blauth W, Gekeler J (1973) Symbrachydaktylien. (Ein Beitrag zur Morphologie, Klassifikation und Therapie.) Handchirurgie 5:121–171
Degenhardt K-H (1972) Poland-Syndrom durch Secale-Alkaloide? Dtsch Ärtzebl 69:3413–3415
Lange M (1937) Grundsätzliches über die Beurteilung der Entstehung und Bewertung atypischer Hand- und Fußmißbildungen. Verh. dtsch. orthop. Ges., 31. Kongr. (Königsberg/Pr.). Z Orthop 66:Suppl. 80–87
Pol R (1921) „Brachydaktylie" – „Klinodaktylie" – „Hyperphalangie" und ihre Grundlagen: Form und Entstehung der meist unter dem Bild der Brachydaktylie auftretenden Varietäten, Anomalien und Mißbildungen der Hand und des Fußes. Virchows Arch Path Anat 229:388–530

Cleft Hand (Chap. 9)

Barsky AJ (1964) Cleft hand: Classification, incidence, and treatment. Review of the literature and report of nineteen cases. J Bone Joint Surg 46-A:1707–1720

Barsky AJ (1958) Congenital anomalies of the hand and their surgical treatment. Thomas, Springfield, Ill
Bauer KH, Bode W (1940) Erbpathologie der Stützgewebe beim Menschen. In: Just G (ed) Handbuch der Erbbiologie des Menschen, Springer, Berlin, pp 105–334 (esp 257–260)
Birch-Jensen A (1949) Congenital deformities of the upper extremities. Det danske Forlag, Copenhagen
Blankenburg H (1967) Spalthand- und Spaltfußbildungen in typischen und atypischen Formen. Beitr Orthop Traum 14:209–215
Blauth W (1969) Die operative Behandlung der angeborenen Fehlbildungen der Hand. Verh. dtsch. Ges. Orthop. Traum., 55. Kongr. (Kassel). Beih zu Z Orthop 106:Suppl. 386–402
Burger L (1928) Doppelte Epiphysenbildung des Metacarpus. (Ein Beitrag zur Physiologie des Knochenwachstums.) Arch Orthop Unfallchir 26:276–286
Grebe H (1964) Mißbildungen der Gliedmaßen (Spalthände und -füße). In: Becker PE (ed) Humangenetik, vol II. Thieme, Stuttgart, pp 179–343 (esp 304–316)
Kelikian H (1974) Congenital deformities of the hand and forearm. Saunders, Philadelphia London Toronto
Klages F, Jacob R (1940) Anatomische und erbbiologische Untersuchungen an einer mit Spaltfüßen und Mißbildungen der Hände behafteten Sippe. Z Orthop Chir 70:265–281
Lange M (1937) Grundsätzliches über die Beurteilung der Entstehung und Bewertung atypischer Hand- und Fußmißbildungen. Verh. dtsch. orthop. Ges., 31. Kongr. (Königsberg/Pr). Z Orthop 66:Suppl. 80–87
Liebenam L (1938) Beitrag zum familiären Vorkommen von Spalthänden und Spaltfüßen. Z Menschl Vererb- u Konstit-Lehre 22:136–149
Müller W (1937) Die angeborenen Fehlbildungen der menschlichen Hand. Thieme, Leipzig
Ströer W (1936) Familiäres Auftreten von Reihen erblicher Hand- und Fußabweichungen. Erbarzt 4:22–35
Werthemann A (1952) Spalthände und Spaltfüße. In: Lubarsch O, Henke F, Rössle R (eds) Handbuch für Spezielle Pathologische Anatomie und Histologie, vol IX/6. Springer, Berlin Göttingen Heidelberg, pp 358–377
Witt AN, Cotta H, Jäger M (1966) Die angeborenen Fehlbildungen der Hand und ihre operative Behandlung. Thieme, Stuttgart

Congenital localized Giantism of the Hand (Macrodactyly) (Chap. 10)

Allende B (1967) Macrodactyly with enlarged median nerve associated with carpal tunnel syndrome. Plast Reconstr Surg 39:578–582
Barsky AJ (1967) Macrodactyly. J Bone Joint Surg 49-A:1255–1266
Ben-Bassat M, Casper J, Kaplan I, Laron Z (1966) Congenital macrodactyly. A case report with a three-year follow-up. J Bone Joint Surg 48-B:359–364
Bernoulli P (1944) Ein Fall von partiellem Riesenwuchs (Macrodactylia simplex congenita). Anat Anz 95:372–395
Blauth W (1972) Möglichkeiten und Grenzen der operativen Behandlung angeborener Handfehlbildungen. In: Blauth W, Koob E (eds) Praktische Orthopädie, vol 3: Die Hand. Vordruckverlag, Bruchsal, pp 243–269
Brooks B, Lehman EP (1924) The bone changes in Recklinghausen's neurofibromatosis. Surg Gynecol Obstet 38:587–595; (cited by Millesi)
Buck-Gramcko D (1971) Fehlbildungen der Hand. Einführung und Grundsätze der operativen Behandlung. II. Kongreßbericht Österr. Ges. für Chir., Verlag Wiener Mediz. Akademie, Vienna, pp 563–577
Buck-Gramcko D (1973) Diskussionsbemerkungen zum Vortrag von D. Schöllner: Behandlung einer exzessiven Makrodaktylie. Handchirurgie 5:97
Clifford RH (1959) The treatment of macrodactylism. A case report. Plast Reconstr Surg 23:245–248
Coninck A de (1965) Mégalodactylie. Ann Chir Plast 10:45–48
Dambrin L (1936) Les macrodactylies. Rev Orthop 23:215–229
Feriz H (1926) Makrodystrophia lipomatosa progressiva. Virchows Arch Path Anat 260:308–368
Fischer H (1880) Der Riesenwuchs. Dtsch Z Chir 12:1–59
Fritzsche H (1955) Zur Symptomatik und Therapie des partiellen Riesenwuchses. Zbl. Chir 80:1200–1210
Gruber GB, Kuss OE (1937) Der angeborene örtliche Riesenwuchs. In: Schwalbe E, Gruber GB (eds) Die Morphologie der Mißbildungen des Menschen und der Tiere, Part III. Fischer, Jena, pp 423–454
Hellmann K (1964) Über die Behandlung der Makrodaktylie. Ann Chir Plast 9:184–186
Hentschen C (1939) Plastische Wiederherstellung riesenwüchsiger Finger durch phalangeale Umkipplastik, Verkürzungsexzision und Weichteilexzisionen. Helv Med Acta 3:166–176
Hopf A (1959) Der angeborene örtliche Riesenwuchs im Bereich der Hand. In: Hohmann G, Hackenbroch M, Lindemann (eds) Handbuch der Orthopädie, vol III. Thieme, Stuttgart, pp 486–488
Iovannovich J, Bartsch G (1971) Zur Klinik und Pathologie der Makrodaktylie. Chir Plast (Berl) 1:1–14
Jäger M (1967) Der angeborene umschriebene Riesenwuchs der Hand und des Fußes. Differentialdiagnose, Kasuistik, operative Therapie. Arch Orthop Unfallchir 61:151–163
Jones KG (1963) Megalodactylism. Case report of a child treated by epiphyseal resection. J Bone Joint Surg 45-A:1704–1708
Kaplan EB (1947) Congenital giant thumb. Bull Hosp Joint Dis (NY) 8:38–44; (cited by Kelikian)
Kehrer FA (1948) Die konstitutionellen Vergrößerungen umschriebener Körperabschnitte. Thieme, Stuttgart
Kelikian H (1974) Congenital deformities of the hand and forearm. Saunders, Philadelphia London Toronto
Langsteiner F, Stiefler G (1935) Über die kongenitalen Hypertrophien (Hyperplasien). Dtsch Z Nervenheilk 138:274–307
Laurenzi V de (1962) Macrodattilia del medio. G Med Milit 112:401–405; (cited by Kelikian a.o.)
Lerch H (1949) Zur Morphologie des angeborenen partiellen Riesenwuchses am Fuß. Z Orthop Chir 78:144–157
Lerch H (1962) Zum Problem des angeborenen, umschriebenen Riesenwuchses. Z Orthop 96:290–298
Massonnoud A (1874) Essai sur la pathogénie de l'hypertrophie bilatérale partielle ou totale du corps. Thèse, Paris
McCarroll HR (1950) Clinical manifestations of congenital neurofibromatosis. J Brit Joint Surg 32-A:601–616

Millesi H (1966) Korrektur der Makrodaktylie bei Erwachsenen durch multiple Osteotomie. Zbl Chir 91:1472–1475
Moore BH (1941) Some orthopedic relationhips of neurofibromatosis. J Bone Joint Surg 23:109–140
Moore BH (1942) Macrodactyly and associated peripheral nerve changes. J Bone Joint Surg 24:617–631
Moore BH (1944) Peripheral nerve changes associated with congenital deformities. J Bone Joint Surg 26:282–288
Müller W (1937) Die angeborenen Fehlbildungen der menschlichen Hand. Thieme, Leipzig
Posch JL (1956) Tumors of the hand. J Bone Joint Surg 38-A:517–539
Schöllner D (1973) Behandlung einer exzessiven Makrodaktylie. Handchirurgie 5:89–92
Thomas HB (1936) Partial gigantism: Overgrowth and asymmetry of bones and skeletal muscle. Am J Surg 32:108–112, 168
Timoney FX (1944) Macrodactyly. Case report. Ann Surg 119:144–147
Tsuge K (1967) Treatment of Macrodactyly. Plast Reconstr Surg 39:590–599
Tucker JM, Carpenter EB (1951) Localized neurofibromatosis with associated overgrowth of an extremity. Equilization of limb length following epiphyseal arrest. J Bone Joint Surg 33-A:103–106
Werthemann A (1952) Der angeborene umschriebene Riesenwuchs. In: Lubarsch O, Henke F, Rössle R (eds) Handbuch für Spezielle Pathologische Anatomie und Histologie, vol IX/6. Springer, Berlin Göttingen Heidelberg, pp 377–389
Wieland E (1907) Zur Pathologie der dystrophischen Form des angeborenen partiellen Riesenwuchses. Z Kinderheilk 65:519–584
Windholz F (1931) Riesenwuchs der Zehen und des Dickdarms. Dtsch Z Chir 232:634–647; (cited by Werthemann)

Pollex Flexus Congenitus (Congenital Trigger Thumb) (Chap. 11)

Bonola A, Morelli E (1972) Le deformitá congenite delle mani ed il loro trattamento. Piccin Editore, Pàdova
Hubenstorf H (1961) Personal communication
Iselin M (1959) Chirurgie der Hand. Atlas der Operationstechnik. Thieme, Stuttgart
White JW, Jensen WE (1953) Trigger thumb in infants. Am J Dis Child 85:141–145
Witt AN, Cotta H, Jäger M (1966) Die angeborenen Fehlbildungen der Hand und ihre operative Behandlung. Thieme, Stuttgart

Camptodactyly (Chap. 12)

Barinka L (1964) Campylodactylia. (A preliminary communication.) Acta Chir plast (Praha) 6:54–60; (cited, a.o., by Kelikian)
Berger A, Millesi H (1975) Spätergebnisse der operativen Behandlung der Kamptodaktylie. Handchirurgie 7:75–79
Bonola A, Morelli E (1972) Le deformitá congenite delle mani ed il loro trattamento. Piccin Editore, Padova
Brüchle H, Merckling D (1972) Ätiologie und Therapie der Kamptodaktylie. Z Orthop 110:89–92
Bunnell S (1959) Die Chirurgie der Hand. Maudrich, Vienna Bonn Bern
Currarino G, Waldman J (1964) Camptodactyly. Am. J Roentgenol 92:1312–1321
Févre M (1936) Camptodactylie (lésions anatomiques d'un doigt surnuméraire atteint de camptodactylie). Ann Anat Path 13:1018–1023
Furnas DW (1965) Muscle-tendon variations in the flexor compartment of the wrist. Plast Reconstr Surg 36:320–323
Landouzy, L. (1906) Camptodactylie: stigmate organique précocé du neuro-arthritisme. Presse méd. 14:251–253; (cited by Kelikian)
Maurer G (1938) Die Kamptodaktylie. Arch Orthop. Unfallchir. 39:365–374
Millesi H (1968) Zur Pathogenese und operativen Korrektur der Kamptodaktylie. Chir Plast Reconstr 5:55–61
Parish JG, Horn DB, Thompson M (1963) Familial streblodaktyly with aminoaciduria. Brit Med J 1963 II:1247–1250
Smith RJ, Kaplan EB (1968) Camptodactyly and similar atraumatic flexion deformities of the proximal interphalangeal joints of the fingers. J Bone Joint Surg 50-A:1187–1203
Welch JP, Temtamy S (1966) Hereditary contractures of the fingers (Camptodactyly). J Med Genet 3:104–113
Wilhelm A, Kleinschmidt W (1968) Neue ätiologische und therapeutische Gesichtspunkte bei der Kamptodaktylie und Tendovaginitis stenosans. Chir Plast Reconstr 5:62–67

Hypoplasias andAplasias of the Radius (Radial Club Hand) (Chap. 13)

Axhausen G (1919) Zur operativen Behandlung von Klumphand und Knickfuß bei bestehendem Knochendefekt (Radius- resp. Fibuladefekt). Langenbecks Arch Klin Chir 111:621–643
Bauer KH, Bode W (1940) Erbpathologie der Stützgewebe beim Menschen. In: Just G (ed) Handbuch der Erbbiologie des Menschen, vol III. Springer, Berlin pp 105–334 (esp 256–257)
Birch-Jensen A (1949) Congenital deformities in the upper extremities. Det danske Forlag, Copenhagen
Blauth W (1968) Erfahrungen in der operativen Behandlung von Klumphänden (Radiusaplasien). Verh. dtsch. Ges. Orthop. Traum., 54. Kongr. (Cologne). Z Orthop 104:Suppl. 439–445
Blauth W (1968) Die Behandlung der Klumphand. In: 4. Monographie über die Rehabilitation der Dysmelie-Kinder (Bundesministerium für Gesundheitswesen, Bad Godesberg, ed). Fränkische Verlagsanstalt und Buchdruckerei GmbH, Nuernberg, pp 105–110 (–114)
Blauth W (1969) Zur Morphologie und Therapie der radialen Klumphand. Arch Orthop Unfallchir 65:97–123
Blauth W, Schmidt H (1969) Über die Bedeutung arteriographischer Befunde bei Fehlbildungen am radialen Randstrahl (radiale Dysplasie). Z Orthop 106:102–110
Hepp O (1962) Die Häufung der angeborenen Defektmißbildungen der oberen Extremitäten in der Bundesrepublik Deutschland. Med Klin 57:419–426

Hippe P (1970) Die Handwurzelossifikation bei Dysmelien. Inaugural dissertation, Tuebingen
Holt M, Oram S (1960) Familial heart disease with skeletal malformations. Brit Heart J 22:236–242
Hopf A (1959) Aplasie und Hypoplasie des Radius („Radiusdefekt"). Die angeborenen Veränderungen des Unterarmes und der Hand. In: Hohmann G, Hackenbroch M, Lindemann K (eds) Handbuch der Orthopädie, vol III. Thieme, Stuttgart, pp 426–429
Lenz W (1963) Das Thalidomid-Syndrom. Fortschr Med 81:148–155
Lenz W (1969) Bone defects of the limbs – An overview. (In: Bergsma D (ed) Clinical delineation of birth defects, Part III: Limb malformations.) Birth Defects: Original article series, vol V/3. The National Foundation – March of Dimes, New York, pp 1–6
Lenz W, Theopold W, Thomas J (1964) Triphalangie des Daumens als Folge von Thalidomidschädigung. Münch Med Wschr 106:2033–2041
Müller W (1937) Die angeborenen Fehlbildungen der menschlichen Hand. Thieme, Leipzig
Riordan DC (1955) Congenital absence of the radius. J Bone Joint Surg 37-A:1129–1141
Riordan DC (1963) Congential absence of the radius. A fifteen year follow-up. J Bone Joint Surg 45-A:1783
Schöllner D (1972a) Die Klumphand bei Radiusaplasie. Pathogenese, Klinik, Therapie. In: Cotta H (ed) Aktuelle Orthopädie, vol 5. Thieme, Stuttgart
Schöllner D (1972b) Behandlungsprobleme bei angeborenen Klumphänden. In: Blauth W, Koob E (eds) Praktische Orthopädie, vol 3: Die Hand. Vordruckverlag, Bruchsal, pp 271–277
Steindler A (1920) Congenital malformations and deformities of the hand. Am J Orthop Surg 2:639–668
Stoffel A, Stempel E (1909) Anatomische Studien über die Klumphand. Z Orthop Chir 23:1–157
Willert HG, Henkel HL (1969) Klinik und Pathologie der Dysmelie. Springer, Berlin Heidelberg New York
Witt AN, Cotta H, Jäger M (1966) Die angeborenen Fehlbildungen der Hand und ihre operative Behandlung Thieme, Stuttgart

Hypoplasias and Aplasias of the Ulna (Ulnar Club Hand) (Chap. 14)

Blauth W (1967) Der kongenitale Femurdefekt. Z Orthop 103, Suppl. 29
Bonola A, Morelli E (1972) Le deformitá congenite delle mani ed il loro trattamento. Piccin Editore, Padova
Degenhardt K-H (1967) Die Bedeutung des Tierexperiments in der Ursachenforschung angeborener Mißbildungen. Wien Med Wochenschr 117:382–386
Hopf A (1959) Die Aplasie der Ulna („Ulnadefekt"). In: Hohmann G, Hackenbroch M, Lindemann K (eds) Handbuch der Orthopädie, vol III. Thieme, Stuttgart, pp 428–433
Kajon C (1921) Angeborener doppelseitiger Ulnadefekt und Pollex bifidus dexter. Z Orthop Chir 41:526–528
Kelikian H (1974) Congenital deformities of the hand and forearm. Saunders, Philadelphia London Toronto
Ke PJ (1937) Der angeborene Defekt des ulnaren Strahles und der angeborene Defekt der Tibia. Arch Orthop Unfallchir 37:42–47
Kühne D, Lenz W, Petersen D, Schönenberg H (1967) Defekt von Femur und Fibula mit Amelie, Peromelie oder ulnaren Strahldefekten. Ein Syndrom. Humangenetik 3:244–263
Kümmel W (1895) Die Mißbildungen der Extremitäten durch Defekt, Verwachsung und Überzahl. Fischer, Kassel
Lausecker H (1954) Der angeborene Defekt der Ulna. Virchows Arch Path Anat 325:211–226
Müller W (1937) Die angeborenen Fehlbildungen der menschlichen Hand. Thieme, Leipzig
Pfeiffer RA, Reinhardt K (1967) Ulno-fibulare Dysplasie. Eine autosomal-dominant vererbte Mikromesomelie ähnlich dem Nievergelt-Syndrom. Fortschr Röntgenstr 107:379–391
Pingel P, Rompe G (1971) Einteilungsprinzipien der Dysmelie, dargestellt am Beispiel der ulnaren Ektromelie. Z Orthop 109:137–144
Reimann-Hunzicker G (1942) Über den angeborenen Ulnadefekt. Z Orthop Chir 73:160–164
Schoenenberg H (1962) Über Mißbildungen der Extremitäten. Bibliotheca paediatrica, Fasc 80. Karger, Basel
Senftleben H (1869) Notiz über eine angeborene Luxation des Radius mit Defekt des mittleren Teils der Ulna. Virchows Arch Path Anat 55:303–304
Werthemann A (1952) Rückläufige Bildungen langer Röhrenknochen in Vorderarm und Unterschenkel. In: Lubarsch O, Henke F, Rössle R (eds) Handbuch für Spezielle Pathologische Anatomie und Histologie, vol IX/6. Springer, Berlin Göttingen Heidelberg, pp 78–103 (esp. 86–89)
Wierzejewski I (1910) Über den kongenitalen Ulnadefekt. Z Orthop Chir 27:101–131 and 504–509

Hereditary Multiple Exostoses (Chap. 15)

Bethge JF (1963) Hereditäre multiple Exostosen und ihre pathogenetische Deutung. Arch Orthop Unfallchir 54:677–696
Blauth W (1972) Möglichkeiten und Grenzen der operativen Behandlung angeborener Handfehlbildungen. In: Blauth W, Koob E (eds) Praktische Orthopädie, vol 3. Die Hand. Vordruckverlag, Bruchsal, pp 243–269
Cocchi U (1952) Multiple kartilaginäre Exostosen. In: Schinz HR et al (eds) Lehrbuch der Röntgendiagnostik, vol I. Thieme, Stuttgart, pp 636–644
Dahlin DC (1957) Bone tumors. Thomas, Springfield, Ill.; (cited by Solomon)
Dominok GW, Knoch HG (1961) Knochengeschwülste und geschwulstähnliche Knochenerkrankungen. Fischer, Jena
Heuk F (1972) Die multiplen kartilaginären Exostosen. In: Haubrich R (ed) Klinische Röntgendiagnostik innerer Krankheiten, vol III/1. Springer, Berlin Heidelberg New York, pp 121–125
Jaffe HL (1964) Tumors and tumorous conditions of the bones and joints. Lea & Febiger, Philadelphia
Lichtenstein L (1972) Bone Tumors. Mosby, St. Louis
Mau H, Siguda P (1974) Angeborene Systemerkrankungen des Skeletts. Chirurgie der Gegenwart, vol V. Urban & Schwarzenberg, Munich, pp 1–18
Solomon L (1961) Bone growth in diaphyseal aclasis. J Bone Joint Surg 43-B:700–716
Solomon L (1963) Hereditary multiple exostosis. J Bone Joint Surg 45-B:292–304
Spjut HJ, Dorfman HD, Fechner RE, Ackerman LV (1971) Tumors of bone and cartilage. In: Atlas of

tumor pathology. 2nd edn. Armed Forces Institute of Pathology, Washington, pp 67–70
Stocks P, Barrington M (1925) Diaphyseal aclasis (multiple exostosis), multiple enchondromata, cleido-craniodysostosis. In: Treasury of human inheritance, vol III/1: Hereditary disorders of bone development. University Press, Cambridge; (cited by Bethge, Solomon a.o.)
Witt AN, Cotta H, Jäger M (1966) Die angeborenen Fehlbildungen der Hand und ihre operative Behandlung. Thieme, Stuttgart

Enchondromatosis (Chap. 16)

Bethge JF (1962) Die Olliersche Krankheit. Pathogenetische Fragen und therapeutische Möglichkeiten. Dtsch Med Wochenschr 87:535–541
Blauth W (1971) Kontinuitätsresektion von Röhrenknochen und plastische Überbrückung von Knochendefekten. Arch Orthop Unfallchir 71:324–338
Blauth W (1972) Möglichkeiten und Grenzen der operativen Behandlung angeborener Handfehlbildungen. In: Blauth W, Koob E (eds) Praktische Orthopädie, vol 3. Die Hand. Vordruckverlag, Bruchsal, pp 243–269
Blauth W, Hippe P (1973) Zur Knochenenchondromatose der Hand. Handchirurgie 5:33–37
Butler ED, Hamill JP, Seipel RS, Lorimier AA de (1960) Tumors of the hand. A 10 year survey and report of 437 cases. Am J Surg 100:293–302
Chrysospathes JG (1929) Beitrag zur sogenannten Ollierschen Wachstumsstörung. Z Orthop Chir 51:177–191
Cleveland M, Fielding JW (1959) Chondrodysplasia (Olliers disease). J Bone Joint Surg 41-A:1341–1344
Cocchi U (1952) Knochenchondromatose. In: Schinz HR, Baensch WE, Friedl E, Uehlinger E (eds) Lehrbuch der Röntgendiagnostik, vol I. Thieme, Stuttgart, pp 644–652
Cocchi U (1964) Knochenchondromatose. In: Becker PE (ed) Humangenetik, vol II. Thieme, Stuttgart, pp 118–123
Dahlin DC (1967) Bone tumors. General aspects and data on 3,987 cases. Thomas, Springfield, Ill.
Dominok GW, Knoch HG (1971) Knochengeschwülste und geschulstähnliche Knochenerkrankungen. Fischer, Jena
Exner G (1950) Chondromatose – Dyschondroplasie – Olliersche Wachstumsstörung. Fortschr Röntgenstr 73:454–463
Fairbank HA (1948) Dyschondroplasia J Bone Joint Surg 30-B:689–704
Frangenheim P (1913) Die multiplen kartilaginären Exostosen und Enchondrome. In: Die Krankheiten des Knochensystems im Kindesalter [Neue Deutsche Chirurgie (Bruns P v ed), vol 10]. Enke, Stuttgart, pp 109–124
Gäde E (1938) Die Dyschondroplasie (Multiple Enchondromatose – Olliersche Wachstumsstörung). Z Orthop Chir 67:321–379
Geschickter CF, Copeland MM (1936) Tumors of bone Am J Cancer; (cited by Dominok and Knoch)
Hellner H (1950) Die Knochengeschwülste. Springer, Berlin Göttingen Heidelberg
Herzog G (1944) Innere oder zentrale Chondrome und Chondromyxome. In: Lubarsch O, Henke F, Rössle R (eds) Handbuch für Spezielle Pathologische Anatomie und Histologie, vol IX. Springer, Berlin; (cited by Witt et al.)
Jaffe HL (1964) Tumors and tumorous conditions of the bones and joints. Lea & Febiger, Philadelphia
Junge H (1949) Über die Dyschondroplasie mit besonderer Berücksichtigung der sog. Halbseitenform (Ollier). Z Orthop 78:130–143
Koob E, Ostendorf U (1972) Behandlungsprobleme bei einer ausgedehnten Chondromatose der Hand. Handchirurgie 4:85–88
Langenskjöld A (1947) Ollier's disease and its relation to other forms of chondrodysplasia. Acta Orthop Scand 17:93–133
Lewis RJ, Ketcham AS (1973) Maffucci's syndrome: functional and neoplastic significance. Case report and review of the literature. J Bone Joint Surg 55-A:1465–1479
Müller E (1937) Die angeborenen Fehlbildungen der menschlichen Hand. Thieme, Leipzig
Narakas A, Verdan C (1970) Osteochondromas of the skeleton of the hand. In: Chapchal G (ed) Operative treatment of bone tumours. Thieme, Stuttgart, pp 20–24
Posch JL (1956) Tumors of the hand. J Bone Joint Surg 38-A:517–539
Schinz HR (1944) Zur Genetik der Exostosis multiplex cartilaginea und der multiplen Knochenchondromatose. Arch Klaus-Stift Vererb-Forsch 19:1
Sharrard W (1971) Cartilaginous dysplasias with proliferation of growth plate chondroblasts. In: Paediatric Orthopaedics and Fractures. Blackwell, Oxford Edinburgh, pp 49–59
Speiser F (1925) Ein Fall von systematisierter Enchondromatose des Skeletts. Virchows Arch path Anat 258:126–160
Spjut HJ, Dorfman HD, Fechner RE, Ackerman LV (1971) Tumors of bone and cartilage In: Atlas of tumour pathology, 2nd edn. Armed Forces Institute of Pathology, Washington, pp 59–84
Spranger JW, Langer LO, Wiedemann HR (1974) Bone dysplasias. An atlas of skeletal development. Fischer, Stuttgart
Takigawa K (1971a) Chondroma of the bones of the hand. A review of 110 cases. J Bone Joint Surg 53-A:1591–1600
Takigawa K (1971b) Carpal Chondroma. Report of a case. J Bone Joint Surg 53-A:1601–1604
Tomaschewski HK, Kruse GH (1970) Unsere Erfahrungen in der Diagnostik und Therapie der multiplen Enchondrome. Beitr Orthop Traum 17:32–34
Truëta J (1957) Trauma and bone growth. Soc. Intern. Chir. orthop. Traumat., Rapports VII. Congr (Barcelona) Brüssel: Imprimerie des Sciences; (cited by Dominok and Knoch)
Weil S (1957) Die angeborenen Skelettsystemerkrankungen: Multiple Chondrome, Chondromatose. In: Hohmann G, Hackenbroch M, Lindemann K (eds) Handbuch der Orthopädie, vol I. Thieme, Stuttgart, pp 232–237
Witt AN, Cotta H, Jäger M (1966) Die angeborenen Fehlbildungen der Hand und ihre operative Behandlung. Thieme, Stuttgart
Zifko B (1966) Behandlung von Frakturen in Chondromen der Hand. Monatsschr Unfallheilk 69:538–543

Subject Index

Italicized page numbers refer to figures or operative examples with accompanying text.
Numbers in parentheses refer to pages which contain discussion pertaining to the term, although the term itself does not appear.

Ivo Pitanguy

Aesthetic Plastic Surgery of Head and Body

1980. Approx. 900 figures, many in color.
Approx. 280 pages
ISBN 3-540-08706-0
Scheduled for publication at the end of 1980

Contents:
Part I: Body Contouring Surgery: Breast and Thoracic Deformities. – Breast Hypertrophy. – Breast Hypoplasia. – Other Deformities: Congenital, Traumatic and Iatrogenic. – Abdominal Wall Deformities. – Gluteal and Lower Extremity Deformities.
Part II: Surgery of the Head and Neck: Facial Surgery. – Face Lifting. – Forehead Lifting. – Eyelid Correction. – The Aging Lip. – Submental Deformities. – The Aging Chin. – Ancillary Procedures. – Congenital and Other Facial Contour Deformities. – Nose. – Ear. – Lip. – Chin. – Atropic and Traumatic Scars. – Other Facial Contour Deformities. –
Part III: Combined Procedures.

H. R. Mittelbach

The Injured Hand

A Handbook for General Surgeons

Translated from the German by T. Telger
1979. 210 figures, 2 tables. XIII, 245 pages
ISBN 3-540-90365-8

Contents:
Functional Anatomy and Diagnostics in Hand Surgery. – Conservative and Operative Phases of Hand Surgery. – Surgery of the Hand. – Anesthesia in Hand Surgery. – Care of Open Hand Injuries. – Amputations. – Fingertip Injuries. – Soft Tissue Injuries of the Dorsal Side: Injuries of the Wrist Extensors, Long Finger Extensor Tendons, and Dorsal Aponeurosis of the Fingers. – Soft Tissue Injuries of the Volar Side: Injuries of the Long Finger Flexor Tendons, Wrist Flexors, and Median and Ulnar Nerves. – Capsular Ligament Injuries of the Finger Joints. – Fractures of the Phalanges and Metacarpus. – Fractures and Dislocations of the Carpal Bones. – Thumb Injuries. – Compressive Nerve Injuries of the Hand. – Transfer Operations for Irreparable Nerve Damage. – Severe Crush Injuries of the Hand. – Foreign Bodies in the Hand. – Infections of the Hand. – Thermal, Chemical and Electrical Injuries. – Hand Injuries in Children. – Sudeck's Disease: Dystrophy of the Extremities. – Ischemic Contracture. – On the Informatory Obligation of the Physician. – Book and Monography on Hand-Surgery. – Index.

H.M. Tschopp

Microsurgical Neuro-Vascular Anastomoses

for Transplantation of Composite Bone and Muscle Grafts
An Experimental Study

With a Foreword be M. Allgöwer
1976. 50 illustrations, some in color. V, 52 pages
ISBN 3-540-07517-8

Contents:
Introduction. – Materials and Methods: Anesthesia and Intravenous Administration. Preparation of the Graft. Preparation of the Recipient Sita. Microsurgical Vessel and Nerve Anastomoses. Grouping of the Animals. Supravital Polychromic Bone Labelling. Examination of the Specimen. – Results: General Remarks. Evaluation of the Muscle Graft. Evaluation of the Bone Graft. – Discussion: General Remarks. Behavior of the Intercostal Muscle Graft. Behavior of the Rib Graft. Conclusions. – Summary. – References. – Subject Index.

Springer-Verlag
Berlin
Heidelberg
New York

MIX
Papier aus verantwortungsvollen Quellen
Paper from responsible sources
FSC® C105338

If you have any concerns about our products,
you can contact us on
ProductSafety@springernature.com

In case Publisher is established outside the EU,
the EU authorized representative is:
Springer Nature Customer Service Center GmbH
Europaplatz 3, 69115 Heidelberg, Germany

Printed by Libri Plureos GmbH
in Hamburg, Germany